THE WORLD OF
BALLET

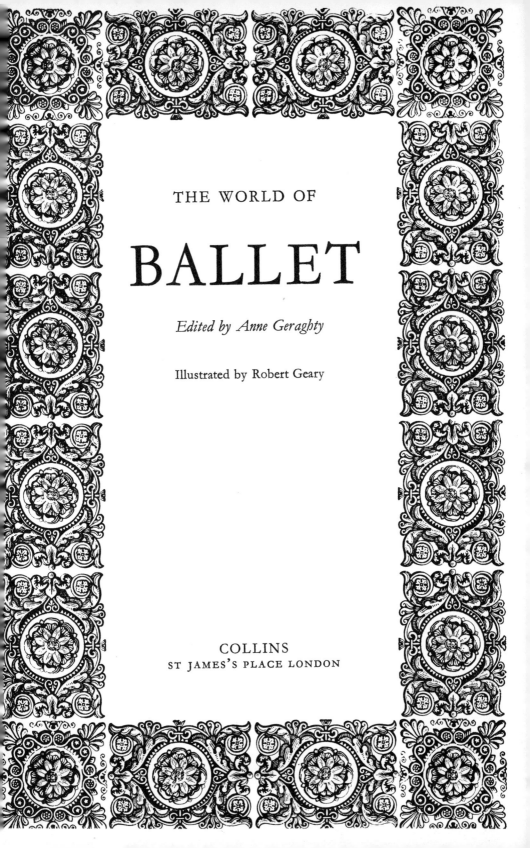

THE WORLD OF

BALLET

Edited by Anne Geraghty

Illustrated by Robert Geary

COLLINS
ST JAMES'S PLACE LONDON

ISBN 0 00 195865 8

The World of Ballet first published in Great Britain in 1970 by William Collins Sons
& Co. Ltd.

This Edition 1972

CONTENTS

INTRODUCTION

This anthology has been collected for your enjoyment: it will tell you a little more about some aspects of ballet that you might not have considered before, and it will also entertain you.

Its purpose is to show you the *real* world of ballet, not the romantic one of so many stories and books. Although not divided sharply into sections, the book has been grouped so that the early articles are concerned with visiting the ballet, and watching it, then they turn to ballet as a professional career; the "mechanics" of creating ballet; and the background and history of ballet through the personalities who influenced its development.

Rumer Godden is a distinguished writer for adults and children, and her article on watching ballet is both beautiful and helpful. It is reprinted from THE YEARS OF GRACE, first published in 1950. No anthology of ballet would ever be complete without a contribution by Noel Streatfeild. A famous children's author, her novel BALLET SHOES has inspired and delighted thousands of children since it was published. She writes here of her first visit to the ballet and tells you something of life and attitudes when she was a small girl. Mary Stacey's article is in complete contrast: *her* visit to the ballet took place only a year ago, when she was nine, and her impressions will be interesting and perhaps shared by many of you.

A few years ago Baron was a famous photographer particularly associated with ballet: his photos included here will show you something of the dancing traditions of other countries and cultures which have also influenced ballet. They have been selected from his books: BARON AT THE BALLET and BARON ENCORE.

Helen Cresswell and Joan Aiken are two of to-day's top writers for children. They were asked to write a humorous ballet story to make a refreshing change from the usual sentimental stories in which the heroine *always* succeeds as a dancer. They both enjoy ballet—Joan Aiken was first inspired by BALLET SHOES, but Helen

Cresswell had to give up ballet when she "grew to be five feet ten inches tall, which would have been quite a handful for Nureyev".

Arnold Haskell is one of the most distinguished and famous writers connected with ballet: a former Governor of the Royal Ballet School, and ballet critic, he has written many books on ballet, including BALLETOMANIA, perhaps his most famous, and FELICITY DANCES, a charming story for young readers. His article was first published in 1950, but it is included here because it is still as relevant to-day.

Clement Crisp is a lecturer and writer on ballet, and his articles on to-day's dancers will help you to appreciate their art when you next see them. The section on famous people in the history of ballet tells you a little of the development of ballet.

Shelagh Fraser is an actress and a writer. Since her sister Moyra grew too tall for ballet, she has always been concerned with the problem of what to do with a ballet training if you don't succeed as a dancer, and in her article she offers many excellent and practical suggestions.

Rudolf Nureyev is a magical name to all modern ballet fans, and in this extract from his biography, NUREYEV, by Alexander Bland, he tells how he first saw ballet and decided to become a dancer, and the difficulties he faced as a small boy living in Russia.

Elaine McDonald is a soloist with the Scottish Theatre Ballet. Her story of how she became a dancer is fascinating because it is *not* like the story-books—she won a competition, but she worked very hard, and then had to face the fact that she would never be a great classical ballerina—so she chose modern ballet.

Robina Beckles Willson used to teach at the Ballet Rambert Educational School, and is now a writer. She feels that in between ballet lessons, ballet is often forgotten, yet there is no reason why you should not invent your own dances to music, and even make up a ballet. Leichner Studios tell you the basic rudiments of stage make-up to help you. When you are making up your own ballet you might wonder who invents the steps for the great ballets you see performed, and how they do it? Elizabeth Malcolm, who has studied ballet at the Royal Academy of Dancing, and choreography at the Institute of Choreology, has written this article to explain the history of choreography, which is also really the history of ballet, and what a choreographer does when he creates a ballet.

Choreographer in His Element is an extract from Bernard Taper's biography of the great modern choreographer, George Balanchine, and helps to illustrate many of Elizabeth Malcolm's points. It is the most difficult piece to read in the whole book but it is worthwhile grappling with it, for it gives you a very real insight into this great man, into the way a modern choreographer works, and into the modern ballet scene.

The Blue Train is the story of the young Anton Dolin, at one time one of our great men dancers. Joan Selby-Lowndes is a very well-known writer of books for young people, particularly connected with ballet and the theatre. This book was first published in 1953 and gives a vivid impression of ballet during the twenties and thirties.

Finally, the cartoons are by Peter Cazalet, a dancer with a good sense of humour!

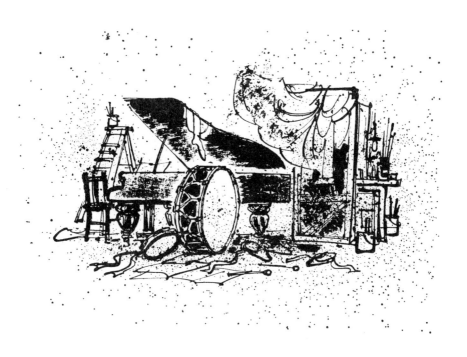

WATCHING THE BALLET

Rumer Godden

"The instruments of music are made ready . . .
. . . and now . . .
up rose the fair ones to the dance
well painted and apparelled
in veils of soft gossamer . . .
The wielder of the little stick
whispers them to their places and the steady drums
draw them through the mazes of the dance."

That was written in China nearly two thousand years ago, but
to-day the wielder of the little stick raises it in a newer flower of
the dance, for the ballet, as we know it, in theatres all over the

world—in New York, London, Paris, Madrid, Moscow, Sydney, Buenos Aires.

Our own Covent Garden is a most exciting theatre; it is truly theatrical with its size and its pillars, its red seats—the mellow red of those Chinese dancers—with its gilt and tier on tier of shaded lights. When those lights dim and go out, tier on tier, and a hush falls on the audience, and there is a crackle of applause as the conductor enters and bows and turns and lifts his baton, his little stick, when the overture begins and swells and fills the theatre, the whole audience is quickened and excited and stirred.

"Quickened" is "shaken into life", and that is what dancing does to us, perhaps what we need. All through the years, since before the days of that Chinese poet, Chang Heng, the dance has been used in magic, in ceremony, in religion; it has colour and movement, vitality, sound and warmth—things that we need to refresh and stimulate us; perhaps this explains the popularity of ballet to-day, when there is so much that is grey and difficult in our lives.

When the curtain goes up—if it is the first time you have sat on that red seat and pressed the backs of your knees down on it with excitement and fingered your glossy programme full of strange names, or if it is the twentieth time you have seen this particular ballet—you will discover riches. I shall tell you some of the ballets you will like: *Cinderella*, of course; *Coq d'Or*, based on a Russian fairy-tale, *Carnaval*, with music by Schumann and a touching Pierrot and a Columbine with her flounced dress decorated with cherries; the second act of *Swan Lake*, with the sad story of the enchanted swan princess; *Prince Igor*, with its vigorous warrior dances; *La Boutique Fantasque*, with its fantastic toy shop where the toys come to life; *Aurora's Wedding* (the last act of *The Sleeping Beauty*), where nursery-tale characters come to the wedding, and you will see the famous dance of the Bluebirds. Later on you will come to the great classical ballets, the whole of *Swan Lake*, the *Sleeping Princess*, *Giselle*, and the more sophisticated ones, such as *Petrouchka*, the newer *The Gods go a'begging*, and the ballets from America that often have great freshness, and those from the new French ballet. Each time you see them you will discover more and more gold—small touches and twists; the strange crowing cry of the dazzling gold cock in *Coq d'or*; the two badly behaved poodles

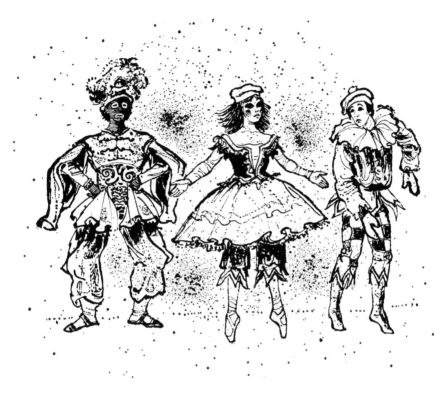

in *La Boutique Fantasque*; the Witch's monkeys in the *Sleeping Princess*; the dreamy, pale-blue tinges in the moonlit skirts of the *Sylphides*. With good ballet it is more interesting to go for the twentieth time than the first—the more you see it, the more you see in it.

But if you go to the ballet you must bring some things with you: the most important, I think, is imagination. Arnold Haskell (who as a writer and critic has done much towards making people understand ballet and who writes for you elsewhere in this book) once wrote of *Petrouchka*: ". . . Your ordinary unimaginative theatre-goer will enjoy it as a brightly coloured nursery tale, the love-story of three puppets. Someone with imagination will read into it the story of the awakening of a soul—and souls are more interesting than puppets." At the end of *Petrouchka* the magician throws down on the stage a toy of straw and rag, but we have seen the poor puppet, the clown, shut in his cell by the cruel magician, tormented by his love for the doll with her rouged cheeks and tin trumpet; we have seen the agony of his dance, and it is no surprise to us when he rises behind the magician on the roof of the booth theatre, as the snow falls and the last eerie strain of his music sounds on and on.

There is one thing about imagination that people are apt to forget—that it is rooted in reality. We all know the Irish fairy-tale of the pot of gold buried at the foot of the rainbow; perhaps ballet seems a little like that, but a rainbow is, after all, a natural phenomenon, the effect of light shining through vapour, and gold is dug out of the earth. It is the same with ballet: its imaginative effect is the result of technique, of that very earthy thing—work. To know about the work is not to destroy the fairy quality, but to make it more real; that is why I think we should learn a little about it, even if we ourselves only do round dancing, or square dancing, folk or ballroom dancing, or no dancing at all: you do not need to be a balletomane to understand something of ballet, but you need to think and feel.

First, let us think what ballet is: it is not only dancing; it is the fusion of several people's work—the work of a choreographer (who designs the steps of the dance), a composer (who writes or arranges the music) and an artist (who designs sets and clothes), and perhaps a poet who writes the story, theme or idea. Each of these works through many other people: the choreographer through his dancers, the composer through his orchestra, the artist through scene-painters, dressmakers and electricians; not to understand this is like expecting gold without a gold-mine, a rainbow without rain.

The best way to understand anything is to imagine you are doing it yourself; imagine that you, a teenage boy or girl, have decided to produce a ballet, as Noel Streatfeild's Sally did in *Party Frock*, using the people and friends you know. Of course, we have to premise certain things: that you know something of dancers and dancing (not necessarily that you dance yourself), and that among your friends are some at dancing schools, some interested in music and painting.

The first thing you will find is that this is very ambitious; everyone will tell you so. "A play," they will say. "Do a nativity play, or something you have written." "But I have *written* it!" (Few people realise that ballets are written.) Still, you have decided, and you begin.

Imagine that you have an idea that you see as a ballet; it may have come from anywhere, from music you have heard (*Petrouchka*, for instance, grew from a theme played by Stravinsky and a conversation about Russian fairs); it may have come from a story—*Spectre de la Rose*—the story of the girl who is visited by the ghost of the rose she wore at the ball that night—came from a Gautier poem; it may come quickly or slowly—Fokine composed the *Dying Swan* for Pavlova in an hour—but let us say that you are fascinated by the idea of a ballet based on the fairy-tale of the Princess whose golden ball fell in the fountain and was rescued by the Frog Prince. You know the story: she promised to share her plate, her pillow, her games with him, and the King, her father, made her keep her word; she hated the frog, but, at last, grew to be sorry for him; and one day she kissed him and he was released from his frog spell and turned back into the Prince he really was. You see the palace garden with gold and silver fountains, perhaps, and white rose-trees with gilded stems; you see the Princess entering, perhaps dancing backwards as she plays with her golden ball; you see her long blue sleeves; slowly the whole story of the ballet begins to come.

Now you must have music, something that gives the idea of that ball in the air; perhaps you know one piece, but are there others of the same composer that match it, that would bring the pathos of the Frog Prince, the sharpness of the Princess's dislike, her melting into pity? It immediately becomes too difficult for you, and you have to call in an expert friend who can arrange music for you, or write it especially for your idea; then he in his turn must find people who will play his music; perhaps, for a home-made ballet, only piano and percussion, but even so, it must be played, and it must be scored so that the drum will come in here, the trills of bells there.

When the music is chosen, the dances have to be arranged, and here again you will need help, this long word of "choreographer", who will arrange the dance pattern of your scenes; if the steps are like words, chains of steps or "enchainments" are like sentences, and from them he will build the whole story of your ballet.

From his idea and the musician's, combined with yours, new things will grow: here is some slow music that gives the idea of a Duenna, a governess for the Princess; the governess goes in; the choreographer, a dancer himself, wants to play the King and he wants a special dance; the ballet is too serious: what about a comic dance? And now you have a gardener who knocks off the King's crown. Soon you begin to wonder who thought of what idea; then you have to find dancers for all these parts, and now, perhaps, you find you have to work backwards, you have to compromise and adjust: your Duenna is too heavy to fit the steps, the gardener may have to double with the butler, and you have to move a dance; the waiting-maid dances better than the Princess; imperceptibly the parts change to fit the dancers as the dancers fit into their parts.

Now you have to set and dress your ballet, and as you don't draw or paint well enough, you have to call in a friend who does, one who can understand your idea of the palace, or the Princess's blue sleeves, of the little pages with the crimson caps; he will bring his people who will carry out his ideas: a friend who can carpenter, another who can paint, a mother or elder sister who likes sewing and cutting out—someone who is interested in electricity and can make spots out of car lamps and footlights, perhaps from bicycle lamps, or contrive candles lit by the page. He again will bring ideas of his own which will add to it; some of them will upset yours, but you will learn how, often, it is best for the ballet to upset them and turn right-about-face. "An artist is always changing his mind," people complain; an artist would not be an artist if he couldn't, and only an artist can produce a ballet.

Then you will start rehearsing, and you will learn many more things, things that every producer of ballet learns, sometimes very bitterly: you will learn what a blessing it is to have properly trained dancers, what their courage and patience mean; you will learn how Henry so-and-so shows off, how Mary so-and-so has an elevation like a young antelope, but seems to have wax in her ears so that she can't hear the simplest beat—and Mary will quarrel with your musician; you will learn how much things cost, in pounds, shillings and pence, in time and trouble; you will learn how to manage people—people who work under you and with you, people above you—in your case parents and grown-ups; you will learn, in your small way, what Pavlova meant when she said, "Those who would accomplish great things have no time to fold the hands"; and one day, in spite of everything, miraculously perhaps, you will probably have your ballet. And now you turn to your audience, to yourself in your seat at Covent Garden, and at once you will realise why it is important for the audience to be responsive.

Did they understand? Did this or that get over? Did they get this or that? Did they know that the King loved his daughter to agony when he was forcing her to keep the promise to the Frog? Did they feel the pent-up longing and feeling in the poor Frog? Did he make them feel it? Did the Princess manage to keep their sympathy when she was so cold and scornful? Did she make them think what it was like to be side by side with a cold, wet, slimy frog? Did they understand what she had to overcome, and he too? Did they like the tenderness of the dance when the Prince was discovered and the Princess shy? Did they see the little parts? The quick, impatient little *relevés* of the Duenna's dance? The page snatching the rose? The gardener scratching his ear? The Princess's poodle? Did they? You see, it *is* important to be responsive, to imagine and think and feel as that Chinese poet felt and thought those two thousand years ago:

"So . . . dance to dance
endlessly they weave . . . break off and dance again.
Now flutter their cuffs like a great bird in flight,
now toss their long white sleeves like whirling snow
. . . in unison
of body, dress and song, obedient
each shadows each as they glide softly to and fro."

TWO CHILD DANCERS

Noel Streatfeild

I was the odd one out in my family. My sisters and brother fitted
far better into the world into which we were born than I did. That
world was vicarages in Sussex. At a very early age I announced to
my family "I don't like vicarages", and this is something I have
never got over, even now I get a claustrophobic feeling if I step
inside a vicarage door.

It was a mixture of things that added up to my dislike of
vicarages. The attitude of the parishioners, which was that a vicar's
daughter should automatically be better behaved than a child who
was not a vicar's daughter. In my case this started me off as a
failure for, as everybody knew, I was worse behaved than most

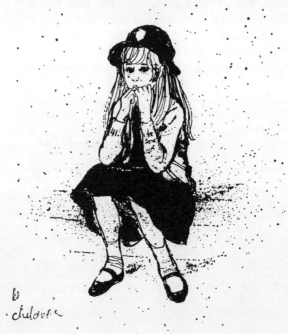

children. Then there was a happy acceptance by my father of poverty, which I detested. Not grinding, starving poverty, but being poorer and worse dressed than all our acquaintances and automatically unable to do the things and have the things which other children took for granted. If only, I thought, my father would roar with rage that a man of his ability should be paid a mere pittance, but no—he accepted poverty almost with gratitude. On top of all this I felt stifled in the vicarage. I felt as I should think a plant feels when it is trying to grow in too small a pot. I wanted? I wanted? I had no idea what I wanted except that it was a bigger, wider world than the one in which we lived. Not getting a bigger, wider world, I was always exploding in one direction or another, with the result that my first school decided I was unmanageable.

To-day it is quite impossible to imagine life as it was when I was a child—or rather as it was lived in our seaside town. I was in the junior school of a large day school which prided itself on its academic achievements. I don't know what happened in the senior school, but in the junior school we were taught in the dullest possible way with practically no artistic training at all. We never heard any music, we knew no poetry except those poems selected for us to learn by heart. We never did any acting and we were never taken to see a play. We learnt no dancing, not even folk dancing, which most schools taught at that time.

On a visit to my maternal grandfather when I was about ten, my eldest sister and I were taken to see an open-air entertainment given by a school. I remember the amazement with which we watched it. It was enchantingly dressed and put on, but most extraordinary of all to us was the gaiety and abandonment when the children sang and danced. Could this really be a school? Could there really be children who in lesson time could learn to dance and sing?

If I was frustrated at school I was lucky in some ways in my home life. My mother was a botanist. From the time we could walk she took us for rambles looking for wild flowers, teaching us their names and how to know plants by sight. She herself painted every specimen she found. Then, in those days, in our type of home games were popular. We came down to the drawing-room after tea and played cards: the old favourites such as Snakes and Ladders and Happy Families, but we were particularly fond of a game called "Who knows?" This was a game in which cards were drawn out of a bag and on each was a question. The players had squared-off sheets in front of them and each time they answered a question correctly they got a card. The first full house of cards was the winner. I cannot tell you how full our brains became with miscellaneous knowledge from playing "Who knows?" and how useful some of that knowledge turned out to be, but not all. Ask any one of us to-day what ink is made of and we shall reply "gum copperash, gum arabic and water". I daresay ink is made of something quite different now—and anyway, who cares?—but most of the general knowledge was of better value than that.

As well we sang. Mother played the piano and we gathered round singing on week-days the songs and nursery rhymes from those lovely old song-books *The Babies Bouquet* and *The Babies Opera*, and on Sundays we sang hymns. The Sunday hymn-singing was one of Sunday's few bright spots for we dreaded Sundays. They started with learning the collect for the day in bed, went on to being heard the catechism after breakfast, then off to matins, then church again in the afternoon. We were allowed no toys nor games, nor to read or have read out loud the same book we were reading during the week. The wonder is that in spite of our Sundays we have all remained Christians. But there is no doubt in my mind that at that period artistically we were starved.

Then, when I was about thirteen, we moved to Eastbourne and were sent to a new and rather more imaginative school, in fact, we all took part in the Greek play *Alcestis* during our first summer term. But even better things were in store for us. Before Eastbourne we had seldom been to a theatre because there were a lot of us and, as I have explained, my father was poor. But when we came to live in Eastbourne a great decision was made. Provided we went out together, I and my two sisters might in future go about on our own. This was amazing news, opening all kinds of doors to us, for you cannot imagine, unless you have endured it, how suffocating it is never to move about without a much older and usually unwilling escort.

As well as being allowed to go out on our own, we three girls unexpectedly found ourselves in the money. We had been existing on sixpence a week pocket money; this sounds ridiculous now, but in those days sixpence had the spending power of half a crown.

But now, without any warning, we were suddenly promoted to
five shillings a week, which was a vast sum to us.

The idea of giving us five shillings a week was that we should
learn the value of money. It was not intended as personal spending

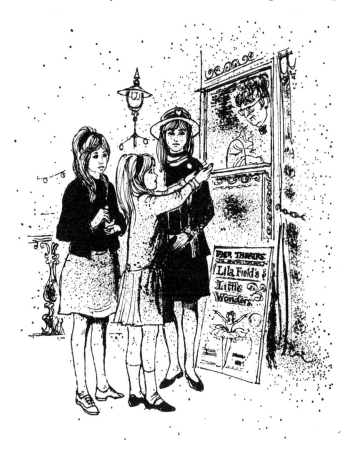

money but was to be used to buy stockings and stamps and pay
bus fares and a lot of other small expenses which, up till that time,
had been paid for us.

I don't remember how my sisters made out, but I know my
five shillings a week disappeared like snow in a hot hand. Masses of
sweets, of course, gay hair ribbons I was not allowed to wear, just
everything and anything I fancied, but, most exciting of all, seats
for the theatre.

It was seats for the theatre which brought magic into my life. We went to see a group of child dancers called Lila Field's Little Wonders. It was one of the Little Wonders who showed me how beautiful classical ballet could be.

Lila Field's company of children danced in the pier theatre—I think twice a year. We three sisters never missed a performance. The programme was made up of solo dances, group dances and little playlets. We never met the child dancers or dared write to them for to us they were creatures apart who would not dream of condescending to talk or write to ordinary, dull children such as ourselves.

Of course, in time, we came to know most of the children by sight and by name. We would notice how they had improved since we last saw them, and were proud when our judgment of a promising child was proved correct by the better parts they took in the plays or by their being promoted to a solo spot in one of the ballets. But there was one child who even my untrained eyes recognised at once as of exceptional talent. This was the child star of the company. Her name was Ninette de Valois—that same Ninette de Valois who many years later was to found The Royal Ballet Company.

Ninette de Valois, when I first saw her dancing, was an aristocratic-looking child with long hair which, in my memory, curled at the ends. To we three sisters, sitting in the cheapest seats in the theatre and therefore far, far from the stage, she looked about twelve. But what a twelve-year-old! How infinitely removed from our gym-tunicked bulging selves. Other wealthier children from our new school had been taken to London to see the great Diaghilev ballets, but even when, breathless and exalted, they had returned and tried to tell us what they had seen it was only words— no fragment of the beauty they had witnessed passed on to us. So we were virgin soil on which to sow a great experience.

The most important name at that time was Anna Pavlova and, indeed, still is to-day. We had never seen her dance, but girls at the new school had picture postcards of her so we knew how she looked. The last part of Lila Field's entertainment, if I remember rightly, took the form of a revue with the Little Wonders appearing as the great stars of the day. Ninette de Valois appeared as Pavlova dancing "The Dying Swan". Perhaps, some might say, it was far too ambitious an effort for a child, that all too many children were styling themselves little Pavlovas, but I doubt if such things matter. What does matter is that Ninette de Valois was given the gift to open another child's eyes to beauty of movement allied to wonderful music. Her dancing of the swan was to me perfection, and when you have the good fortune to see perfection as a child, it changes your life.

Many girls and boys who have had the luck to see great dancing at an early age are fired with ambition to become dancers themselves. This happened to me, but I suffered from no delusions. I was the wrong shape. I had the wrong legs and, fighter though I was for what I wanted, I knew this had me beat. Not by the wildest stretching of my imagination could I see my father either paying for me to learn classical ballet or even, should I talk a godparent into feeling generous, allowing me to learn. He had never, I think, seen great dancing, but he had seen dancers on their *pointes* at charity performances and he thought it horrifying because they showed too much leg. Showing too much leg was in those days considered by many to be a sin.

With more sense than I usually showed, I accepted that I could never be a dancer, but that I could and would study dancing, not physically but through books. At that time books about classical ballet were few and far between and hard to come by, but with help from school-fellows I read all I could lay hands on, including a mass of articles from magazines.

Slowly I trained my eyes to know what to look for and my ears to listen, so that I should be ready when the day came when I was grown up and earning enough money to take myself to watch real ballets.

As things turned out when I grew up and was earning money, which I would have dearly loved to have spent on seats for the ballet, there was no ballet to watch. Diaghilev was dead.

To-day you can write down "Diaghilev was dead" without feeling as though you had written "Dancing was dead", but at the time that was how it felt, for without Diaghilev there was no ballet. But though there were no ballet companies there were dancers. All over the world little girls—and occasionally little boys too—were slaving away in studios exactly as though when they were trained there were ballet companies which they could join.

Then there was a ballet company. A Colonel de Basil had learnt that though, because of the revolution, it was no longer possible to get dancers from Russia, the great Russian dancers who had escaped were teaching, largely in Paris. So Colonel de Basil went the rounds of the French studios and discovered three brilliant child dancers. Tamara Toumanova, Irina Baronova and Tatiana Riabouchinska. I think Baronova was twelve when I first saw her dance, Toumanova thirteen and Riabouchinska perhaps two years older. These three girls were the nucleus of a magnificent ballet company.

I must have been fated to be taught to learn to love ballet by children. Of those three I think Baronova taught me the most. For just as the child Ninette de Valois had left an indelible mark on my memory with her interpretation of "The Dying Swan", so Baronova gave me something I shall never forget when she danced in a ballet called *Présages* to the music of Tchaikovsky's fifth symphony.

All great dancers have moments of perfection when what makes them great seems to fuse together: their dancing, their technique, their musicality, and something so beautiful is arrived at that for a second you stop breathing. Baronova often gave me such moments.

Of course there have been other dancers since who have moved me past speech. Margot Fonteyn and Ulanova are two, but it so happened that it was the two children—Ninette de Valois and Baronova—who first showed me what classical dancing could mean and so it was they who influenced my future life.

If I had been less engaged in scraping enough money together to watch the de Basil Company and instead had kept my ear closer to the ground, I would have learnt many things to interest me, all stemming from the child that was Ninette de Valois.

Ninette de Valois, now grown up, was a girl of vast determination, talent and vision. Her dream was of an English ballet company. How she brought that dream to life is a long story—far too long to tell here—and I, from stupidity, missed some of the early stages at which I could have been present. When I woke up to what had been going on and now was actually happening, the Vic-Wells Company was established at Sadler's Wells Theatre.

It was a wonderful experience to see what is now The Royal Ballet Company growing up. Whenever I could possibly manage it I was at Sadler's Wells. When the war came I was on night work and seldom had an evening off, but when I did I was at The New Theatre. This was the wartime home of the Vic-Wells Ballet. The Company danced there accompanied by two pianos, and though the wardrobe grew shabbier and shabbier and almost all the men were called up, for me and for many it was our ballet which kept our souls alive in our darkest hours.

For some years I had been writing adult novels. Just before the war a publisher had asked me if I would attempt a book for children "about the stage". She said, "I think children will like to read about child actors." At first I said, "No, what I like writing is adult novels." Then suddenly I saw what such a book could mean to me. I would let one child in the book be an actress, but one should be a child dancer. A child of startling talent such as I had seen in Ninette de Valois and Baronova. I would give my fictional child dancer as a present to the child me who had so longed to be what she could never be. So I sat down and wrote the book. It was about three children, only one of them was a dancer. This did not matter to me. Still pleasing myself, I called the book *Ballet Shoes*.

A VISIT TO
THE BOLSHOI BALLET

Mary Stacey (aged nine)

Crash! went the orchestra. The curtains rose to reveal the scene of a Christmas party. The Bolshoi Ballet had begun.

I was at Covent Garden to see the *Nutcracker*, danced by the most famous ballet company in the world—the Bolshoi Ballet.

Covent Garden is in the heart of London and is famous for two things. One is the fruit, flower and vegetable market where people from all over England come to buy their greengroceries. The other is the Royal Opera House. It is odd to feel that whilst in the splendour of the Royal Opera, with its chandeliers and fitted carpets, only a few yards away in the early mornings the sounds of barrows and people shouting "come buy my fresh flowers" are heard.

Well, here I was in the Upper Slips, feeling very grand and high and mighty.

The party on the stage is being given by Masha and her brother. The conjurer appears and brings all the dolls to life to play with them, but they disappear. To console her the conjurer makes her a present of Nutcrackers. Her brother breaks the toy accidentally. The conjurer chases the boy away and tries to mend it, but does not succeed.

It is now night. Masha comes down to see the wounded Nutcracker. To her surprise and delight the toys grow and come to life: the tin soldiers march into the room under the Nutcracker's command.

Suddenly, from under the floor, mice appear, led by King Rat. The Nutcracker alone confronts them. Masha manages to fling a lighted candle among them. The mice disappear in fear. The field of battle is deserted except for the Nutcracker who lies motionless on the floor. Masha and the dolls rush to him. A miracle occurs—

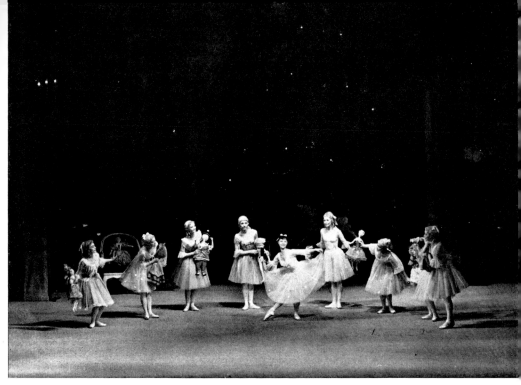

Ekaterina Maximova as Masha at her Christmas Party in the Bolshoi
Ballet's production of *The Nutcracker*

Galina Ulanova, formerly one of the greatest ballerinas of the Bolshoi
Ballet, instructs Ekaterina Maximova and Vladimir Vasiliev at a
rehearsal for *The Nutcracker*

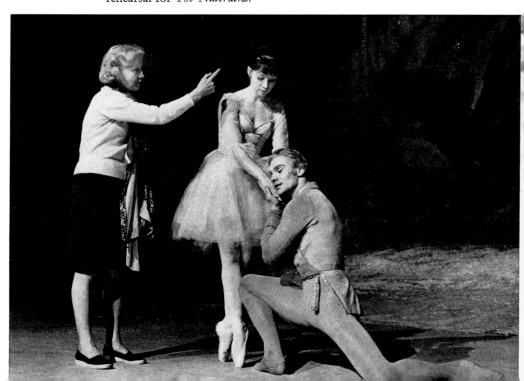

instead of the ugly and amusing toy there stands in front of her a young and handsome prince. He takes her to his land. And so begin Masha's adventures in the land of the Christmas Tree.

The Russian dancers managed to portray a very wonderful and exciting dream to the audience, especially the Nutcracker Doll. He was so doll-like and managed to appear so floppy when he was wounded that I really thought he *was* a doll.

Ekaterina Maximova, as Masha, danced really well. She showed her feelings in graceful and romantic dancing, and she was so good that I felt what she felt. When she thought the Nutcracker Doll was dead, I wanted to cry. The Rat King with his ruby red eyes was an excellent villain. On his second appearance he climbed half-way up a curtain and looked round evilly. I was scared and felt like hiding under a chair, but instead I sat and laughed nervously. The men dancers were so strong that they tossed the ballerinas up in the air as easily as wink. Everyone leaped across the stage and made it look easier than it actually is, so much so that I wanted to go and join them.

The costumes were gorgeous. The dolls wore brightly coloured national costume, which made them stand out, especially the Spanish dancers. The Nutcracker Doll and Prince were in bright red. The Rat King wore a rat's head with a purple cloak, and the Hours wore sky-blue with beautiful gold wings.

I liked this ballet because it is the sort of thing little girls do dream about, and I have often imagined I will meet the Nutcracker Prince, bold, handsome and brave, because he is the sort of man I would like to marry.

STORIES
FROM THE BALLET

Swan Lake

Music by Tchaikovsky
Choreography by Petipa and Ivanov

The young Prince Siegfried was celebrating his twenty-first birthday with his friends and the local peasants in front of the old grey castle. His special friend Benno, and his tutor Wolfgang, were with him, and for a while the young Prince was able to put aside his worries and responsibilities as heir to the throne.

Unfortunately, at a particularly rowdy moment the Princess-Mother paid them an unexpected visit, extremely displeased to see her son and his courtiers mingling freely with the peasants. Coldly, his mother reminded the Prince that on the following evening he must fulfil his duties as heir and choose a bride at the State Ball held in his honour. Then she turned and swept back to the castle.

The Prince felt depressed, as if his last hours of freedom and happiness were ebbing away. He rejoined the festivities with sudden desperate vigour, and the merry-making continued until sunset. The peasants began to leave and the Prince stood sadly apart, alone. The soft red rays of the setting sun were slanting across the castle walls as Siegfried gazed at the darkening fields and woods that would one day be his kingdom. A flock of wild swans flew low over the castle and across the meadows to a distant forest, and on a sudden impulse Benno suggested that Prince Siegfried should join him and hunt the swans.

By midnight the hunting party had arrived at a lake, deep in the heart of the forest. Benno and the huntsmen sighted the swans and dashed after them, but the Prince preferred to remain alone, thinking, watching the moonlight on the water and listening to the night breeze in the reeds.

He watched a swan glide across the lake towards him. It reached the bank nearby, and was suddenly transformed into a lovely young girl. Prince Siegfried stared in wonder as she moved slowly towards him, as graceful on land as the swan had been on water. The girl explained that she was the Princess Odette and with some faithful companions she was doomed under the spell of a wicked magician to spend her life as a swan, only regaining her natural form for a few hours at night. The sorcerer watched over them constantly, either in his own twisted shape, or as a great grey owl. Prince Siegfried, horrified, asked Odette if there was any way she could escape her grim fate. Only, Odette told him, by the promise of marriage from a young man who had never plighted his troth before. It must be a young man whose love for Odette was as faithful and deep as her love for him.

As Odette finished her story the magician leaped down before them, his eyes flashing with malice, his owl-wings poised to attack Siegfried. Odette pleaded with him not to harm the Prince, but Siegfried impulsively raised his bow to shoot the evil creature. The sorcerer towered over Siegfried ready to destroy him, but Odette flung herself forward and stayed the Prince's hand. The magician departed in a rage, swooping among the nearby trees, a sinister owl shape through the branches.

The little glade by the lake was filled with swan-maidens, floating across the moonlight, half flying, half dancing. As they glided through the trees, Benno and the huntsmen caught sight of them, and in the dim light saw only the shape of swans. They raised their crossbows to shoot while the swan-maidens trembled in fear. Prince Siegfried, drawn by the mystical, wonderful sight of the flock of swan-maidens, hurriedly appeared and ordered his men not to shoot.

Delicately Odette begged the Prince for protection, which he gladly agreed to give. Never had he seen such sweet beauty, and as the swan-maidens danced with their Queen, Siegfried felt transported to a world of dreams and unearthly happiness. Odette slipped quietly away, and the Prince followed, anxious not to lose her.

The swan-maidens continued their dancing, watching with amusement the antics of four little cygnets, and after a time a puzzled Siegfried joined them, still searching for Odette. Suddenly she appeared again and Siegfried declared his love for her. When Odette expressed her own love for him, Siegfried solemnly promised to marry her and save her from the sorcerer's spell. In tender happiness they danced together, until the first grey light of dawn crept across the lake. Though Siegfried tried to hold Odette, she slipped from his arms, already part swan again, her winged arms fluttering, her slender neck bending this way and that as she returned to the lake with her swan-maidens. Siegfried remained, a lonely figure, on the shore, watching the swans disappear across the water.

The following night the castle glittered with the splendour of the State Ball. Only the Prince seemed melancholy amid such excitement, and a little preoccupied as he and his mother greeted the guests. The Princess-Mother ordered Siegfried to dance with each of the six royal maidens she presented to him. Then he must choose one for his bride. Though each princess was pretty and charming, Siegfried hardly noticed them, for his thoughts were only of Odette.

The dancing ended. The Prince now faced the formidable task of either choosing one of his six partners or explaining to his unsympathetic mother about the Swan-Queen. But before he could do anything there was a sudden bustle and commotion. Two uninvited guests were announced: the wicked magician, now in human form and calling himself Baron von Rothbart, presented to the court his daughter, Odile, who by his magic seemed to be Odette herself. Yet there was a sinister difference in her hard flashing eyes, her showy brilliance. She was dressed entirely in black, her dress embroidered heavily with diamonds, a glittering crown in her hair. But Siegfried saw only the Odette of his dreams in her looks and smiles and was certain he had found his Swan-Queen again.

The Ball continued: everyone buzzed with rumours and gossip as they watched the Prince dance on and on with the beautiful, unknown Princess. A few guests noticed with surprise a delicate white swan beating its wings in distress against the windows. It was Odette, not yet able to assume her true form, beseeching Siegfried to be faithful to their love. But the false Odile kept the Prince's attentions fixed on her alone. Never once did he lift his eyes from her face. As midnight neared, von Rothbart hovered closer, and Odile increased her affectionate looks and smiles for the Prince. Infatuated, Siegfried asked for her hand in marriage. Leering with triumph, the Baron made him swear that Odile was his only true love. As he did so, before the whole court, Siegfried suddenly looked up and saw the distressed Odette outside the window. He had forsaken her. With mocking laughs, von Rothbart and Odile vanished, and as the court was plunged into confusion, Siegfried rushed from the castle in a desperate search for Odette.

In the forest, by the lake, the swan-maidens waited exultantly for their Princess, certain that Prince Siegfried would break the magician's spell and free them all. But Odette arrived, distraught and weeping, her hope and joy shattered. She gazed longingly at the dark waters of the lake, wanting to drown herself while she was still in human form, but her companions gently restrained her. A distant growl of thunder warned them that a storm was approaching, and the first heavy drops of rain began to fall. Shafts of lightning lit the tiny clearing, and Odette saw Siegfried stumbling through the trees, calling her name in anguish. He begged her forgiveness for his unwitting betrayal and they were joyfully reunited. But the magician appeared, grinning his revenge: Siegfried must fulfil his oath and marry Odile, and Odette must return to her swan form. The lovers decided to die together while there was still time. Von Rothbart vanished, determined to thwart this plan with all his mighty powers. But Siegfried and Odette, with one last embrace, cast themselves into the rain-torn lake. Von Rothbart appeared again but it was too late. The joint sacrifice of Siegfried and Odette had broken the spell. His powers vanquished, the evil sorcerer fell dead.

The storm slowly died out, and the swan-maidens clustered round the bank, but as daylight gently awoke the world, they realised they were free from enchantment. And across the water they saw Odette and Siegfried journeying hand in hand to a world of eternal happiness.

*   *   *

Swan Lake *was first staged at the Bolshoi Theatre, Moscow, in 1877, with Karpakova as Odette/Odile, and was not a success. After the success of the* Sleeping Beauty *at the Maryinsky Theatre it was decided to revive* Swan Lake *too, in 1895, though Tchaikovsky did not live to see the*

*triumph for he died of cholera in 1893. Petipa and Ivanov were responsible
for the revival, Petipa arranged Act I and most of Act III, and Ivanov
the remainder. Act II was produced at Tchaikovsky's memorial service.*

*The ballet was first performed in London by a Russian company in a
shortened version based on the first two Acts in 1910. Diaghilev's Ballet
presented another two-Act version (Acts II and III) at Covent Garden
with Mathilde Ksheshina and Nijinsky.*

*The first truly English production was when Act II was presented by
the Camargo Society at the Savoy Theatre with Olga Spessiva and Anton
Dolin in 1932. The full-length ballet entered the Vic-Wells repertory in
1934, with Alicia Markova in the leading role. As this version preserved
the original choreography of Petipa and Levana, it was the one remounted
by the Royal Ballet when they designed a new production of the* Sleeping
Beauty *in 1963, with David Blair and Margot Fonteyn.*

COPPELIA

Music by Delibes
Choreography by Ivanov and Cecchetti

Many, many years ago scholars and alchemists were much more
learned in the magical arts than we are to-day. One of them, Dr.
Coppelius, was a very clever toymaker, who could make dolls so
lifelike that when he wound them up they could move their arms
and legs, and even walk and dance. His greatest ambition as a
magician was to bring one of his dolls to life.

He had produced a doll so realistic that from a distance people
really thought she was a young girl. He called the doll Coppelia,
and he would place her on his balcony, supposedly reading a book,
but when anyone passed by the wily old doctor would turn a key
so that Coppelia nodded and smiled to them, looked from side to
side, and waved her hands. She never spoke, of course, but this
reserve, together with her pretty face, excited the admiration and
curiosity of the young men of the town.

Opposite the house of Dr. Coppelius lived Swanilda, a young
and popular girl in the town, who had become suspicious and
jealous of Coppelia. She felt there was something odd about this
haughty young girl who never spoke but only bowed and stared

with her hard little blue eyes. Besides, Swanilda had a nasty feeling that her own sweetheart, Franz, was paying too much attention to this girl.

One morning, Swanilda, filled with curiosity, decided to try and speak to Coppelia and discover a little more about her. She approached the balcony where Coppelia was sitting, apparently reading. Swanilda made some polite greetings—but received no answer. She went a little farther and curtsied and smiled, but still there was no response. Swanilda grew annoyed and started to perform the most ridiculous antics, but Coppelia ignored her and kept her eyes on her book. In a fit of temper Swanilda shook her fist and stormed back into her house.

As the door slammed behind her, Franz appeared, and with a guilty look behind him at Swanilda's house, rushed eagerly towards Coppelia's balcony and stood gazing rapturously at her. Then he began to throw kisses to her and clasped his hands over his heart to show his fervent love. Old Dr. Coppelius saw him through the window and, overjoyed at the success of his marvellous doll, stretched out his hand surreptitiously to turn the key. To the delight of Franz, Coppelia suddenly began to nod and bow to him, and he was more entranced than ever.

After a short while the doctor removed Coppelia in order to preserve the air of mystery about her, and the disconsolate Franz turned away. He was met by an irate Swanilda, who had seen his protestations to Coppelia. She hardly had time to storm at him when a group of young friends came running into the little square and started a noisy dance. They were interrupted by the Burgo-master who announced that there would be a fête to celebrate the presentation of a bell to the town. The Duke would present dowries to all those who were betrothed, and the Burgomaster teasingly asked Swanilda if she would be amongst them. Mischievously, Swanilda tested Franz's faithfulness with an ear of corn and was distressed when the test failed. The Burgomaster hurriedly tried to reconcile the couple and persuaded all the young people to dance for him, but Franz, feeling confused and unhappy at Swanilda's anger and Coppelia's aloofness, soon departed.

Just after the Burgomaster had left the square, old Dr. Coppelius appeared from his house for one of his rare walks through the town. He looked so comical with his black hat and long coat, his spindly legs and ungainly walk, that the young people started to tease him wickedly. They danced round him and tried to make him join them, jostling the poor old man hither and thither. Angrily waving his stick, he managed to get rid of them, but as he pulled out his handkerchief to mop his brow the big black key of his house fell to the ground. In his agitation the doctor failed to notice and went on his way. But Swanilda and her friends pounced on it with glee. Now, at last, they could discover the unknown secrets and mysteries of the old man's toy shop. Now they would really be able to meet his stuck-up daughter, Coppelia.

Swanilda unlocked the door and she and her friends crept fearfully into the house. At that moment Franz returned—he had seen Dr. Coppelius leave and decided that he would improve his acquaintance with Coppelia.

The toy shop was a strange, dark place filled with deep cupboards, musty books and lots of tall, still figures staring silently at Swanilda and her friends, frightening them into momentary confusion. They soon realised that they were only looking at dolls and found the clockwork apparatus to set the dolls in motion. They had a Scottish doll dancing a jig, a Spanish doll the flamenco, Chinese, Oriental and Crusader dolls all dancing while they laughed and tried to join them.

Swanilda approached one of the cupboards and, flinging it open, started in astonishment at finding Coppelia. So she was only a doll after all! Swanilda walked round, poking the doll, and slipped Coppelia's shawl round her own shoulders. She was just about to try on all her clothes for a full imitation when the door was flung open, and with a roar of rage Dr. Coppelius rushed in. He drove the young people out, but Swanilda slipped into Coppelia's cupboard and shut the door.

Wearily the old man sat down in his chair to rest. His attention was suddenly caught by the sound of footsteps. He stayed quiet until the intruder appeared. It was Franz! Coppelius pretended to be one of his own dolls and sat quietly until Franz got inside the door. Franz peered round the room anxiously looking for Coppelia. He even poked the old doctor to see if he were real or just a toy.

When Franz was right inside the toy shop the old doctor jumped up and seized him by the ear, determined to teach the impertinent youth a lesson. As Franz pleaded for mercy, pouring out his love for Coppelia, the doctor had a better idea. He had discovered in his ancient books of magic that the transfer of a human spirit into a doll would bring it to life, in the way that he had always dreamed. He decided to experiment with Franz.

He gave the boy a glass of wine, into which he slipped a strong sleeping draught. Soon Franz lay sleeping peacefully, and the doctor started to chant spells over him.

By this time Swanilda, peering frantically from the cupboard, had devised a plan to save Franz and teach the doctor a lesson. Before he could go too far with his spells she stepped stiffly out of the cupboard dressed in Coppelia's clothes.

Dr. Coppelius was terribly excited. After so many years of dreaming, here was his own creation, walking, smiling and alive. With pride and delight he encouraged her to run, dance, jump: to do any thing she wanted. But things soon got out of control. The doctor watched in horror as she tore up his book of magic. Then she mocked him, and when he tried to scold her she ran round breaking the dolls. Crash! Smash! In vain the doctor tried to pacify her. He gave her the lovely Spanish shawl from the broken doll and she flung herself into a wild Spanish dance. He tried the Scottish shawl and she started an even wilder jig.

The noise and commotion roused Franz, and he sat up slowly, rubbing his eyes. Delighted to see him safe and unharmed by magic, Swanilda ran across and hugged him. Dr. Coppelius was now completely bewildered, and distraught, and when Swanilda flung open the cupboard and revealed the limp doll slumped on her chair, he could only collapse with a moan. Franz now realised how foolish he had been to fall in love with a clockwork doll and he begged Swanilda to forgive him. She did this gladly, and as their friends arrived, anxious to know what had become of the couple, they all departed in high spirits, leaving poor old Coppelius disconsolately surveying his wrecked toy shop.

Later, at the fête, the Duke gave all the betrothed couples, including Swanilda and Franz, purses of gold. Coppelius doddered in, angrily complaining that his dolls had been broken and a lifetime's work ruined. The Duke managed to pacify him with an extra large bag of gold. Then a masque of the Dance of the Hours was performed in honour of the wedding of Franz and Swanilda.

*   *   *

Coppelia was performed for the first time at the Paris Opéra in May 1870. It was a magnificent occasion graced by the Emperor Napoleon III and the Empress Eugenie. Revised from a tale of Hoffmann, the ballet was the corporate effort of Delibes, Saint Leon, the choreographer, and Charles Nuitten who produced the scenario. The first Coppelia was a young Italian girl of fifteen, Guiseppina Bozzacchi, and the whole production was a magnificent success.

Sadly, within two months the Franco-Prussian war broke out, Paris was besieged and the Opéra closed. Bozzacchi died of smallpox in November.

In France much of the original version has been preserved. An arrangement by Ivanov and Cecchetti was produced in St. Petersburg in 1894, and it is this version which forms the basis of the Royal Ballet's production.

Coppelia was first performed in Lendine, produced by Alexander Genée for his niece Adeline in 1911. Acts I and II were performed at Sadler's Wells in 1933, with Lydia Lopokova as Swanilda. It was first danced at the Royal Opera House in 1946, with Margot Fonteyn and Robert Helpmann (Coppelius), and revived again in 1954.

GISELLE

Music by Adam
Choreography by Marius Petipa

In a small Rhineland village lived Giselle. She was much admired for her good looks, her high spirits and her gay dancing, but she had two particular suitors: Hilarion, a young peasant boy, had loved Giselle for a long time and hoped to marry her, but he had become increasingly resentful of the rival attentions of a handsome young stranger to the village. This was Count Albrecht, a wealthy noble whose castle towered above the village and the surrounding forests and pastures. He was already betrothed to Bathilde, the cool, dignified daughter of the Duke of Courland, but having seen Giselle on one of his hunting expeditions, Albrecht had fallen desperately in love with her. Knowing what an unsuitable sweetheart he was for a simple village girl, but heedless of future unhappiness, he decided to disguise himself as a peasant named Loys in order to win her love. With the aid of his young squire, Wilfred,

Albrecht used to arrive secretly at a deserted cottage, discard his fine clothes and his sword, and attired as a simple peasant go forth to meet Giselle.

Albrecht easily won the love of Giselle and their meetings were full of joy and tenderness. Giselle was delighted to discover that Albrecht shared her passion for dancing, and they were soon acclaimed by the other young villagers for their graceful dancing.

Hilarion grew very jealous of the happiness of Giselle and Loys, until, hearing that they were betrothed, he could bear it no longer. Rudely thrusting into one of their gayest dances, he reminded Giselle of his own steadfast love for her and warned her against Loys, an unknown stranger whom he feared would only bring her unhappiness. But Giselle had fallen too deeply in love with Albrecht to listen and, confident of his own feelings for her, she begged Albrecht to send Hilarion away.

The couple were joined by the other young peasants, who were ready to celebrate the grape harvest, and soon Albrecht and Giselle were leading the rejoicing. Their gaiety disturbed Giselle's mother, Berthe, who shared Hilarion's distrust of the handsome stranger, and she was not at all pleased to see her daughter wasting her time with such an unsuitable partner. Scolding Giselle, she reminded her of the sinister legends of the Wilis, the ghosts of young girls, too fond of dancing, who are betrayed in love and die of a broken heart. Each night they rise from their graves to dance, and should they encounter any man, they remorselessly revenge themselves by dancing him to death.

Albrecht listened carelessly to such village tales, but suddenly the sound of hunting horns brought him to his senses, and with a hasty farewell to Giselle he hurried off to join his hunting companions. Hilarion followed him, determined to find out his rival's secret.

The hunting party arrived in the village—it was the Duke of Courland and his daughter, who, having lost Albrecht, needed rest and refreshment. Berthe ordered her daughter to serve wine and food to the noble couple. Bathilde was enchanted with the grace and beauty of Giselle, and hearing that she, too, was betrothed gave the girl a present of her own necklace. Delighted, Giselle broke into a happy dance, and was crowned Queen of the Harvest by the other villagers. The Duke and his daughter entered Berthe's cottage for a rest, leaving the villagers to continue their celebrations. Giselle was soon joined by Albrecht, satisfied that he had lost his hunting companions and anxious once more to claim Giselle as his own true love.

Suddenly Hilarion burst among them, waving Albrecht's sword which he had discovered in the cottage and on which he had recognised the Count's noble crest. His desire for revenge overcame any feelings of sympathy for Giselle, and he rushed forward to tell her his discovery and, in unmasking Loys, to destroy her idyllic love.

At first Giselle refused to believe him, but Albrecht could not deny it, and when Bathilde emerged from the cottage, disturbed by the fuss and claimed Albrecht as her fiancé, she flung herself in her mother's arms sobbing hysterically. Attempts to soothe her failed, and suddenly she threw off her necklace in disgust and broke into a wild, whirling dance, her mind numbed by shock, her reason gone. Her troubled friends watched helplessly as she pathetically re-lived her love affair with Loys, eloquently repeating the steps of their happiest dances together. Then, as Albrecht tried to soothe her, she realised how cruelly she had been deceived, and in a sudden fit of despair she seized his sword and tried to stab herself. Brokenhearted, she faltered a few more steps and fell dying to the ground.

Giselle was buried in a lonely grave in the forest, a spot avoided by the superstitious villagers after sunset because of the legends of the Wilis. One night, Hilarion, returning home late, caught a glimpse of wraith-like figures and hastened to warn his friends that the fearful ghosts had appeared. As midnight struck, Myrtha, the Queen of the Wilis, summoned her maidens to dance. Using her supernatural powers, she brought Giselle from her grave to join their terrible rites, so that henceforth she, too, was doomed to dance from midnight to dawn, and seek revenge on any man they found. The shimmering, graceful figures, clad in soft white dresses, glided away through the trees to seek their victims.

With slow, sorrowing steps, Albrecht searched the forest for the grave of Giselle. Bitterly reproaching himself for deceiving her, and causing her death, he had decided to lay a wreath of lilies on her grave and keep a night vigil in atonement. He approached the white cross that marked her grave and, kneeling, prayed and wept for the young girl he had truly loved. After a time he rose, wearily, and turned to go: but there stood Giselle, as beautiful as ever. Full of joy they danced together once more, except that Albrecht could never quite grasp Giselle in his arms—for she always eluded him, would teasingly vanish and then reappear elsewhere.

Suddenly a tormented and terrified Hilarion appeared, harried and pursued by mocking Wilis who compelled him to dance on and on with them until, as he stumbled with exhaustion, they drove him into a deep dark lake nearby.

Giselle anxiously tried to protect Albrecht—but it was too late. The Queen had seen him and now condemned him to the same fate. Giselle whispered to her lover to cling to the cross, over which the Wilis have no power, but the angry Queen asserted her control over Giselle as a Wilis and coldly commanded her to lure Albrecht from the protection of the cross by her exquisite dancing. The agonised Giselle could not disobey, and slowly started to dance so movingly that Albrecht could not resist: too soon he eagerly joined her.

In that haunted glade they danced with unequalled ecstasy and beauty, danced only for each other, their love reaching heights they had never known before. The other Wilis surrounded them, whirling into wilder and wilder dancing, until Albrecht began to falter in exhaustion. Desperately Giselle tried to sustain him, but the contemptuous Queen ordered her to continue the dance. On and on they whirled, while Albrecht vainly tried to keep step with his beloved Giselle, hoping to win her for ever, yet knowing his strength was ebbing fast. He began to stumble, to sway, to sink, knew he could hardly last longer, but still Giselle compelled and entreated him. Mists formed in front of his eyes and in agony he stretched his arms out to Giselle. He knew he could last no more. But now the first pale light of dawn flickered into the glade and the Wilis drew back, slowly fading through the trees, and taking Giselle with them. Albrecht was left alive—but alone.

* * *

Giselle, *the greatest ballet masterpiece of the Romantic period, was first created at the Paris Opéra on 28th June, 1841, and was soon being performed all over Europe and in America. Théophile Gautier, the poet and a perceptive ballet critic, wrote the scenario in collaboration with a professional dramatist, Saint-Georges, taking his inspiration from the Slavonic legend of The Wilis.*

The first London performance of Giselle *was at Her Majesty's Theatre on 12th March, 1842, but it was an almost forgotten ballet in Western Europe when the Diaghilev Ballet presented it in 1910 with Karsavina and Nijinsky, and Paris then found it old-fashioned.*

Giselle *was first performed by the Royal Ballet (then the Vic-Wells Ballet) at the Old Vic on 1st January, 1934, with Alicia Markova and Anton Dolin. It was first danced at the Royal Opera House, Covent Garden, on 12th June, 1946, with Margot Fonteyn and Alexis Rassine, and is now frequently performed there.*

THE NUTCRACKER

Music by Tchaikovsky
Choreography by Petipa and Ivanov

In a large house in the centre of a little German town, about a hundred years ago, Councillor von Stahlbaum and his wife were giving a magnificent Christmas party for their two children, Fritz and Clara. The rooms were a blaze of lights, the atmosphere full of excitement, as the guests began arriving through the snow with their gay, mischievous children.

Inside the house the grown-ups were decorating the Christmas tree with candles, sparkling stars, bells and baubles, crackers and presents. The children simply could not bear to wait a moment longer to see it and burst into the room. The grown-ups began to hand out the presents as the children crowded eagerly round: toys, sweets and charming surprises. Clara was delighted with a pair of pretty dancing slippers.

Dr. Drosselmeyer arrived at the party, an old friend of Councillor von Stahlbaum, but his spindly arthritic legs, his bent back and long nose gave him such an odd appearance that the children were terrified at first. Dr. Drosselmeyer was a kind old man, though, and he soon won his young guests' friendship, for from nowhere—or so it seemed—he produced some life-size dolls and made them dance.

Clara put on her new slippers and gave a little dance of thanks for Dr. Drosselmeyer. He was charmed by her dance and gave her a handsome Nutcracker, shaped like a soldier. The children were

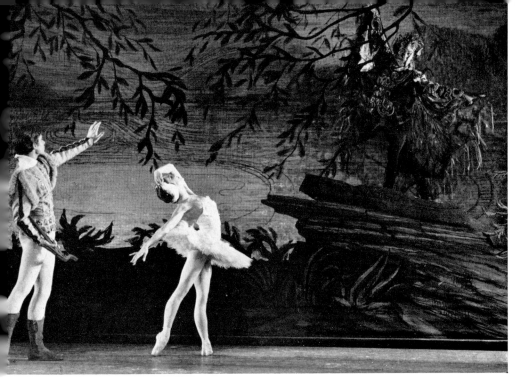

Swan Lake: Odette (Shirley Graham) protects Siegfried (David Wall) from the Magician (David Gordon)

The Royal Ballet in *Swan Lake:* Prince Siegfried dances with Odette and her swan maidens

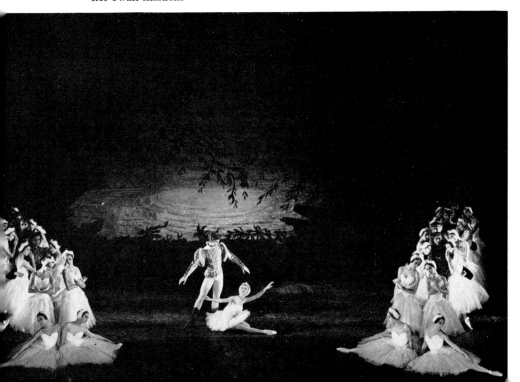

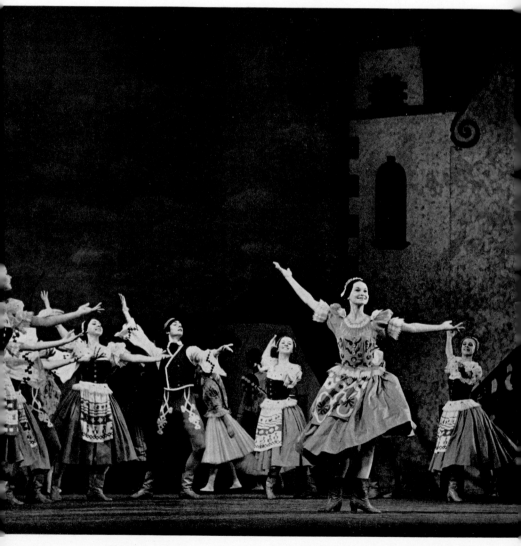

The Royal Ballet in *Coppelia*: the young people of the town dance
noisily together

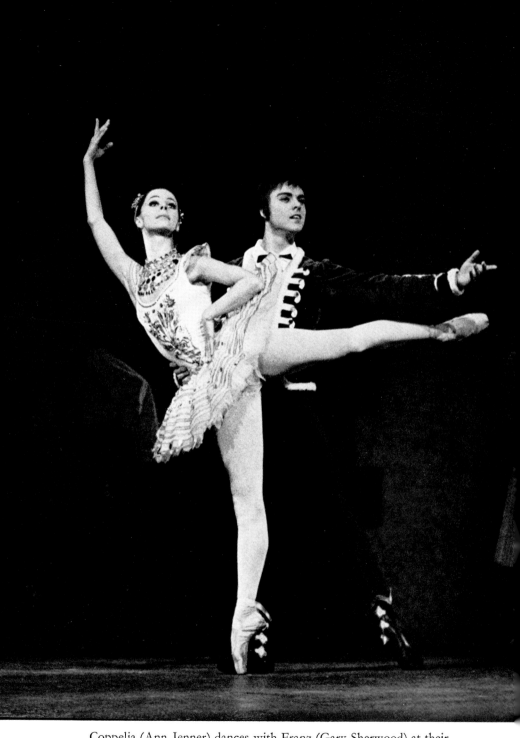

Coppelia (Ann Jenner) dances with Franz (Gary Sherwood) at their wedding

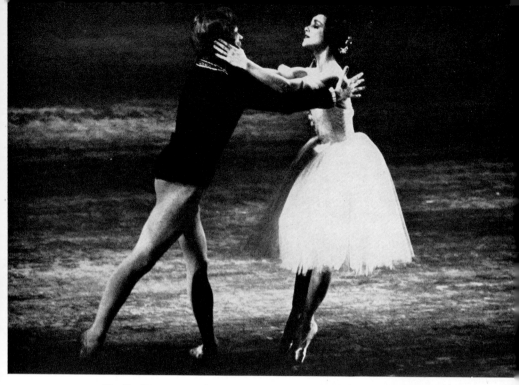

Giselle (Doreen Wells) compelled by the Wilis lures Albrecht
(David Wall) away from the safety of her grave to dance with her

The Sleeping Beauty: Aurora (Svetlana Beriosova) dances with one of her
suitors on her sixteenth birthday

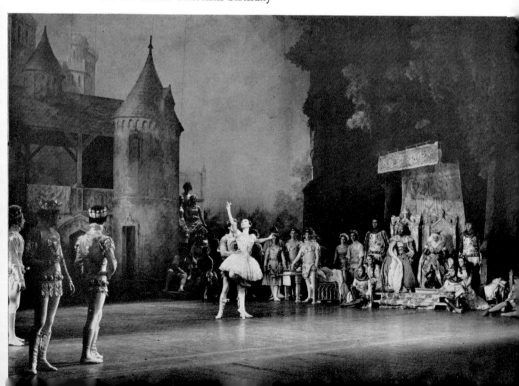

fascinated and the old man showed them how the doll really could crack nuts. To Clara, the Nutcracker seemed almost real, and she hugged it and played with it. Franz, her brother, soon became jealous and teased and mocked her. Then he snatched the doll, but Clara tried to grab it back, and in the struggle the Nutcracker was broken: no longer could he raise his arms and crack nuts. Clara sobbed, and her father, ashamed at his son's bad behaviour gave him a beating, while Dr. Drosselmeyer comforted Clara. The guests began to say good-bye and go home through the crisp winter snow, and sleepy Franz and Clara were carried up to bed.

Later that night Clara crept down the stairs to the darkened drawing-room to play with her beloved Nutcracker. The room seemed strange and mysterious in the dark, and as Clara approached her doll she was startled by the malevolent beady eyes of two large mice, who silently vanished. Safely in a big arm-chair at last, Clara started to talk sleepily to the Nutcracker. The clock struck twelve, and she was startled to look up and see Dr. Drosselmeyer—but a different, agile Dr. Drosselmeyer, who smiled at her but did not speak. He made the Christmas tree grow bigger and bigger before her eyes and the candles burn brightly once more. Then he was gone and Clara heard sudden scuffling movements. She watched in excitement as the dolls began to come to life, including her dear Nutcracker, who saluted and kissed her hand.

A mass of beady eyes peered across the room, a hundred mousy tails went flick-flack, flick-flack ominously along the floor, and Clara and the Nutcracker realised they were about to be attacked by an evil mouse army. The dolls hid in terror but the brave Nutcracker summoned the toy soldiers and a fierce battle began. Clara crouched in her chair and held her breath as a duel between the Mouse King and the Nutcracker started. The cunning mouse was almost victorious when Clara suddenly acted— and threw her shoe at the Mouse King. He was distracted just for a moment—and the Nutcracker darted forward and killed him.

In his moment of victory over the Mouse King, the Nutcracker was transformed into a handsome Prince, dressed in silver and white. He commanded the walls of Clara's house to disappear with a wave of his hand, and suddenly Clara found she was standing in a forest of glittering snow. The Prince was bringing a dazzling fairy towards her: the Fairy of Ice and Snow, who persuaded Clara to dance with her. It was a magical dance for Clara. She felt like a snowflake as she whirled and jumped and floated in the fairy's arms. Then the Nutcracker Prince took Clara and flew with her over mountains, vast plains and glittering rivers to the Kingdom of Sweets, where the sweet, delicate Sugar Plum Fairy reigned.

The graceful Sugar Plum Fairy invited Clara to sit on her throne and watch the festivities in her honour. And a wonderful carnival began, one that Clara would never forget, with entertainments and dances by strange Arabs, fiery Spaniards, fast-whirling Russians and many more, oh, so many more that she could hardly keep count. Then a galaxy of soft, colourful flowers appeared and danced a gentle waltz.

The Sugar Plum Fairy and the Nutcracker Prince danced a graceful duet for Clara and then invited her to join them all in a final waltz. But Clara felt terribly sleepy—she couldn't keep up, her eyes were closing, she couldn't keep up, she couldn't keep up, she couldn't . . . then she suddenly opened her eyes. She was back at home. There stood the dark Christmas tree, the toys scattered on the floor, the Nutcracker lying at her feet. Had it all been a dream? Clara wondered.

Another version of this ballet exists, retained in Russia, by the Bolshoi Ballet:
Clara is called Masha, and when the Nutcracker fights the Rat King he is wounded, lying motionless on the floor. Masha rushes to him as the mice flee, and the Nutcracker rises from the floor, a handsome Prince—while Masha herself seems suddenly older, more beautiful—a Princess! They go to the land of the Christmas Tree, but the wicked mice pursue them. As Masha and the Prince approach the beautiful Star of the Tree, the Rat King leads his army in another attack. The Prince vanquishes him for ever and then, with the dolls, he and Masha celebrate their victory. But a new day dawns and Masha awakes to find herself alone at home, a little girl with her Nutcracker doll.

*　　*　　*

The Nutcracker *was the third and last of the great ballet scores which Tchaikovsky composed for the Imperial Theatres in Russia. It was planned as a successor to the* Sleeping Beauty. *At first it had little success, but it has become one of the classics of ballet.*

Based on a French version of a story by Hoffmann, the choreography was devised by Petipa and continued after his illness by Ivanov. The original production was first performed at the Maryinsky Theatre in St. Petersburg in 1892, but the set and costumes were found dreary in the first act and vulgar in the last. But largely because of Tchaikovsky's music, the Nutcracker *continued to be occasionally revised. It was first produced for the Vic-Wells Ballet in 1934. The Royal Ballet's version, based on that of the Bolshoi Ballet, was first performed in February 1968, but the customary version told here is produced every year by The Festival Ballet.*

THE SLEEPING BEAUTY

Music by Tchaikovsky
Choreography by Petipa

In a magnificent fairy-tale palace a lavish christening feast was in full progress. King Florestan and his Queen were so delighted at the birth of their baby daughter, Princess Aurora, that they had invited the most famous and important people in their kingdom to be present.

Anxiously the Master of Ceremonies checked that all the guests had arrived, and when everyone had honoured the little Princess in her golden cradle, they stood aside for the most important guests of all. For the King and Queen had asked the Fairies to be Godmothers to the Princess, hoping each Fairy would bestow her special gift upon her and give her their powerful protection.

In a dazzling group they arrived. Each one first enchanted the guests by her graceful dancing, and then waved her wand over the tiny Princess. The Fairy of Beauty was first, and then came the Fairies of Honour, Modesty, Joy, Song and Temperament. The delighted royal parents were sure that their lucky daughter would have all the qualities to make her happy and beloved throughout her life.

The Lilac Fairy, the most powerful and beautiful of all, stepped forward. Her gift would be the last and the most important, and everyone waited, hushed and expectant. Suddenly a roll of thunder

shook the palace, and as the lightning flashed a terrible creature
stormed through the frightened guests and stood before the King
and Queen. It was the wicked Fairy Carabosse, angry and insulted
that she had not been invited to be a godmother. With trembling
hands the Master of Ceremonies looked down his long roll of
names, but Carabosse snatched it from him and threw it on the
ground. The Fairies gathered round the cradle to protect Princess
Aurora, but Carabosse pushed them aside, hissing that she would
still bestow a present, but it would be one to make the King and
Queen regret their rudeness. Everyone shivered with horror
as Carabosse peered in the cradle at the sleeping baby. With a
triumphant smile she turned and announced that at some future
date the Princess would prick her finger on a spindle—and drop
dead.

The anguish of the King and Queen was pitiful to see, and all
the guests were confused and distressed: could none of the
Princess's powerful protectors help her?

Carabosse had forgotten one person: the Lilac Fairy, who had
not yet made her gift to the Princess. Helplessly, Carabosse writhed
in rage as the Lilac Fairy promised that Aurora would not die, but
fall into a deep sleep for a hundred years from which she would be
awakened by a Prince's kiss. She waved her wand over the golden
cradle and slowly peace and happiness returned to the Court.

*   *   *

Princess Aurora grew into a beautiful and charming girl, beloved
by everyone. On her sixteenth birthday King Florestan arranged
grand celebrations, and four princes, the Prince of the North, the
South, the East and the West came to woo her. In the palace
gardens the guests joined in gay country dances, and no one was
more graceful and happy than the Princess herself.

As she danced she noticed an old woman working a strange
object she had never seen before. Aghast, her friends recognised it
as a spindle, although the King had banished them from his kingdom, hoping to forestall the fatal curse of Carabosse. Aurora was
fascinated and the old woman handed her the spindle and showed
her how to work it. She spun it a little, and then a little more—and
was so delighted she whirled into a gay little dance, teasingly resisting the attempts of her friends to remove it. Suddenly she stopped

with a little cry of pain—she had pricked her finger. As the King and Queen rushed forward in alarm, Aurora stood dazed for a few seconds and then sank to the ground, unconscious.

In a flash of triumph Carabosse appeared, mocking the weeping royal parents and rejoicing that her curse had come true. But as she vanished the Lilac Fairy entered to fulfil her promise. Gently and sweetly she cast a spell of sleep over the Court, and as everyone settled in a deep slumber round Princess Aurora, the Lilac Fairy used her magic to make tall trees of an enchanted forest spring up around the palace, concealing it from sight.

*   *   *

A hundred years went by and young Prince Florimund entered the forest on a hunting expedition. Despite the gaiety of his companions, the Prince was moody and reflective, brooding romantically on his ideal dream of love. The hopeful attempts of a young countess to win his attentions were ignored, and at last, after some lively dancing, Florimund impatiently ordered his friends off to join the hunt while he remained alone to dream.

After a short time he felt restless and impelled to walk on and on through the forest, as if some hidden force was driving him on, preventing him from quietly lingering on his thoughts. The Lilac Fairy appeared before him and showed him a vision of the Princess Aurora sleeping peacefully on her couch, as young and beautiful as at the moment she had fallen under the spell. The Prince gazed at her eagerly, and watching his interest, the Lilac Fairy summoned the vision to dance with him. Passionately, the Prince danced with the graceful girl, but all too soon the lovely creature vanished. The disappointed Prince implored the Lilac Fairy to lead him to the place where the Princess slept for he was now deeply in love with her: she was the ideal love of his dreams.

The Lilac Fairy commanded the Prince to follow her and led him through dense and tangled creepers, prickly bushes and overgrown paths to the heart of the forest where the palace stood.

It was an eerie sight inside—shrouded in dust and cobwebs the whole palace slept: servants, courtiers, King and Queen, grouped like stone statues around the soft white couch on which Aurora lay. Moved by her exquisite beauty, the Prince bent and gently kissed her—and immediately the spell was broken. The awakened Princess gazed tenderly at her Prince, filled with increasing love for him. Slowly the Court stirred and stretched. The King and Queen, roused from their long sleep, felt light of heart and full of gratitude to the Prince, and gladly consented to give him their daughter in marriage.

The wedding of the Princess Aurora and Prince Florimund was celebrated with great joy and splendour. The Lilac Fairy came with the other Fairy Godmothers, as fresh and sparkling as ever. They were joined by many famous characters from the Land of Fairy-Tales: among them Red Riding Hood and the Wolf, Puss-in-Boots and the White Cat, Harlequin and Columbine, and the Blue Birds. They danced and entertained the guests, and each new couple seemed more brilliant than the last, but when Princess Aurora and Prince Florimund appeared, their lyrical dancing dazzled everyone.

As for old Carabosse, she and her wicked magic were never heard of again, and Princess Aurora and Prince Florimund lived happily ever after, as all fairy-tale Princes and Princesses should.

*   *   *

The Sleeping Beauty *was first performed before the Tsar of Russia at the Maryinsky Theatre in St. Petersburg in 1890, who was not very impressed. "His Majesty treated me very haughtily," wrote Tchaikovsky in his diary. However, the ballet soon became very popular, but it was not until thirty years later in 1921 that Diaghilev brought it to the West, to the Alhambra Theatre, London. Surprisingly, audiences failed to respond to the magnificent production he staged, but after the war the Royal Ballet revived it, and the ballet has become a popular classic.*

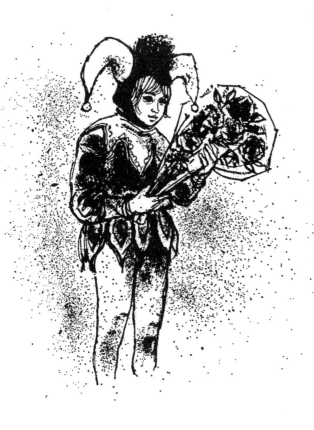

THE UGLY SWAN

A Modern Fairy Tale, with apologies to Hans
Christian Andersen, the Master.

Helen Cresswell

This story, like all good fairy-tales, begins with a christening, and
the heroine is a girl who was called Pavlova Jenkins. The really
sad thing about her name is that it was a mistake. Her parents were
ordinary people for whom plain British names were quite good
enough, and the thought would simply never have entered their

heads. Even their Dalmatian ran to nothing more exciting than Spotty.

Names are very odd things. People have a strange tendency to grow like their names, so that they come to fit them like gloves— which is why, on the whole, plain ones are best. A name like Joy, for instance, must take a good deal of living up to. So you see, Pavlova Jenkins began life, as we all do, handicapped by her name. The only difference between her and us is that her handicap was worse.

The baby was christened when she was three months old, and the names that had been decided upon were Ann Rosa. Aunt Sophie, Mrs. Jenkins's sister, was to be godmother.

The little party set off for church in high spirits, the ladies wearing large hats and the gentlemen their dark suits and quietest ties. No one had the least inkling of the disaster that was to befall them.

The Jenkinses' baby was the only one to be christened that afternoon. It was three o'clock and the vicar had just been woken from the nap he took after his Sunday dinner. This could have been partly the trouble. The vicar was a little deaf and a little vague at the best of times, and a meal of roast beef, Yorkshire pudding, roast potatoes, brussels sprouts and carrots, followed by treacle tart and custard, seemed to have had the effect of making him a little deafer and a little vaguer than usual. If there had been several babies for christening that day I fear that the vicar would have mixed them hopelessly. Girls would have been named Gregory, boys Rosalie, and letters written to the bishop. As it was, he made only the one small but fatal slip that was to send our heroine through life a Pavlova.

All went well till the family gathered round the font. Mrs. Jenkins handed the baby over to Aunt Sophie who held it gingerly away from her, not being used to babies. The vicar had just launched into the ceremony when above his drone came the loud, unmistakable drone of a bee. The Jenkins family peered nervously about them. However solemn the occasion, nobody wanted to be stung. Someone in the Jenkins family had once died of a bee sting so they were naturally nervous of all striped insects and even avoided eating honey as far as possible. As Mrs. Jenkins was fond of saying, "You never *know*."

The bee settled on the edge of the font. It was a particularly large one and Mr. Jenkins was sorely tempted to bang his hymn-book down on it and finish it off. But it hardly seemed either the time or the place. The bee began to walk tiptoe round the stone brim. The eyes of the Jenkins family followed it, step by step. The vicar's voice stopped. Mr. Jenkins gave his wife a sharp dig.

"Amen," he said loudly.

"Oh, yes, amen," she agreed.

The vicar started another prayer and the bee took off again. Mr. Jenkins said afterwards that it was the ladies' hats that were really to blame.

"It must have thought it was in the Botanical Gardens," he told them severely.

His theory was probably right. Mrs. Jenkins sported a few daisies and Grandma Jenkins's hat was of silken petals, but it was Aunt Sophie's that really rioted. And it was Aunt Sophie, you will remember, who was holding the baby.

To begin with she managed very well. The vicar asked her various questions and she replied quite promptly, as well she might, for she had rehearsed the scene quite fifty times during the previous week. But as the service progressed the bee began to hover ominously about the brim of her hat, and what with having to keep one eye on the baby, one on the bee and one on her place in the service sheet, Aunt Sophie began to crumble.

Both hands were fully occupied with the baby, so she was powerless to swat, flap or otherwise discourage the invader. All she could do was roll her eyes up, round and sideways in an effort to keep as close a track of it as possible. When it went out of sight she listened for the buzz, and plotted its position from that.

The service mounted to its climax. The bee matched the vicar, drone for drone. And just as the vicar asked the vital question the bee, probably excited by an imitation petunia dangling just above Aunt Sophie's left ear, zoomed in. Things happened so fast that it is difficult to analyse exactly what happened then. The theory arrived at later was that Aunt Sophie started to say, "Please, some-one—get that bee off!" or words to that effect, but remembered her obligations as a godmother in time and managed only to get out the "p" of "please". So what she then said to the vicar, in a high, strangled voice, was "P-ann Rosa!"

Even this would not have been irredeemable had not the vicar, just before his nap, been browsing through the colour supplements where an article about ballet had particularly caught his eye. So that when Aunt Sophie cried "Pannrosa!" at him, the name Pavlova (which was more or less how it sounded to him) seemed the most natural name in the world and he dipped his finger in the font and wet the baby's forehead, saying, "I name thee Pavlova," without so much as turning a hair. The Jenkinses were all so mesmerised by the bee, which was stalking the font again, that only Grandma Jenkins noticed anything amiss at the time, and as she said afterwards, "You hardly liked to take the vicar up at a time like that—and in his own church."

Then the baby began to cry and the bee (who, you will have guessed by now, was a bad fairy in disguise) buzzed off to suck the nettle flowers among the tombstones, its wicked work worked. It was only when they stopped on the way home to admire the christening card the vicar had beamingly handed them that the mistake was discovered. There, inside a border of cherubs and forget-me-nots, was the fateful word, clearly written in the vicar's large curly copperplate. They stared disbelievingly, peering over one another's shoulders.

"We shall have to go back and tell him!" shrieked Mrs. Jenkins, waving the baby for emphasis. "I never heard of such a thing! Pavlova! *Pavlova!* As if I'd call my baby that—nasty foreign name!"

Mr. Jenkins stood awkwardly fingering the christening card.

"Aren't you going to do something?" she cried. "Aren't you going to *complain?*"

"I don't really think it's the kind of thing you can complain *about,*" said Mr. Jenkins worriedly. "I mean, it's not like taking a pound of bacon rashers back to the butcher, is it?"

"Bacon rashers!" cried Mrs. Jenkins, fiercely hugging the bewildered baby.

"When it's done, it's done, isn't it?" went on her husband. "Like getting married. You just can't go back after a wedding and tell the vicar you've changed your mind, can you?"

He sounded almost wistful, and Mrs. Jenkins shot him a sharp look.

"I think it's quite a pretty name, Maggie," ventured Aunt Sophie timidly. "Dainty sounding."

Mrs. Jenkins gave her sister a murderous glance and Aunt Sophie turned the same shade as the dangling petunia that had been the cause of all the trouble. The party then started glumly back to Dunroamin, where they ate a silent tea and tried to avoid looking at the cake, which bore the legend "For our darling Ann Rosa" amid a border of pink icing rosebuds.

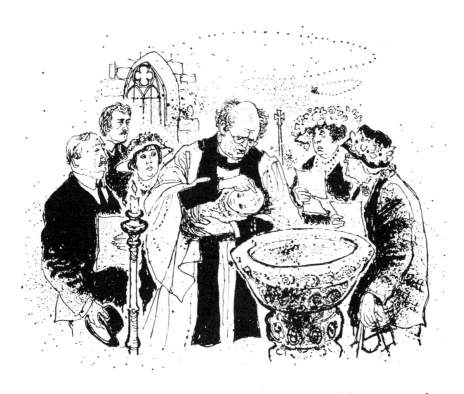

That evening Mr. and Mrs. Jenkins discussed the matter after the guests had gone. The question was whether to ignore what was written on the certificate, and call the baby Ann Rosa willy nilly, or whether to grit their teeth and stick to the Pavlova. Surprisingly, Mrs. Jenkins decided on the latter course. Or perhaps not surprisingly, as she was a person with a great respect for law, order and the printed form, and felt that once the name had actually been entered on a register, particularly a *church* register, it was really irrevocable and beyond her power to change.

Then another surprising thing happened. In the days that

followed people would peer over the edge of the pram to see the baby on her pink blankets kicking her chubby legs, and say,

"Is it a girl? What's her name?"

And when Mrs. Jenkins told them, half defiantly, they would cry,

"Oh, how sweet! What a pretty name!"

By the end of a fortnight Mrs. Jenkins had become resigned, by the end of a month she was half-convinced that she had chosen the name herself in the first place. After three months the fluffy rabbit on Pavlova's pram cover had been exchanged for a swan, and Mrs. Jenkins had decided that the baby had "dancer's legs". She was able to recognise these by virtue of having watched (at least till she had dropped off) a performance of *Giselle* on the television—a thing she would never have dreamed of doing in the past, having much preferred the Black and White Minstrels.

She borrowed a book about Pavlova from the library and was much impressed by it. Next time a ballet was shown on television she woke the baby and propped her up facing the screen. Pavlova had wakened refreshed, and gurgled and waved her arms high spiritedly throughout the performance. Mrs. Jenkins was ecstatic.

"It's as if she *knows*!" she cried. "It must have been fate, that bee in the church. And to think we might never have known!"

"Steady on, Maggie," her husband said. "There's no use going planning things for the child while she's still in her cradle. She'll have to make up her own mind."

"As if I would!" cried Mrs. Jenkins indignantly. "Of course I wouldn't *dream* of influencing her. She shall do exactly as she pleases. You know my views on mothers that push children."

Mr. Jenkins said no more, and Mrs. Jenkins did not refer to "fate" again. But she made sure that Pavlova never missed a television performance of *Coppelia* or *Les Sylphides* during the next few years and was very fussy about having her daughter's feet fitted for shoes. By now she had read enough books about ballet to know that ill-fitting shoes during childhood spelled death to any hopes of later dancing the lead in *Swan Lake*.

At three years old Pavlova was enrolled in a tots' dancing class run by a Miss Linley in the local church hall. Pavlova would thud about the floor with twenty or so other toddlers to the strains of "The Teddy Bears' Picnic", played somewhat erratically by Miss

Linley herself, who would shriek encouragement over her shoulder between bars. Sitting on a hard-backed chair and watching with the other mothers, it would sometimes seem to Mrs. Jenkins that this was a far cry from Sadler's Wells and the *Sleeping Beauty*. But she would comfort herself with the thought that this was only the beginning, and watch carefully for signs that Pavlova was beginning to appear less heavy on her feet than her contemporaries. They really all were very heavy on their feet indeed. When Miss Linley got on to "Do You Know the Muffin Man" and "The Grand Old Duke of York", the floor positively shook.

"But it's all helping to develop her little muscles," Mrs. Jenkins would think happily, counting stitches in her knitting. "And developing her poise and posture."

At five years old Pavlova was enrolled in a "proper" ballet class, run by a Miss Carter who was dark and Spanish-looking, with her hair done up in a large black chignon. She looked very much more like a prima ballerina than had Miss Linley, who had been given to handknitted woollies and untidy perms. Miss Carter wore a very short black satin dress and black fishnet tights and had the most impressively muscley legs. Mrs. Jenkins was so excited that she took Pavlova straight off and bought her first real ballet dress, in pale blue. It was not easy to fit Pavlova, because she was what her mother called "well made". What she really was, was fat. She was also unusually tall for her age.

After two months at Miss Carter's Academy Pavlova was moved into the next class. The reason Mrs. Jenkins gave for requesting this move was that Pavlova was "repeating" work she had already done at Miss Linley's. It also had the advantage that among the six-year-olds Pavlova looked less enormous and at times her mother could almost persuade herself that she was graceful, if not actually dainty.

Mrs. Jenkins no longer stayed to watch the classes. This was a "proper" school, and no such cosiness was encouraged. So it was not until the dancing display at the end of the year that she was able to watch her daughter going through her paces. Of course, she knew that Pavlova learned the five positions, and Mr. Jenkins had photographed her in all of them in the back garden. But when she saw Pavlova actually up there on the brilliantly lit stage, twirling and gliding at last in what seemed to Mrs. Jenkins like the manner born, her eyes flooded until Pavlova's new dress swam into a rose-pink blur.

After that, Mr. Jenkins was asked to put up a barre in the garage so that Pavlova could practise at home. The neighbours would hear her on summer evenings, and her "one and, two and, three and, four and," would echo over the gardens and they would smile knowingly at one another. One day, they were sure, Pavlova Jenkins would be famous. Her mother's faith was infectious, and besides, if anyone did have any doubts, there was her name—and who could argue with that?

But what of Pavlova herself? The truth of the matter is that it did not even occur to her to doubt her destiny. Her destiny was in her name, and she accepted it. Sometimes, perhaps, she would sigh wistfully as she went into the garage for an hour's practice on a summer evening, while the rest of the children in the road ran in the park, played hide-and-seek and French cricket. Sometimes, too, she would look at her reflection in the glass and wish that the round, sandy doughnut perched on the back of her head could be un-pinned sometimes and her hair fall blissfully free, or even—most daring of all thoughts—be cut off. But on the whole she did not fight against her fate and hardly even recognised her own vague feelings of uncertainty or sadness.

As to Mrs. Jenkins, if she had ever had any such feelings herself, they were dispelled once and for all one day shortly after Pavlova's sixth birthday. It was a hot day, and Pavlova was in the garden skipping while Mrs. Jenkins had a quiet snooze in the sitting-room. There was a knock at the front door and Mrs. Jenkins jerked into life. She got up, automatically untying her apron as she went, and opened the door.

A gypsy stood there, swarthy-skinned and black-eyed, like an apparition between the neat twin tubs of geraniums and lobelia.

"Oh!" cried Mrs. Jenkins.

"Clothes pegs, lady, clothes pegs, see. Buy some, lady, buy a dozen, only a shillin'."

Mrs. Jenkins stared at the wooden clothes pegs.

"But—" she faltered. She didn't want the pegs. She used plastic ones, all different colours, and had a bag full of them in the kitchen.

"Wait," she said. She went into the kitchen and fetched her purse, still only half-awake. "Never turn a gypsy away," her mother had always told her. "If you turn them away, they'll give you *the eye!*"

"Here." She held out a shilling and the gypsy smoothly exchanged it for a bundle of pegs. But she did not go. She put down her basket and looked straight into Mrs. Jenkins's sleep-blurred eyes with a hard black gaze.

"I'll tell your fortune," she said softly. "I'll tell you your luck, lady, look in the ball and find your luck for you."

"Oh no! No thank you!" cried Mrs. Jenkins. She stared back at the gypsy like a hypnotised rabbit and wondered frantically if this long black gaze was the "eye" her mother had talked about. "Really—I really don't want—" her voice trailed off.

"Cross my palm with silver," said the gypsy softly. It was half an invitation, half a threat. "There's only silver'll clear the mist from the ball . . ."

"Oh dear, is there? Oh dear! Well, here you are, then."

She fumbled into her purse and fished out all the small silver and passed it over into the smooth, ready palm, hoping that there would be enough to "cross" it with, whatever that meant. The gypsy became suddenly business-like. She dived into her basket and came up with a crystal ball that she cupped between her palm and looked into so fiercely that Mrs. Jenkins found herself staring at it too, almost as if she expected to find it suddenly full of swimming goldfish.

At that moment Pavlova appeared round the corner of the house, red-faced and puffing heavily. A sudden inspiration flashed into Mrs. Jenkins's befuddled mind.

"Tell hers!" she cried, and pointed to Pavlova. "Don't tell mine—tell hers!"

The gypsy glanced swiftly in the direction of the pointing finger.

"I'll ask the ball for the little one," she agreed, and rapidly glued her eyes back on the crystal.

"The mists is clearing, it's the silver at work, the mists . . ."

"Mummy, who's that funny lady with the glass ball?"

"Sssssh!" hissed Mrs. Jenkins fiercely. "Quiet! Listen!"

"Oh, there's luck in the mist, there's luck a'coming for the little lady, and there's green grass I see and luck all over. And there she is and all in white, she's all in white and jumping and flying, and the people shouting and yelling and clapping and oh, there's fame that the ball's telling me, fame and fortune and luck for the little lady."

Abruptly she stopped, lowered the ball and stowed it back in her basket among the pegs.

"Oh, but—is that all?" cried Mrs. Jenkins. "Couldn't you see anything else? All in white, you say?"

"The ball has shown and I have spoke," said the gypsy. "The mist rises, and the mist falls."

"Yes, I suppose it must," agreed Mrs. Jenkins, "but couldn't you just see—"

"If the ball was all, we should all be kings," said the gypsy enigmatically over her shoulder. "Good day, lady, and luck for you both."

"Oh, good morning. I mean afternoon. Thank you. And good luck to you too!" called Mrs. Jenkins after the rapidly retreating figure. "Oh dear, she's gone. Run and shut the gate after her, will you, Pavlova, she's left it open. Oh dear—what an afternoon! What was it she said—all in white . . . people clapping . . . Thank you, dear. Now run off and play. Mummy wants to think."

She thought, in fact, for most of the afternoon, so that by the time Mr. Jenkins came home that night the story she had to tell him was very much more exciting than what had actually happened, and the gypsy's predictions and Mrs. Jenkins's own hopes had been so neatly dovetailed that they were inseparable. She left out the bit about "the green grass" because it didn't seem to fit in, and expanded the bit about "all in white" into what was virtually a description of the last act of *Swan Lake*.

Mr. Jenkins, nevertheless, was unimpressed.

"Lot of rubbish!" he said when she had finished. "I'm surprised at you, Maggie. Never thought you believed in all that rubbish!"

"Oh, but I *don't*!" cried Mrs. Jenkins. "Heavens, of *course* I don't. But you must admit it's very strange. I mean, she didn't know a single thing about us, and yet she saw all that. You must admit it's strange . . ."

Mr. Jenkins, however, was not prepared to admit even that, and the subject had to be dropped. But for Mrs. Jenkins the gypsy's words seemed to be those of Fate itself, a bright promise that her own dreams for Pavlova would one day become real.

At the age of nine Pavlova took the leading part in Miss

Carter's end of term concert. Miss Carter had herself composed a ballet to fit the music of one of Benjamin Britten's lesser known works. She had a strong feeling that Pavlova Jenkins ought to be one of her star pupils, but none of the major (or even minor) classical roles really seemed to fit her exactly, and so she had ingeniously written a part that would.

The ballet was entitled *Punch and Judy*, and Pavlova herself danced the part of Punch. She enjoyed prancing about the stage brandishing her truncheon, with her bells in a feverish jangle, and her *pas de deux* with the policeman in the last act practically brought the Scout Hall down. (Literally, too.) The part also disguised her weakness in the pirouette, since if she fell over sideways in executing the step (as she frequently did) everyone thought it was deliberate and extremely funny. There were seven curtain calls, and Mrs. Jenkins was ecstatic.

She had picked some flowers, tied them with pink ribbon and encased them in cellophane, and at the end went round to the stage-door to present them. As it happened, the photographer from a local paper had gone round in the hope of finding a picture for a fill-in on the back page, and was duly rewarded. Next day there appeared a large picture of Pavlova, still in her Punch costume with the hat at a rakish tilt over one eye, clutching at the bunch of flowers with one hand and holding the other outstretched with the fingers in arabesque position. The caption read "Local Pavlova plays the Fool". This Mrs. Jenkins found annoying. It was obvious that the photographer had not taken the trouble to watch the performance, or even look at the programme, and had taken the costume for that of a jester. When Mrs. Jenkins cut out the picture to paste it in her scrapbook, she snipped the caption off first. It did not seem worthy of posterity.

That was the year when Pavlova began to play tennis. The young man who lived next door and whose sister was Pavlova's best friend, was a very good player. He had started to coach his sister, so Pavlova went along with them. At first Mrs. Jenkins had been dubious about this, thinking that perhaps Pavlova might strain some muscles, or even develop the wrong ones. She consulted Miss Carter, who assured her that the danger was very slight.

"It will be good for her," she said. "It might help to—" she hesitated, "to fine her down a little."

By now Pavlova was not so much fat as extremely sturdy. She was also the tallest in her class by half a head.

"She's got a good long reach," said the young man next door enthusiastically. "And packs no end of a punch."

Mrs. Jenkins had winced ever so slightly. This was not quite the sort of compliment that seemed to apply to a future danseuse. Pavlova obviously enjoyed her tennis, so her mother said nothing. She did not buy her a tennis dress, though. Pavlova did not even notice. She went swinging happily down to the courts most days, wearing her pink garden shorts and black gym shoes. Soon she would be leaping and racing about the court, lost in pursuit of the elusive ball, thrilling to the feel of a well-timed shot, purposely taking the ball on her backhand to strengthen it. All through the summer she played, and right through the winter too, on the hard courts, measuring herself against any opponent who came to hand —some of them nearly twice her own age.

Mrs. Jenkins knew nothing of this. She merely thought that Pavlova was "knocking about" and enjoying herself.

"Those ballet classes have certainly done her some good," the young man told her in the spring. "I've never known a kid her age like it. She'll have to enter the tournament next month."

"Tournament?"

"Junior Section," explained the young man.

"But is she good enough?"

"Good?" he echoed. "Have you *seen* her?"

Mrs. Jenkins had not seen her. She said nothing and went back indoors to her sewing machine. She was making a white dress for Miss Carter's concert. Next day they tried it on.

"Your shoulders!" cried Mrs. Jenkins in dismay. "Just look at them! And I cut it exactly to the pattern! Look how it pulls!"

Pavlova stared at herself in the full-length mirror. This was supposed to be the dress that would prove, at last, that she was a swan born. She saw a round, anxious face topped by a sandy bun. She saw narrow white straps straining over square, sunburned shoulders. She caught sight of her feet, still in their black plimsolls, and nearly let out a giggle. But then she saw her mother's face reflected behind her own. An enormous misery descended. She just stood, arms dangling, staring, while her mother clucked and tugged and did things with pins.

Afterwards she changed into her shorts and came slowly down-stairs, where her mother was enveloped in white net.

"I'm just off for a game of tennis, Mum," she said.

Mrs. Jenkins looked up. She saw her daughter standing awk-wardly in the doorway, big, clumsy and miserable. Then she looked down at the cascading net.

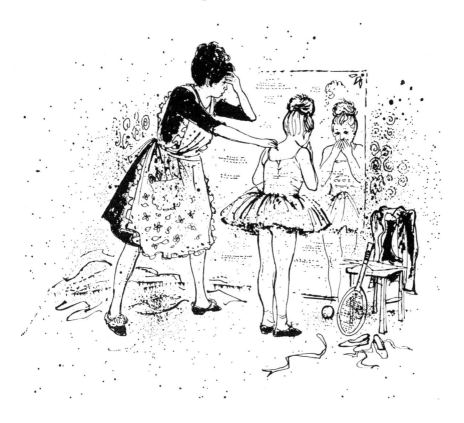

"Wait a minute," she said. "I'll come with you."

Pavlova stared. Together they walked along to the park.

"Want a game, Pavlova?"

The girl who spoke was at least fifteen. Pavlova nodded. Mrs. Jenkins sat in a daze and watched them play. A knot of spectators gathered and she overheard remarks.

"Just look at that kid! Can you beat it?"

"Isn't that big one a Junior County player?"

Mrs. Jenkins had watched Wimbledon on television. This had not taught her very much, but at least enough to know that her daughter was winning, that the bigger girl was scoring hardly a point. In her present dazed state, Pavlova, leaping and flying about the court, arms outstretched, legs scissoring, looked suddenly more like a ballerina to Mrs. Jenkins than she had ever done in her flimsy dresses, gallantly going through her set dances. Mrs. Jenkins knew then, quite certainly, that here, between the dusty tramlines, and not on a chalked stage behind the footlights, her daughter was at home.

When the game was over Pavlova came over to her mother, watching anxiously for signs of disapproval. She would know now for certain that it was playing tennis that was developing her shoulders.

"You play very well, dear," said her mother at last. "I never realised."

"I love it," said Pavlova simply.

"You ought to have a proper dress, if you're going to take it up," she went on. "A nice short white dress. I'll make you one."

Pavlova stared. Her mother stared back. Not a word was said, and yet they both knew.

"Pity it can't be net," said Mrs. Jenkins at last. "It looks as if I'm going to be stuck with a few yards."

She was never very good at making jokes. Pavlova laughed at this one, though, and felt an enormous weight lift from somewhere between her well-developed shoulders and fly off somewhere up among the elms, as if it had wings. In the same moment, a thought struck her.

"I'm not a swan, after all!" she thought exultantly. "*I'm an ugly duckling!*"

*   *   *

All this happened three or four years ago. So any time now you can start watching out for the name Ann Jenkins at Junior Wimbledon. Because that was another thing Mrs. Jenkins discovered that spring. Names *can* be changed. It's perfectly easy. Did you know, for instance, that the real name of Lydia Sokolova, who made famous the role of the Chosen Maiden in *Le Sacre du Printemps*, was Hilda Munnings? And that would never have done . . .

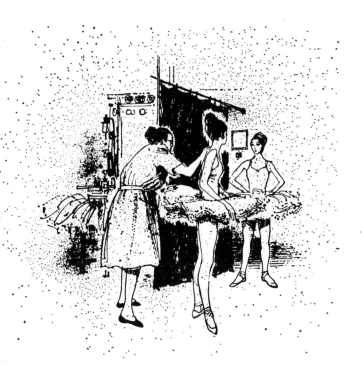

BALLET AS A CAREER

Arnold Haskell

When you watch a great ballerina, a Markova or a Fonteyn, in her filmy white dress floating across the artificial moonlight of the stage, it seems so natural and so effortless. All true art must give this illusion of ease. It is only the clumsy amateur who reveals the enormous effort of attainment. Every time a Markova or a Fonteyn dances, a score of small girls, some of them not so small, say to themselves: "How wonderful it must be to dance so easily to this beautiful music and then to bow to the applause of a large audience, to receive the brightly be-ribboned bouquets of flowers, to sign autograph albums at the stage-door."

There is a kind of magic that even the oldest of us feel as we sit in the auditorium and look out at what is happening across the row of footlights, that bright barrier between two worlds, the world of reality and the world of make-believe. Should that sense of magic ever disappear, the theatre itself would die. But magic is not enough. Those on the other side of the barrier from the audience are working people who require discipline, skill, good health, and as practical an outlook as the hospital nurse, the schoolteacher, or shorthand typist.

Some of my readers may feel that in trying to make a bridge between darkness and light, reality and fairy-tale, I am spoiling something, just as if I explained exactly how it was that the conjurer produced a rabbit or a dove out of an empty top-hat. I do not feel that, because no amount of explanation can ever damage genuine art. In any case, I am prepared to take that risk.

ii

There are at this moment in Britain some fifty thousand children who are learning ballet dancing. By no means all of them really want to go on the stage. However, a vast number do, and they are the very ones who cannot afford to live in a fairy-tale world. It is for them that I am trying to build a really solid bridge over those treacherous and deceptive footlights.

Here, then, is the main foundation of my bridge. There are at the most—and this is an optimistic figure—five ballet companies in Europe that can find employment for the fully trained British dancer. Let us say on an average that each company employs forty dancers. Five × forty = two hundred. That is a very simple sum and a very important one. It means that not more than two hundred would-be dancers can find regular employment in ballet at any one time. That may still seem a big figure, but we have not yet finished with our arithmetic. If, for some reason or other, in every company six girls a year leave and have to be replaced, we have thirty vacancies a year available for newcomers. Bear with my arithmetic for just one more moment. In our five companies some four girls may be given leading roles; that is, twenty out of two hundred. The rest remain in the *corps de ballet* or very near to it.

These are depressing figures, but I have not set out to depress you. It is important to speak the truth in order to build this bridge that may carry you into the sylph's enchanted glade as solidly as possible.

You have seen how few are the chances of success. Therefore it is necessary to handicap yourself as little as possible. Every step must be a wise one. The trouble is that it is very difficult to be wise between the ages of eight and ten when the whole thing starts.

Try first of all to think of the dancer as someone who is playing a musical instrument, a fiddle, a 'cello, an oboe, or a piano. That is exactly the case, only the dancer's musical instrument is her own body. This instrument must be made before it can be played upon. It takes time and skill to make a musical instrument. That is the reason why the dancer must start at so early an age, while the body is still supple and the bones pliant. The ideal age is around ten, while, after twelve, every additional year is a handicap; you have already seen how serious the slightest handicap can be.

Now just because the body of the ten-year-old is so very supple and can be bent into so many shapes, it is extremely important for the teacher, our instrument-maker, to be an expert. Unfortunately, there are very few experts; there are equally few people who can make a perfect violin. The very first thing that the teacher will have to decide is whether you are built in the right way for ballet training. Have you a straight, strong spine, well-proportioned neck and shoulders, the right legs and knees, a strong instep, and toes that will be able to support the weight of your body? I would have been more precise had that been possible, but these things cannot be put down on paper, though they can be seen by the eyes of a sensitive and experienced person. Even so, they may need checking by a trained anatomist. Sometimes knock-knees or bow legs can be cured by ballet training, and two of our best-known ballet dancers originally suffered from defects that remained after infantile paralysis. The teacher has, in fact, to ask herself the same question as the fiddle-maker; is this material of the right type for me to make it into a musical instrument? If the answer is yes—for the time being, for the pupil may later grow too heavy or too tall—the next step is one of method—the method that all good teachers require, whether their subject is geography or domestic economy. The teacher must proceed slowly and, it may seem, far too slowly for her eager pupil. No honest teacher, for instance, will let her pupil rise on to the tips of her toes before the age of eleven or without two years of pre-liminary training, and then only for a very short proportion of the lesson.

Oh, those tips of the toes, or "points" as they are called. To many they seem the sole aim and beauty of ballet, the main in-gredient in the magic spell. How many girls write to me that they practise for hours in front of a mirror, and how many wrecked feet I see every month! How many dance competitions encourage youngsters to struggle on to wobbly toes, and how many wrecked feet; how many school shows produce their rickety fairies, and how many wrecked feet!

I feel very angry about this, and no wonder, when year in and year out I add up the wasted talent, to say nothing of the deformed joints, that turn so many people against ballet.

Alas, I cannot tell you how to choose that exceptionally rare person, the perfect teacher; but I can tell you that if your teacher is treating you in the way I have mentioned, you had better leave her at once.

Then there are examinations; yes, even the sylphs can be examined, incongruous as it may seem. And here I may be able to help you a little by putting examinations in their right place; and a very useful place it is. First of all, the examination is valuable because it allows a competent authority to look at the work of the teacher, perhaps to stop her ruining those feet. Had you ever thought that your teacher was being examined at the same time as yourself, and far more severely? But that does not really concern you. What does concern you is the lesson that can be learnt from an examination, and the reason for taking it in the first place. Let me deal with that last point right away. Even if you get honours at every stage, it is not going to help you in a ballet company. As the great Diaghilev once said to a girl who boasted of honours in an examination, "Do you propose to dance with your certificate pinned to your costume?"

But if you ever reach the ballet company—and you know how few do—your examinations will be indispensable to you if you become a teacher. That is not the only reason for their value, though it is a practical one. An examination from time to time does help you to sum up what you have learnt and also gives you a tidy mind. It underlines your shortcomings—shortcomings that have become so familiar to your teacher that both of you may take them for granted. A successful pass, however, is no indication at all that you are going to be equally successful on the stage. Rejoice when you pass, but keep your head; you are going to need it later on. An examination is a useful check from time to time and nothing more. But to work with only an examination result in mind is dangerous. It takes all the joy and artistry out of dancing. Therefore, it is important not to cram, not to take the major ballet examinations too young. If you begin them around the age of fifteen, you will then take them in your stride, you will know what they are all about and you will profit by them. A fifteen-year-old of average ability who has already swept through her "majors" with honours is rather a pathetic sight; in knowing too much about steps, she risks forgetting altogether about dancing.

iii

So far I have written about dancing as if it depended on the body alone and was not an art of expression. I have, in fact, written about the instrument and have not yet mentioned the player. It may be a very dull way of doing things, but in writing about art too many people do the reverse. They like to imagine that the artist is created by the touch of a magic wand; they forget the maddening scales, the fiddle scrapings and the vocal gymnastics. In ballet they forget the muscle-aching exercises that must go on by the hour, year in and year out, before there is something for an audience to applaud.

Let us say that you have been one of those whose instrument has responded to a daily lesson over a number of years. The early effort has vanished and you are beginning to take a real pleasure in movement, the same sort of pleasure that you took when, before you had a lesson in your life, you danced to a gramophone. The instrument is made, all but for a little varnish; the tuning must go on for the rest of your stage life. How are you going to play it?

You will soon begin to realise that you, the dancer, are not

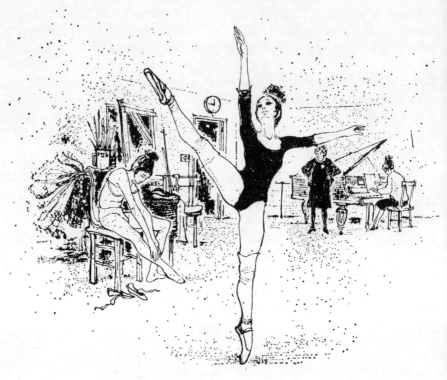

alone in ballet. The very first person you will notice is your class pianist. Music is to be your constant companion for the rest of your life. First of all the music tells you when to begin, when to pause, when to stop. It issues certain definite commands, simple ones at the start. As rhythm grows more complicated you will need to make a deeper study of its structure. Dalcroze Eurhythmics is an excellent system, learning to play the piano is also a great help. Rhythm, however, is by no means the whole story. The more good music you hear, the more you develop, not only your knowledge but your response to it and the greater dancer you may become. All other things being equal, it is the response to music that separates the great dancer from the merely competent one.

A dancer has to wear costume—the costume of a country or a period. In one evening you may have to visit Spain (*The Three-Cornered Hat*), eighteenth-century England (*The Rake's Progress*) and a modern Glasgow slum (*Miracle in the Gorbals*). You must therefore know something of style, which is a combination of history, geography and art appreciation. In other words, your ordinary school work is important, whether you fail to cross the bridge or whether you succeed. Should you fail you will be equipped for other work, and should you succeed you will have the background and material so necessary in creating a role.

iv

By the time you are seventeen, after seven years of hard training, you should know whether you are one of the very few fortunate ones qualified to take up ballet as a career. It is a hard life, more strenuous physically than that of a hospital nurse, requiring the same rigid discipline, but, if you have the vocation, equally rewarding.

I have made the comparison between nursing and ballet deliberately, because films like *Red Shoes* give an altogether glamorous and false view of the position. For one great artist there are hundreds doing a hard job competently. And both the nurse and the dancer have aching feet by the end of their day!

The picture I have painted may seem such a gloomy one that you may well ask why take up dancing at all. Whether you ask it or not, I feel I must answer.

First of all, dancing is fun, it is healthy, it makes you graceful. Then it is an admirable education for a whole number of activities. If you take up dancing and are well trained from the start you have not wasted your time, even if you are not one of the lucky ones. You only lose if you fail to realise the truth, if you put all your eggs in one basket and think of yourself as a tragic failure when you are turned down at an audition. I have seen so many minor tragedies brought about by this inability to look facts in the face. Too often parents and teachers in trying to be kind only succeed in being cruel. A shock is hard to bear, but there need never be a shock. I always try to tell young dancers the truth as I see it. If you can enjoy the work for its own sake, then you must be the gainer. Apart from ballet there is the teaching of dancing, and every other branch of the stage, the films and television. Ballet training is the finest foundation for every one of these. And if your path does not lie in that direction, you will enjoy the performance you watch all the more keenly for your training.

FAMOUS DANCERS OF TO-DAY

Clement Crisp

Margot Fonteyn

In 1934, when Margot Fonteyn made her first appearance with the Vic-Wells Ballet as a snowflake in *The Nutcracker*, no one could have guessed that either the company or the beautiful dark-eyed girl would have achieved the greatness that we know to-day. Fonteyn's career is almost the history of the Royal Ballet itself; she is a great classical ballerina because Dame Ninette de Valois insisted from the very first that her Vic-Wells Ballet should be properly based in the classical traditions of the masterpieces of the Imperial Russian ballet, particularly the ballets of Marius Petipa.

When the Vic-Wells Ballet started in 1931 it was fortunate that there was a ballerina available to dance these classics: Alicia Markova. As a young girl, Markova had danced for the Diaghilev Ballet—hence her Russianised name, and her participation was vital in the productions of *Giselle*, *The Nutcracker* and *Swan Lake* that were put on during the first three years of the Vic-Wells Ballet's existence. These ballets are the great showpieces and training grounds for classical dancers, and they help both dancers and audiences to understand the wonderful riches of classic ballet. But in 1935 Alicia Markova ended her association with the Vic-Wells Ballet, and Ninette de Valois saw that in the sixteen-year-old Fonteyn she had a potential ballerina. Each succeeding year saw the development of Fonteyn as a classical dancer. A great challenge in her career came in 1939 with the production of *The Sleeping Beauty* at Sadler's Wells; the role of Princess Aurora confirmed Fonteyn as a ballerina, and it almost became her "signature" ballet, as it was for her company. When the Sadler's Wells Ballet (as the Vic-Wells Ballet became called) moved to Covent Garden in 1946, *The Sleeping Beauty*, in an opulent new production, opened the season. The ballet, with Fonteyn in the leading role, became a symbol of the excellence of what is now our national ballet.

One other influence has shared in shaping Fonteyn's career—and the career of our national ballet: Sir Frederick Ashton. When he joined the company in 1935 Ashton soon noticed the qualities of the young Fonteyn, and she became the inspiration for many of his finest works. The relationship between a ballerina and the choreographer who works with her is an extraordinary one; each reacts upon the other, and Fonteyn's abilities inspired Ashton, while his choreography shaped and developed her powers. They have worked together for twenty-five years, on ballets as different as *Cinderella*, *Symphonic Variations*, *Daphnis and Chloe*, *Sylvia*, *Marguerite and Armand* and, supremely, *Ondine*, and together they have created some of the most important and beautiful ballets of our time.

Fonteyn's greatness has always been the perfection of her classical dancing; other dancers have been more brilliant in performing certain dazzling and difficult steps, but great classical dancing demands qualities of elegance, dignity and an absence of mannerisms that are rarely all found in one dancer. Fonteyn has them. She is also the most musical of artists—this means that her dancing seems directly inspired by the ballet's score, so that both the choreography and the drama of the ballet are shown to be perfectly at one with the music. Everything she dances looks clear, powerful and totally convincing, and her dancing conforms always to the very demanding rules of the classical style; it is the mark of the very finest dancers to be able to do this, and Fonteyn achieves it perfectly.

RUDOLF NUREYEV

When Rudolf Nureyev made his first appearance in London it was obvious straight away that he had "star quality". His appearance had been surrounded with a tremendous amount of publicity and excitement, for he was a member of the great Leningrad ballet company that takes its name from its home theatre, the Kirov. When the Kirov Ballet first visited the West in 1961 they danced in Paris before coming to Covent Garden. In Paris Nureyev decided that he wanted to stay in the West and he ran away from the company. He hit the headlines at once, and three months later he made his London début at one of the annual Gala performances that Dame Margot Fonteyn organises for the Royal Academy of Dancing, of which she is President.

Sir Frederick Ashton had composed a short dance especially for him, and Nureyev dashed on stage to roar like the wind through this brief solo. There, unquestionably, was "star quality", and since then this amazing dancer—often in partnership with Dame Margot Fonteyn—has won audiences all over the world and become the best-known male dancer of our time. He has unusual qualities as a dancer: an extraordinary natural physical gift that was superbly trained at the Kirov school (which produces the most beautifully trained and stylish classical dancers in the world). Add to this Nureyev's magnetic stage personality that means that everything he dances becomes compulsively watchable, and you can understand why his appearances have excited such public attention. He is always an exciting dancer, with a daring brilliance about much of what he does on stage.

However, Nureyev is a choreographer and producer as well as a dancer, having made versions of several ballets that he knew in Russia, notably the lovely Kingdom of Shades scene in *La Bayadère*, and *Raymonda*, two superb Petipa ballets that have become important additions to the Royal Ballet's repertory. He has also made an entirely new version of *The Nutcracker* for the Royal Ballet, and stagings for foreign companies of *Swan Lake* and *The Sleeping Beauty*, in all of which, characteristically, the role of the leading male dancer has been revised and expanded.

LYNN SEYMOUR

The very special magic that happens when Lynn Seymour dances is the result of a combination of two wonderful qualities that are rarely found in one ballerina: a very beautiful way of moving so that every step she takes is soft and flowing, and an extraordinary acting ability. When this young Canadian-born graduate of the Royal Ballet School first appeared on stage it was obvious that she was a uniquely gifted dancer. Soon ballets were being created specially for her. Kenneth MacMillan, the Royal Ballet's brilliant young choreographer, chose her as leading dancer for many of his best ballets, and when Sir Frederick Ashton created *The Two Pigeons* he cast Lynn Seymour as the young girl who is deserted by her true love.

It is the MacMillan ballets that have best shown us what a marvellous talent Lynn Seymour has. MacMillan was inspired by her fluid way of moving, by the beautiful line of her long legs and the arch of her feet, as well as by her ability to make her movements dramatically exciting. He first cast her as the girl in *The Burrow* (a ballet about a group of people hiding from danger in an attic), and in 1960 he gave her a wonderful role in *Le Baiser de la Fée* (*The Fairy's Kiss*). This was a ballet about a young man who left his beloved on their wedding day because a fairy had chosen him for herself. MacMillan provided a great duet as the centre of the ballet in which the young man and the girl dance together, and in this Lynn Seymour displayed her superb powers: her softly flowing movements and the flawless line which is one of the most important qualities in a dancer.

The next year MacMillan devised a totally different ballet for her: *The Invitation*, a tragic story of a girl who is the victim of a terrible assault which destroys all her chances of future happiness. This role gave Lynn Seymour the chance to reveal herself as the finest dramatic artist in British ballet. In 1965 came the greatest challenge of her career: the role of Juliet in MacMillan's *Romeo and Juliet*. The role was created for her and it owes everything to her way of acting and dancing; everything Juliet does in the ballet —from her first meeting with Romeo at a party to her tragic death in the tomb—is inspired by Lynn Seymour's gifts. The ballet offers a portrait of this wonderful dancer.

In 1966 Lynn Seymour left the Royal Ballet to go and work with MacMillan in Berlin for three years with the ballet company there. Berlin's gain was a sad loss to British ballet, which can ill afford to lose this superlative dancer.

MARCIA HAYDEE

It is one of the curious facts about contemporary ballet that Germany should have gained a very lively and interesting classical ballet tradition during the past twenty years. Even more curious is the fact that many British choreographers should have gone to work in Germany, including our two finest young creators—John Cranko and Kenneth MacMillan. MacMillan spent only three years in Berlin, but since 1961 John Cranko has worked in Stuttgart and has built up one of the finest companies in the world in a very short time. He has also guided and developed the career of one of the finest dancers of our time: Marcia Haydee.

Born in Brazil, a pupil for a time at the Royal Ballet School, Marcia Haydee went to Stuttgart in 1962 and since then she has been revealed in the ballets that Cranko has staged there as a thrilling classical ballerina. Her slender physique, her dark-eyed beauty, recall to many people the memory of the purest and most aristocratic of Russian ballerinas of this century, Olga Spessivtseva; certainly, Haydee's dramatic strength and the delicate "poetic" quality of her dancing make her a ballerina whose every performance is to be treasured by those fortunate enough to see her.

She has been widely hailed in the great classic ballets: her *Giselle* and *Swan Lake* are celebrated, and John Cranko has also created three long ballets for her—*Eugene Onegin*, in which she is unforgettably touching as a young girl whose love for a man is cruelly rejected; *Romeo and Juliet*, in which she is a wonderful Juliet, though very different from Kenneth MacMillan's creation for Lynn Seymour; and most recently as the high-spirited Kate in *The Taming of the Shrew*, in which she has shown herself to be a brilliant comedienne.

Alas, she has been seen all too rarely in London, but she has danced at Covent Garden in a great role that Kenneth MacMillan created for her in *The Song of the Earth*. This ballet uses the music, and the words, of a symphony for two singers and orchestra by Gustave Mahler, and it tells of the beauty of the world around us, the joy people find in it, and the inevitability of death that must end that joy. But the ballet is not ultimately a sad one because death also means a renewal of life, and the central role of the work is that of a woman (created by MacMillan for Haydee) who must express in her dancing all the mixed feelings of joy and loss and the acceptance of death.

It is a tremendously difficult part, both technically and because the dancer must interpret and express such serious and difficult

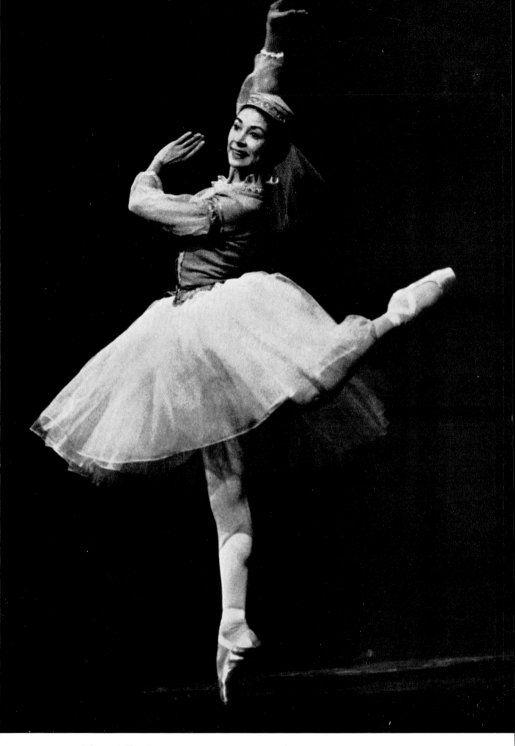

Margot Fonteyn

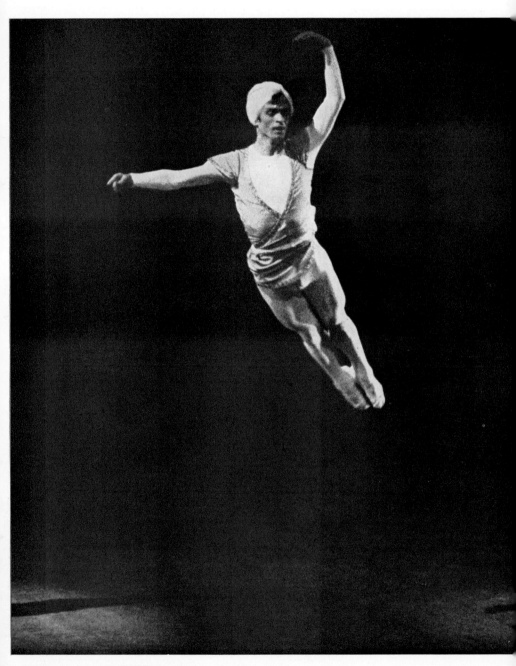

Rudolf Nureyev

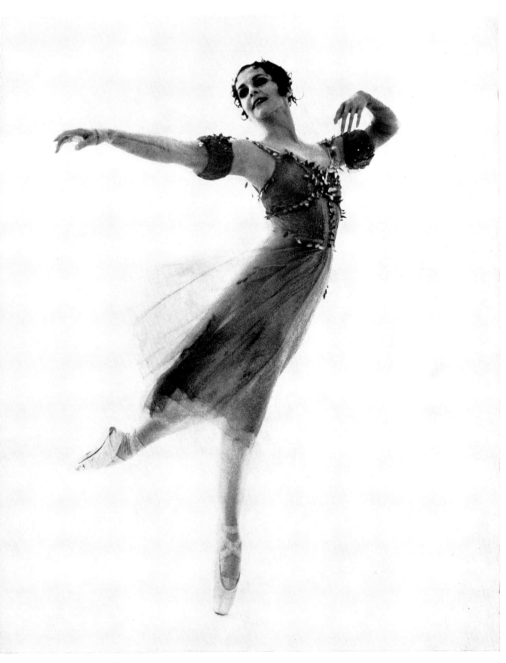

Lynn Seymour

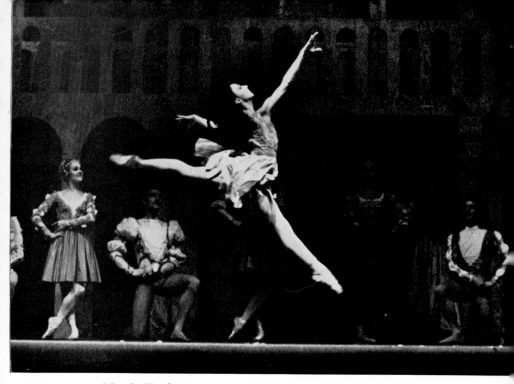

Marcia Haydee

Anthony Dowell

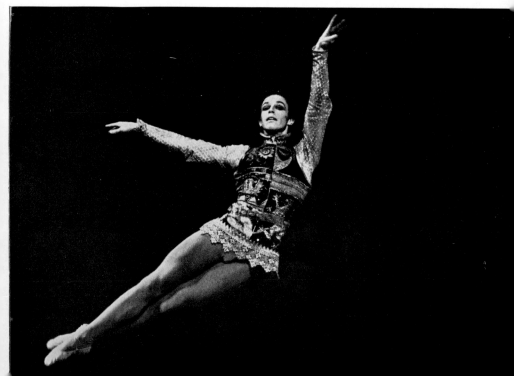

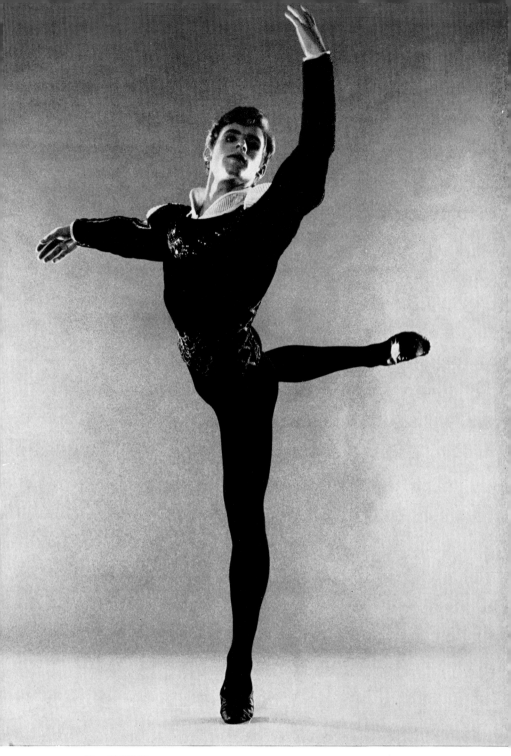

David Wall

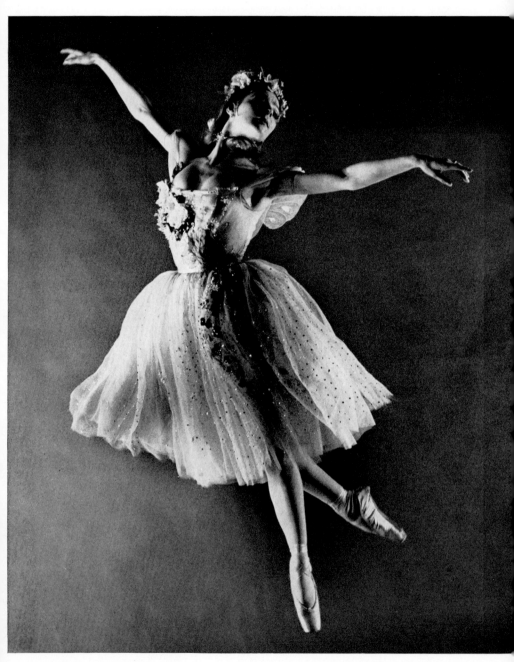

Antoinette Sibley

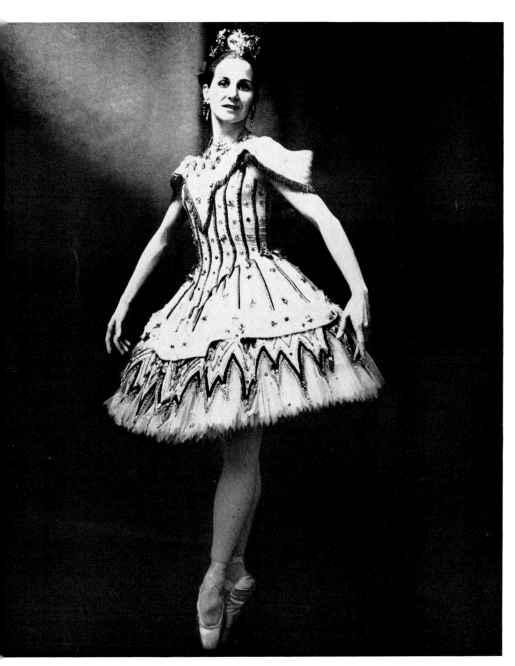

Merle Park

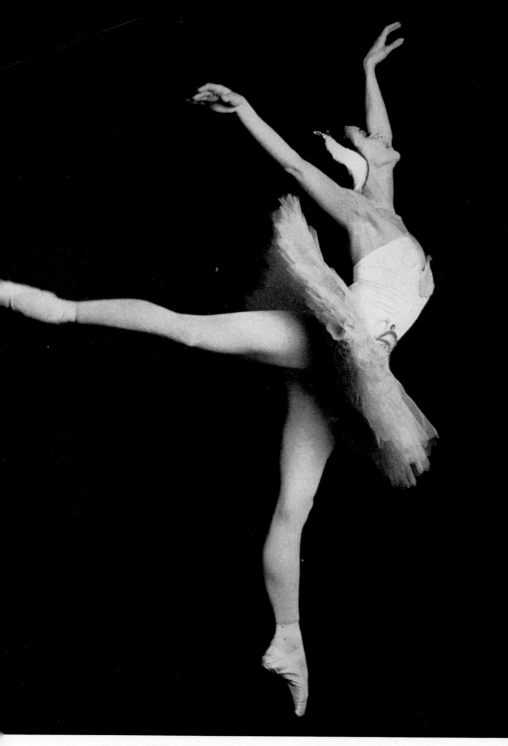

Doreen Wells

emotions; Marcia Haydee does it to perfection, and in return the ballet shows the wonderful elegance of her dancing, her sensitivity and her ability to convey emotion to an audience with absolute sureness. It is a ballet that moves members of the audience to tears; Haydee's greatness lies in the fact that she can suggest all the beauty of a work to her audience, a quality that only the finest dancers possess.

Two Male Dancers:
Anthony Dowell and David Wall

It is one of the chief tragedies of ballet in the West that there are far fewer young men who want to make their career in dancing, while in Russia it is a calling that is viewed with respect and admiration. Hence the magnificence of so many Russian dancers and the relative weakness of some of the male dancing in Europe.

There is still a strange myth among many Englishmen that dancing is not sufficiently "manly"—though you have only to consider the tremendous athletic training that a male dancer undergoes and notice the strength and virility that are needed to dance in ballet (including carrying ballerinas across the stage without showing any muscular effort) to see how foolish the myth is. The male dancer is an athlete, but he is taught during the whole seven or eight years of his schooling (and throughout his professional career) to hide difficulties and to move with ease and grace. The jumps and leaps and beaten steps that a man performs in ballet, and the skills that a boy acquires during his ballet training, are far beyond anything that a professional athlete could accomplish.

In Russia and Denmark there has always been a great tradition of male dancing; in the rest of the world the shortage of good male dancers is still a most serious problem for ballet. Britain has produced some fine male dancers in this century: Anton Dolin started his career with the Diaghilev Ballet and went on to become one of the most famous principal dancers of his time. In the Royal Ballet David Blair set new standards of virtuosity and brilliance, which are vividly seen in the part of Colas in *La Fille Mal Gardée* which was created for him and is a dazzlingly difficult role that he dances with faultless ease and with great dramatic power.

In the next generation of dancers in the Royal Ballet there are two outstanding young artists who are carrying on this tradition: Anthony Dowell and David Wall. Anthony Dowell works with the company resident at Covent Garden and he is one of the most accomplished and elegant male dancers anywhere in the world. He dances most of the principal male roles in the classic repertory, and his partnership with Antoinette Sibley is hailed—notably in New York—as some of the most exciting dancing to be seen in the world to-day. Dowell's dancing is distinguished by elegance and purity of style; steps are performed with all the clean perfection that the classic dance demands. In Sir Frederick Ashton's ballet based on Shakespeare's *A Midsummer Night's Dream*, Dowell dances Oberon, and you have only to watch the scherzo (the scene in which Oberon summons up a mist to confuse the lovers lost in the forest) and you will see an amazing male variation—the name given to a solo dance in ballet—built on turning and spinning steps which demand the greatest brilliance and lightness. In another ballet created for him, Antony Tudor's *Shadowplay*, Dowell showed remarkable dramatic skill as well as beautiful dancing in a most difficult role.

Antony Tudor also created a ballet for another fine young male dancer, David Wall, who is the leading dancer of the Royal Ballet's Touring Section. Wall is even younger than Dowell, and in Tudor's *Knight Errant* he has a role that tells us a great deal about his tremendous abilities. He is called upon to act quite as much as he has to dance; in fact, he has to "carry" the ballet—without his presence it would be far less exciting—and he makes it a thrilling experience in the theatre.

In his brief years with the Touring Section, David Wall has gained a great reputation as a principal male dancer; he has interpreted all the leading male roles in the classical repertory and shown that he can present them in a fresh and exciting way. It is one of his outstanding gifts to be able to make the princes of classical ballet seem real and convincing as people. In *Swan Lake* and in *Giselle* there are few dancers to match him because he brings to the leading roles such vitality, such strength and presence (a word that conveys the dancer's ability to seem the focal point of the ballet) that they take on a new and exciting life for his audience. In *La Fille Mal Gardée* he is the best possible successor to David

Blair, and in the *Two Pigeons* he is now unsurpassed as the young painter.

With two dancers as gifted as Dowell and Wall, and with the promise of some interesting and even younger artists following in their steps, there is the hope that in a few years' time our male dancers will be as many (they are often as good) as our young ballerinas.

ANTOINETTE SIBLEY

I have just come from Covent Garden where I have been watching Antoinette Sibley dance Aurora in *The Sleeping Beauty*. Her performance was dazzling; light, youthful, radiant and so effortless that it looked as if Miss Sibley—like Eliza Doolittle in *My Fair Lady*—could have danced all night. What audiences never see, and sometimes, I am sure, never realise, is the years of hard work, the constant practice that has gone into giving a ballerina the skill to seem so effortlessly brilliant on stage. The dancer, like the musician, is an artist who must work every day to keep in practice. Dancers go to class regularly every day right up to the last day of their stage career; they work as hard when they are established stars (probably harder) than when they were young students at ballet school learning their craft. The dancer's career is really a search for perfection that can never be attained, and a dancer never stops learning until the day he or she stops dancing. Like every other ballerina, Antoinette Sibley's lightness and brilliance are the result of unceasing hard work and dedication, plus the vital factor of the natural physical gift of a beautifully shaped body. Because the Royal Ballet is a company which is firmly rooted in the great traditions of the classical ballet, its ballerinas are accustomed from a surprisingly early age to undertake the extremely taxing roles of the classic repertory: Aurora in *The Sleeping Beauty*; Odette/Odile in *Swan Lake*; Giselle, as well as the leading roles in the full-length ballets of Sir Frederick Ashton.

Antoinette Sibley, one of the galaxy of bright young stars produced by the Royal Ballet during the past ten years, has had great success in this repertory. She danced her first Odette/Odile role at the age of twenty, her first Aurora just two years later, and these early triumphs confirmed that she was destined for fine things. The succeeding years have seen her extending her powers in many different roles: as Cinderella, Clara in *The Nutcracker*, Juliet in MacMillan's ballet, and several more. Her dancing has never lost the youthful lightness and charm that endeared her to audiences when she made her first appearances, though maturity has of course deepened and strengthened her interpretations. In the tremendously demanding double role of Odette and Odile she has been widely hailed for the tragic intensity of her dancing, and the Aurora I have just seen was danced with brilliance. In the Rose Adagio of the first act, where Aurora dances with her four princes who have come to woo her, Antoinette Sibley balanced so long and with such poise that the audience gasped in amazement. Her most recent created role was as Dorabella in Sir Frederick Ashton's *Enigma Variations*. The ballet is about the composer Elgar and about the friends whose musical portraits he drew in his *Enigma Variations*. Ashton chose Antoinette Sibley to dance the young girl Dorabella, whose friendship for Elgar was so important to the composer; the role shows Sibley as a delightful and fleet-footed girl: it is a lovely tribute by a choreographer to an enchanting and gifted dancer.

MERLE PARK

When Sir Frederick Ashton made his great comedy ballet, *La Fille Mal Gardée*, in 1960, he created the leading role of Lise (the daughter who manages to marry the man of her choice despite her mother's precautions) for Nadia Nerina, who was the most brilliant technical ballerina in the Royal Ballet. The role was a dazzlingly difficult one, a combination of humour and technical fireworks that made tremendous demands upon its interpreter; it set a standard of dancing that few people thought could be rivalled for years. In fact, within a very short time several Royal Ballet ballerinas had danced the role with great success, and now it is a popular role with many artists; but Merle Park was the first dancer after Nadia Nerina to accept the challenge of the part, and she showed a wonderful technical skill in it. From the very first Merle Park had demonstrated a remarkable ability to sail through the most difficult steps with ease; her early successes were as Swanilda in *Coppelia* and in the most taxing variations in *The Sleeping Beauty*. She danced with ever-increasing technical and dramatic skill leading roles in many short ballets, and gradually extended her range even further to include the major classics: Aurora in *The Sleeping Beauty*, and *Giselle*, as well as the role of the young girl in *The Two Pigeons*.

To-day, as a leading ballerina of the company, she sets her dazzling technique at the service of a wide range of roles, and her two most important created parts show something of her skill. When the English choreographer Antony Tudor made his return to Britain after thirty years in America, he chose Merle Park to interpret the mysterious Celestial in his first ballet for Covent Garden, *Shadowplay*. It was a role calling for rare physical abilities as well as dramatic gifts; the Celestial is one of the creatures who appear to the hero of the ballet and who form part of the series of incidents which are to be vital in showing him what the world is like. Merle Park danced with tremendous force and subtlety, notably in two *pas de deux* in which the Celestial tried to dominate the boy.

A totally contrasting role was that of Clara, the heroine of Rudolf Nureyev's version of *The Nutcracker*. Here she impersonated the young girl whose magical adventures are caused by the gift of a Nutcracker Doll at a Christmas party. Nureyev made Clara a full-scale ballerina part, and Merle Park was particularly exciting in the two extremely difficult *pas de deux* that Nureyev wrote for Clara and the Nutcracker Prince. Merle Park is a very exciting dancer to watch because of her remarkable speed and brilliance, even in a small role like the Autumn Fairy in Ashton's *Cinderella*, where she dazzles the audience by her phenomenal accuracy and lightness in a variation that seems to whirl and dash across the stage like leaves blown in the autumn wind.

DOREEN WELLS

The Royal Ballet is a large and complex organisation. Londoners who go to watch the company at the Royal Opera House, Covent Garden, tend to forget that there is another Royal Ballet that spends most of the year taking ballet round the country in long tours that include many of the large cities of Britain. In recent years this

Touring Section of the Royal Ballet has also had a season in London in the spring, so that the Covent Garden audience can have the opportunity of enjoying the ballets and the artists who spend so much of their year at work outside the capital.

Touring ballet is a hard life, complicated by many factors—not least the constant travelling that means that dancers may have no real home for six months at a time and must live out of suitcases. New theatres, new "digs" to stay in, new audiences, new stages to work on—sometimes far below what they should be—all this requires a dedicated and enthusiastic artist to be a member of a touring ballet company. The Royal Ballet Touring Section is a wonderful company, and its leading ballerina, Doreen Wells, is yet another member of that splendid group of artists who have come to the forefront of British ballet during the past ten years. Doreen Wells is a heart-warming and enchanting ballerina; a lovely technique is linked to a charming and fluent style of dancing. Everything she dances looks fresh, graceful, sincere, and she has shown herself to be equally effective as Aurora in *The Sleeping Beauty*, as a tragic Giselle, and as Odette and Odile in *Swan Lake*.

In the ballets made by Sir Frederick Ashton, she has been outstanding in *The Two Pigeons* and *La Fille Mal Gardée*. In the first of these she finds a great deal of humour in the early scene when the young girl is posing for her artist boy-friend and finds it impossible to keep still—much to the painter's annoyance. When a troupe of gypsies comes into the painter's studio and proceed to show off, one gypsy girl steals the affections of the painter. Doreen Wells is at first terribly funny as she quarrels with the gypsy, mocking her vulgar dancing, and later when the painter leaves her for the gypsy, she is immensely sad and pathetic. (The ballet ends with a happy *pas de deux* for the lovers in which Doreen Wells is excellent.) In *La Fille Mal Gardée* Doreen Wells is probably the best interpreter to-day, finding a vast amount of humour and naughtiness and fun in the part, it is a role in which she has been called "adorable", and this perfectly conveys the charm and bounding lightness of her performance.

She dances all the leading roles in the repertory with success, and audiences outside London are enviably fortunate to have more opportunity of seeing this delightful ballerina than the followers of the Covent Garden company.

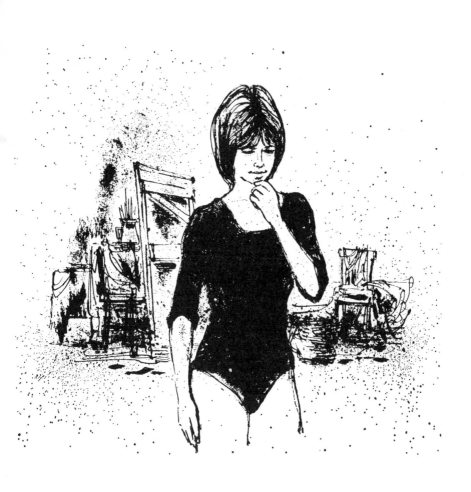

"TO DANCE
OR NOT TO DANCE?"

Shelagh Fraser

I am an actress who has never danced a step of classical ballet but
have been surrounded by dancers, attended innumerable classes,
rehearsals, dress rehearsals, and as many performances. If I had

the necessary credentials I could take a Beginners' Class with confidence.

Why? Because my sister, Moyra Fraser, won a scholarship to the Sadler's Wells Ballet School, eventually becoming a soloist in the Royal Ballet, dancing such classical roles as the "Lilac Fairy" in *The Sleeping Princess*, "The Queen of the Wilis" in *Giselle*, and in the modern ballets created a wide variety of characters, notably the tragi-comic spinster "Hen" in Robert Helpmann's *The Birds*. But alas, she grew and grew until she was too tall for a Prima Ballerina, the peak of a dancer's career.

In her case there was a blessed alternative—a gift for mime and acting, especially comic roles. Frustrated by the handicap of her height, she started voice and singing lessons and finally launched herself into the more commercial world of musicals and revue. Her first speaking part and real success was, "The Ballerina", in *The Song of Norway*, at the Palace Theatre. After that it was plain sailing. She starred in a series of revues, including the famous *Airs On A Shoe String*, with Max Adrian and Betty Marsden, establishing herself as a dancing comedienne, a clown with a ballet dancer's grace of movement. She appeared at the Old Vic with Maggie Smith in *The Merry Wives of Windsor*, in *Camelot* at Drury Lane, while films, television and broadcasting she took in her stride. Leaving the ballet had paid off; its severe classical training gave her endless advantages over rival actresses. For her musicality and ease of movement enabled her to dominate the stage, physically.

It is a great mistake for young dancers to regard the ballet as the be-all and end-all of their career. Moyra never regrets leaving. It was too restricting for her adventurous, versatile talents; too heart-breaking, too rigid in its dedication, indifferent to anything and everything outside. Moyra made many friends, and had unforgettable moments of artistic satisfaction, not least, the thrill of dancing at Covent Garden Opera House, but her real gifts developed when she left the ballet.

My own experience of ballet is that of the professional onlooker. I am a straight actress, my world a very different one, and this has given me strong views on the pros and cons of studying for ballet. If you are an actor, no matter what age, there are always good parts to play. As you grow older, you simply play older people, and your career is a continuing one, often becoming more successful—some actors only come into their own when they are well over forty. The films suddenly discover them, or they achieve a great television success as Andrew Cruikshank did in *Dr. Findlay's Case Book* at quite a late stage in his career. Providing you are a good actor, anything can happen at any time.

Alas, not for a ballet dancer. Even the greatest must stop dancing the leading roles between thirty-eight and forty. Some companies forcibly retire their stars and permanent dancers, offering them teaching positions or the smaller mime roles. If they prove unsuitable for these, their contracts are terminated.

Then what happens? How do you make use of your talents and fame? How do you earn your living? How do you keep a family and children? It is an alarming prospect and the greatest disadvantage of becoming a ballet dancer. In fact, teachers and dancing organisations should take far more trouble to educate young students to the idea that they must have other things and plans growing alongside their ballet training. They should do as much as possible to ensure a broader career outside ballet itself. For when you are seventeen, you never think you will be forty—you will be dead by then!

Then there is the matter of your physical appearance. Actors are cast according to their physique. A fat actor plays a fat man, a tall, thin actress plays tall, thin women. No problem. But classical ballet insists on a near perfect physique for its interpreters. The standards are very high. Even the most promising students are rejected if they are too small or grow too big, and while they may get into the Corps de Ballet, they may be allowed no further because of their imperfections. In the Bolshoi Ballet, the physical standards are even higher. From twenty-five twelve-year-old students only five will be chosen to go on to the next term. Naturally England has fewer potential ballet dancers to choose from and such perfection is not always possible. Therefore certain dancers are chosen with some imperfections provided their talent is outstanding.

If you are looking forward to a round of parties, entertainments, plenty of friends, hobbies and holidays—give up all idea of the ballet immediately.

Actors have a private life and, when not actually rehearsing or

performing, time to themselves for sport, hobbies, seeing their
friends, holidays, and so forth. A dancer might just as well be in a
nunnery. Performances every night, going to bed late, exhausted.
Yet up again at eight for the compulsory early morning classes,
followed by long, nerve-wracking rehearsals, with just enough
time for tea and to get ready and made up for the evening's performance . . . Long, regular tours, sometimes spending just one
night in each town; rumpled and crumpled, packing and unpacking.
A tiring life with precious little time for fun in the world outside.

If I have drawn a gloomy picture, it is meant to be a helpful
one! Far better know what you are in for before you start. As one
dancer said: "Deciding whether to study ballet is like listening to
those people who tell you that if you marry that man or woman,
you are doomed . . ." And what do most of us do? Take no notice
and marry them!

So, become a ballet dancer by all means. It is an exquisite form
of art, absorbing to study, superbly satisfying to perform. If you
decide to say "Yes", and I hope you do, have the courage to face
the fact that by the time you are forty you must stop active dancing
and be able to branch out in other directions. Bear this in mind
from the beginning and do everything possible to make it easier
for you to change over, to achieve equal success and satisfaction in
other theatrical fields. But what other fields? What would I do in
your place? What have my many dancing acquaintances done?

A good ballet training is never wasted and if, at the end of it
you are not accepted by a leading company, it will be of help to
you in every other theatrical medium . . . in teaching, acting,
modelling (Barbara Goalen, one of the greatest models, started as
a ballet dancer), and there is also producing, writing choreography,
films and television. Study every aspect of the dance: the notation
of steps, the history of dancing all over the world. Learn the
rhythms and steps of modern dancing, jazz, Greek dancing, the
Martha Graham American school of dance. See theatre plays, good
films, musicals, study singing and voice production—the method
of breathing tends to make a dancer's voice thin and breathy. Study
one instrument, acquire a genuine musicality which is essential for
a ballet dancer.

Some of the best advice for potential ballet students comes from
the skilled people who treat their numerous injuries. A friend of

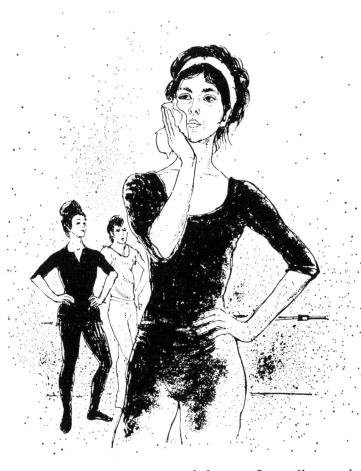

mine, Miss Wareing, has treated dancers from all over the world. Kindly, sympathetic, she knows the heartbreaks and listens willingly to their troubles as she is dealing with a twisted ankle, a torn ligament. In fact, she can tell you more about your future career than almost anyone. She insists that the youngest student be made aware of the discomfort and severe muscular pains they must learn to endure. These come from exercising unusual muscles and every part of the body in a way no normal person will ever do— certainly no actor. Dancers must stretch their bodies beyond ordinary limits, just as a leading athlete.

Miss Wareing advises studying anatomy to make you aware of your muscles and limbs and where the strains will fall. She does not insist on physical perfection, saying that there is only one Margot Fonteyn in a generation, but that you must have a well-proportioned body with strong feet, long neck, be neither too short nor too tall. She believes that a good dancer must first learn to relax, complete physical mobility is what matters. Massage helps this, and to keep your body fluid and soft. Manipulation is only necessary for real injuries.

She believes that you should find yourself the best teacher available and the earlier you start, the better. When you are nine is ideal. Miss Wareing names Margot Fonteyn as the most disciplined person she has ever met and stresses the importance of this. As a ballet dancer you must learn to do exactly as taught, overcome faults, improve any physical disability. Whatever happens to you, a ballet training will keep you fit and well, and I know one musical comedy dancer who was cured of polio by studying ballet. She is now a star. Finally, Miss Wareing says that no decision can be reached as to your physical suitability until you are in your teens. But, if you are rejected, console yourself with this fact. Even if classical ballet is not to be your career, there are many other forms of dancing to choose from and fulfil your wish to dance. In all these, your long ballet training will be tremendously helpful and give you great advantages.

With so many heartbreaks, hazards, difficulties and setbacks beyond your control—why take it up at all? Because if you have sufficient spirit and the will never to admit defeat, there are many, many good things as well. Real and exciting rewards.

Gerd Larsen, Royal Ballet star, travelled from Norway to join. Secretly preferring to act, she now laughs at her early struggles in the *corps de ballet*, desperately trying to remember the correct sequence of intricate steps in *Swan Lake*, my sister Moyra prompting her from behind, hissing in her ear as they all swept round the stage—"No, no, Gerd—quick, this way, now left, two turns, up stage, jêté, jêté!"

Gerd was a success, but when offered a leading teacher's job with the company she accepted with pleasure and loves every minute of her work. Her acting talents have been developed in playing the occasional but important character parts, not least of these, her quite brilliant "Carabosse", the Wicked Fairy, in *The Sleeping Princess*. She is the only woman I have seen play this part.

Her full life includes conducting rehearsals, directing and advising the company's television performances and films. In association with Sir Frederick Ashton, she adjudicates the auditions deciding which of the Royal Ballet school's students shall join the company, ruthlessly weeding out the unsuitables. Even if they get into the *corps de ballet*, they will not necessarily prove strong enough to be given solo parts. People like Gerd are hard task-masters, and both technical and physical standards have never been higher. She learned in a tough school under the legendary Dame Ninette de Valois, founder of the Royal Ballet, and knows only too well that dancers must have the intelligence and humility to take harsh criticism . . . As my sister Moyra wryly remarks—"Survive the ballet and you can survive anything—even a shipwreck!"

But even when they reject young dancers, Gerd Larsen and her colleagues are tireless in their efforts to help place them in other jobs, recommending them to film producers, as models and as actresses. Many are found lucrative openings and an entirely new career outside the ballet, succeeding in a way impossible without the classical training. It gives you a grace and deportment that makes you outstanding wherever you go. According to Gerd, there is a stamp and "chic" about a ballet dancer's figure which enables her to pick them out in any gathering, and she will quote actors who are proof of this . . . Vanessa Redgrave, Maggie Smith, Christopher Gable (Royal Ballet star, recently turned actor), film star Deborah Kerr, also from the Royal Ballet. Claire Bloom had a classical ballet training. There are many others.

Gerd Larsen believes that a large permanent company is the only real future for the young student, and in it they can have a varied and wonderful life, meeting interesting, famous people of all nationalities. All Hollywood turns out to welcome the ballet when it arrives, and its tours go from Athens, to Mexico, New York, California, Rome, Paris and Beirut. Its members literally see the world in a way only millionaires could afford, fêted wherever they go. She loves the life and considers that a ballet training gives you an added success in your social life and the confidence to enjoy every moment of it. So—there is a good side to the picture!

These are some of the professionals who spend their lives in ballet, realise the disadvantages, make fullest use of the advantages. And they are right in that dancing gives you mental speed and alertness, an all-round education and the ability to study every form of art.

Leslie Edwards is another senior member of the Royal Ballet now turned teacher and ballet master. Like Gerd, he used a great flair for acting to create vivid character studies and cameos in ballet when the time came to give up dancing the more arduous roles. The first few classes which Leslie took as a teacher gave him the idea for something which has paved the way for a new outlet to his long career. As he watched the young dancers, talked to them about their hopes and ideas, he found out how many of them longed to create ballets of their own and how little opportunity there was for this. Mounting a new ballet is expensive and a beginner's failure could be a costly gamble. Few companies are rich enough to risk it. Gradually he worked out a way in which he could help and by so doing develop his own creative future. He formed a small group of dancers who wished to be choreographers, and rehearsed with them after work had finished at Covent Garden. New ballets were slowly composed, the dancers giving their services willingly and rehearsing long hours to build a whole programme which could be their shop window.

One momentous Sunday night an experimental show was given at Guildford's Arnaud Theatre to an awe-inspiring audience led by Fonteyn, Ashton, de Valois, all the leading stars of ballet. The evening was a triumph and "The Royal Ballet Choreographic Group" was born. That first evening several extremely promising choreographers were discovered and they were away to a flying start. Under Leslie's patient, ever-encouraging direction, they have gone from strength to strength. More public performances were given, and the final honour has come with some of the new ballets being performed by the Royal Ballet at Stratford and Covent Garden.

In fact, what has happened to Leslie Edwards is a typical example of the way in which a good training can develop in so many other sides of the theatre . . . Ex-dancers John Cranko and Kenneth MacMillan now run famous companies abroad and are brilliant choreographers. Kenneth MacMillan is to succeed Sir Frederick Ashton as Artistic Director at Covent Garden. And there is Gillian Lynne—restless as a dancer, she found her niche in the wider world of the commercial theatre. Intelligent, intensely musical and creative, she first became a musical comedy star, and more recently famous for directing and choreographing shows such as Tommy Steele's *Half A Sixpence*, *The Matchmaker*, TV series (including Topol's show) and operas.

Royal Ballet Prima Ballerina, Beryl Grey, is now artistic head of the Festival Ballet company, full of ideas and with the authority to carry them out . . . Sir Robert Helpmann has the most versatile of talents—film star (*Chitty Chitty Bang Bang*), Director of the Australian Ballet, of *Camelot* musical, of plays . . . television actor, Shakespearian actor.

They are all fine examples of dancers whose careers did not finish when they were forty but whose talents and dedicated training helped them to even greater heights.

A great family friend, Brenda Hamlyn, trained with my sister and as a leading dancer with the Rambert company she went all over the world, ending up in Italy, where one job led to another. By the time she had been Prima Ballerina at the leading opera houses, La Scala, Milan, the open-air arena at Verona, Rome and Florence, she had fallen in love with Italy and married her Italian husband, photographer Rafaello Bencini.

One day Brenda went with him to see possible studio premises at the Palazzo Racasoli in Florence. As they wandered round a vast room with seventeenth-century frescoes, high ceilings and glittering chandeliers, she made a lightning decision—there would never be such beautiful surroundings for a dance studio! She had five more years of dancing ahead of her, but this was an opportunity she must not miss. Her husband went without his photographic studio for the time being, and his wife became a teacher. In a few weeks "The Brenda Hamlyn School of Dance" was opened, and to-day Brenda is the proud head of Florence's leading school of dance. She has 150 pupils (including mothers), and London examiners fly out to take the examinations in the Cecchetti method.

Brenda Hamlyn is a realist and she never regrets her decision. Under her sympathetic guidance, her pupils will be fully prepared to use their training in the best possible way—even if they are not good enough for a permanent ballet company. And I agree with her views on dancing . . . While encouraging the idea of taking it up, she stresses the disappointments and hardships of her own career but thinks that if you have the smallest success, the sense of achievement is great and that you reach fantastic artistic heights. And when dancing stops, there are many exciting things you can do, not least teaching, which she loves. She smiles cheerfully when she says that the discipline of ballet teaches you to deal with every side of your grown-up life . . . "A nine-thirty class every morning prepares you for anything!"

I must be honest—an actor's life is simpler, pleasanter, but not nearly so self-disciplined. It would be better for all actors if it were. As a result, ballet dancers are tougher, less vulnerable than we are, and therefore better equipped to take necessary criticism and set-backs.

But, as in Brenda's case, be it dancer or actor, impulse and chance fashion our careers more than we care to admit. And Alfred Roderigues is the first to agree. Now celebrated director of plays, operas, revues and musicals, with his own television series, he soon tired of the almost religious atmosphere of ballet, feeling that even a fanatical, devout spirit is not always sufficient and humorously states—"You need a group of blessed spirits at your birth, con-ferring the priceless gifts of soul, stamina and shape. You must be best 'cream' . . . To be milk is unacceptable, for an ordinary member of a company simply helps and prepares the 'chosen ones' (Fonteyn and Nureyev) to dance on their dedicated way to (so he considers) a most artificial paradise!" He thinks that the monastic seclusion of the ballet is as inbred as the Pharaohs and maybe will last no longer than they did. Old Petipa and Diaghilev are still the main bloodstream of the ballet, which he dislikes. These rigid classic traditions should be broken, new forms discovered, and he, for one, thinks that the old classics have had their day and should only be performed as museum pieces on special occasions. He has only found his ballet training useful when actually doing choreo-graphy for a ballet . . . His interests are very modern, highly imaginative and concerned with the "real theatre" as he sees it; music of every kind and country, dancing from everywhere. The ballet for him was merely a stepping-stone to these things.

As an actress I agree with him, for in my side of the theatre things are changing all the time, methods of acting, plays, design, films—all breaking away from out-dated, stuffy traditions. Were I a dancer, I would wish to rebel against the old order. I would want to be in a company which was modern, vivid, using "dancing" in

the broadest sense of the word . . . I would want to use a general
love of the theatre, music, dancing and art and combine them all.
I disagree with Roderigues in that I am sure, as a dancer, a long
ballet training would be invaluable . . . Agnes de Mille, Jerome
Robbins (*West Side Story*), Herbert Ross, and Larry Oakes of
Oliver, are ex-dancers who have brought great musicals to life
with their originality and knowledge of the dance.

I have been directed in a film by Wendy Toye and in a play by
Sir Robert Helpmann and was impressed by their characteristic
dancer's capacity for long hours, hard work, strict theatrical
discipline, attention to detail and, above all, by their punctuality!
All learned in the ballet and never forgotten.

New audiences have been attracted to ballet by television, and
the person largely responsible for this is another ex-Royal Ballet
star, Margaret Dale, who has strong views on the future of ballet.
She reminded me that in Russia and Denmark a dancer has a
pension on retirement. Ours have nothing and she feels that dancers
should do everything to resist pressures put on them by their
teachers and organisations to keep "pure". In other words, to
study nothing but ballet. She advises students studying every form
of dance to safeguard their very uncertain future. And that regular
companies should have a special person who does nothing but
advise young dancers and look after their well-being in these
things—organises mutual pension schemes in which the artists
make a contribution as well . . .

Strong-minded, forthright, Margaret Dale thinks that dancers
must look after themselves and not be pampered and spoilt by the
apparent security of a big permanent company. She has always
been independent, self-contained, and when she found that just
being a dancer was not enough (she had so many creative urges
that she had no idea what to do with), she tried her hand at choreography—a flop. This was a hard lesson and taught her the limits
of her ability . . . Standing in for Ninette de Valois, she recon-
structed an old ballet for television, as she was the only one who
knew it. Through this, she met Sir George Barnes and gave him
her views on televising ballet properly. Amused, he told her to get
in touch with him if she ever wanted a job. The years passed and,
tired of dancing and with a choreographic flop behind her, she
contacted him again. He said he would train her as a director if she

could get leave from the ballet. Being Margaret Dale, she did. And being Margaret Dale, she succeeded and, in my opinion, is the only person who has ever been able to bring ballet to the screen in a really exciting, imaginative way.

If all I have said and told you hasn't entirely put you off and you are still wanting to be a ballet dancer, pay a visit to "The Dance Centre" in Covent Garden one day. Even if you don't study there, you'll want to go there if you are a dancer. And in the crowded restaurant you will meet dancers from all over the world, of all ages; talking dancing, practising, rehearsing, studying, learning of auditions . . . For dancers it is one of the best new developments and started by two dancers who wanted "a side line". They have converted an old warehouse into a vast Dance Centre containing large airy studios, snack bar, showers, changing rooms, reception hall manned by a very helpful staff, and in the future there is to be a swimming pool as well. It has filled a great need in the dancing world. Young teachers who have not the money for their own premises can simply hire a studio, put their name up on the big notice board, with their times and the type of dancing they teach, and away they go. You may learn Indian, Spanish, Jazz, West Indian and classical ballet dancing. There are classes in mime and movement, and special classes for actors. There are beginner's classes, children's classes, advanced, private and professional's classes. It is cheap, it is good. Leslie Edwards rehearses his Choreographic Group at the Dance Centre. Brenda Hamlyn has refresher classes there when she comes to London and meets old friends. And night and day the staff answer inquiries, take bookings, organise and advise.

Actors have little opportunity to take much physical exercise and as it is important to keep supple and limbered up . . . I asked Gerd Larsen what I should do . . . "Go to the Dance Centre and find a suitable beginner's class!" was her immediate answer. So— off I went, swinging back and forth to a West Indian rhythm, and soon I started a beginner's class in ballet. I watched a trial one, given by Roger Tully, an ex-dancer who is an inspired teacher . . . The ages of the pupils ranged from nine to nearly ninety, and every Saturday morning at ten o'clock they learn the first stages of ballet. After all I have told you, I thought I had better try for myself and see what it feels like to be really stiff and aching.

So there—if I haven't put you off altogether, and I hope I haven't—are a few examples of people I know who have managed to make dancing their whole life instead of a very brief career which must come to an abrupt and frustrating end when you are too old to dance in *Swan Lake* or *Giselle*.

Take it up by all means, but know what you want to do when you stop.

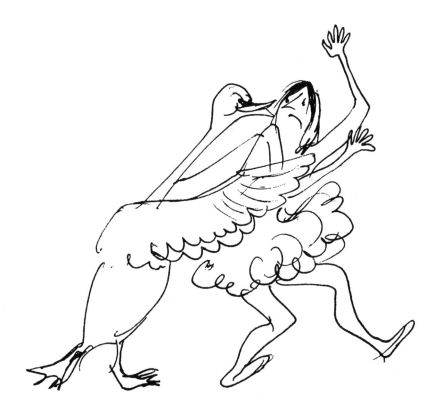

THE DAWNING
OF AN OBSESSION

An extract from "Nureyev" by Alexander Bland

As with most children, my early irresponsible years came to a stop
when it became time to go to school, and I remember very vividly
that first day at Kindergarten. At that time we were so totally
lacking in everything that I literally had no suitable clothes—no
coat, no shoes, in fact nothing to lend me the appearance of a
normal child. Mother had to carry me to school on her back and I
was acutely, painfully aware of the bizarreness of the situation. I
was a proud child and poverty as humiliating as ours caused me a
very real mental anguish. On that first day Mother dressed me in
my sister Lida's coat—and there is nothing more calculated to
make a small boy of six feel foolish than having to wear his sister's
clothes. Arrayed in a little girl's cape complete with "wings", I
looked and felt like a clown.

My entrance into the kindergarten was far from triumphant.
The moment they saw me all the children started to sing aloud in
Tartar: "We've got a bump in our class, we've got a bump in our
class." I didn't know Tartar well in those days. After spending
my first three years in Moscow, some Bashkir words were still
without meaning to me. When I came home I asked Mother for an
explanation. She told me not to worry. However, she finally did
explain that the word "bump" meant—a beggar. I didn't really
feel upset, I seem to remember, by the fact that on my first encounter with a group it had spontaneously rejected me. Nevertheless, my abnormal aversion from being bullied or pushed around
probably dates from that time. A push with the slightest hint of
rudeness can make me instantly feel like a rearing horse, quivering,
snorting and refusing to move.

I think that the insult at school would have upset me much
more had I not been conscious of something else which made an

even greater impression: it was on that first day that I became aware of class differences. I realised with a shock that many children at school were much better off than I was, better dressed and, above all, better fed. Those kids probably came from solid Ufa families who had not led our unsettled life, evacuating Moscow for what we thought would be only a short time and leaving most of what we owned behind us.

I got the impression that some of the children were immensely rich. Later, I came to realise that my idea of extreme wealth meant simply never to be hungry. My deductions, for a child, were really extremely logical: most of those children in class never ate all that was given to them, but with me the situation was radically different. Almost every morning I would arrive in class late. Every morning the teacher would demand to know the reason why. And I, surprised that she didn't understand my problems, would always give her the same answer: "But I can't come to class before having breakfast . . ." And she would reply: "Don't you understand that you're supposed to eat here?" Then, all I could do was to mumble: "Well, I just wasn't ready in time, that's why." She'll never understand, I simply can't let that chance pass me by. Especially as we never knew what was going to happen about dinner at home.

And indeed, that same year, I remember coming to class one morning and fainting there from hunger. There had been nothing to eat at home since the previous morning. Mother had gone on one of her food-hunting trips with Rosa and all I could do was to try and sleep through the evening. Next morning I woke feeling dizzy and fainted in school.

But when the time came for me to start my first year at the real school—I was seven, then—I loved it from the start. I steadily became the best pupil, thanks to an unusual capacity for grasping everything the first time I heard it. Everything my teacher said I memorised there and then during the class and never had to study my lessons again at home. Soon, that sponge capacity for soaking up everything I heard was going to be applied to dancing and I would become the worst pupil in the class. But that time had not quite arrived.

Still a very solitary child, I spent all my leisure time either listening to the music endlessly poured out by our radio until I

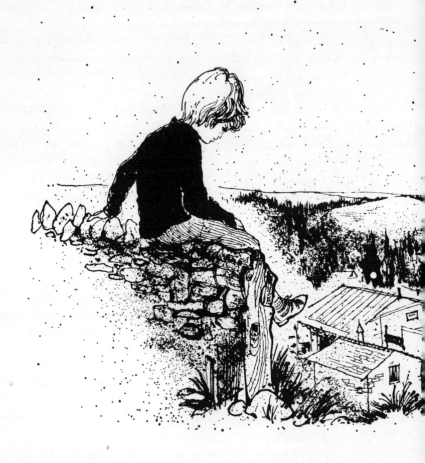

would become drunk with its sensations—or climbing up to my private observation point.

I had found, not very far from our house, a little hill, from the top of which I would watch for hours the people of Ufa going about their work. The scene on Saturdays used to amuse me the most: small groups of men walking briskly along Ufa's main streets in their bathrobes—even, sometimes, in their pyjamas—on their way to the weekly steam bath. Some even carried a little broom of

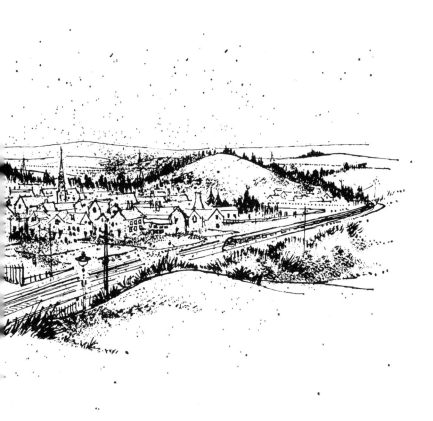

birch-tree twigs in their hands with which to beat themselves after
the bath.

But another reason for choosing that particular vantage point
was that there I dominated the Ufa Railway Station. I would sit
there motionless for hours, watching. For several years of my life
I think I went there every day, simply watching the trains slowly
starting and getting up speed. I loved the sensation of being driven
somewhere else by those wheels; I was more attached to that

railway station than to school, or even to home. In later years in Leningrad before creating a role in a new ballet I would often go to the station and just look, until I could feel the movement become part of me, and I part of the train. That helped me somehow in my dancing though I can't say exactly how.

But by now I was seven, and the time was drawing near for my real, unique passion to invade my heart, my body and my whole life. One day at school I was shown how to dance to the music of simple Bashkir folk songs. I didn't realise immediately just what intense pleasure I was soon to know from the act of dancing. But that first year the sonorous Bashkir folk songs set my senses reeling and filled me with delight. Once back from school I would sing and dance all the afternoon at home until it was time to go to bed.

Mother, despite her never-ending worries, couldn't help but notice my unusual inclination for both music and dancing. Often during that first year friends would come and say to her: "Rudi's got a natural talent for dancing . . . it's a gift . . . you ought to send him to the Leningrad Ballet School." (Children enter this school at the age of six or seven and stay until they are about eighteen, when they are fully-fledged dancers.) Or they would say: "What Rudi needs now is to start a classical training under good teachers." Mother would nod, smile and say nothing. Leningrad indeed! Why not the moon? Who was going to pay for that!

Meanwhile our school groups of boys and girls performing Bashkir dances had expanded. We had quickly gained a small reputation in Ufa and the school used to send us to hospitals to entertain wounded soldiers back from the front. I used to look forward to those small concerts and gradually dancing became more and more dear to me. It was "my" world. All that time I learned no other kind of dance but that shown to us in class. I could remember every step. It was enough for the teacher to show me the dance once and it was literally engraved in my memory and in my body. Everything which was shown to me seemed to pass directly into my very blood.

I think it was already then, at the end of the war, that I became sickened, once and for all time, by praise. Every friend of our family was constantly telling my parents that I was so gifted, "really born to dance", that I simply had to study in Leningrad. Apparently nowhere else would do. I believed it, and from then on that belief never left me. Although still such a small child, all I could think of was Leningrad, Leningrad . . .

From that time, too, dates an unshakable conviction that I was moving towards an already fixed destiny: that of a dedicated dancer. It was on New Year's Eve, during that first year of studies, that I saw a real ballet performance for the first time. Still, to-day, I vividly remember how dazzled, fascinated and moved to the core I was with what I saw.

In Russia every Republic has one, and sometimes two, ballet companies. (I think there must be thirty-three now in Russia.) It is the same with Philharmonic orchestras, the same with theatres. I'm sure that in no other country in the world is there such a passionate interest in music and ballet as in Soviet Russia. Anyway, that performance on New Year's Eve at the "national" Ufa Opera starred a "national" ballerina, Nazredinova, who, through my maturer judgment to-day, I still consider a beautiful dancer. She was to dance a Bashkir ballet entitled *The Cranes' Song*, to my childish eyes a most dramatic and poetic work. Our Ufa Opera, in those days, was particularly brilliant, sheltering as it did many evacuated artists from the Moscow Bolshoi and the Leningrad Kirov. But even without those outside contributions from our two greatest theatres, I consider the Ufa Ballet Company at least as good as, say, the de Cuevas Company which I was to get to know later.

My first encounter with ballet, which was going to fill my entire life from then on, was unorthodox. It was love at first sight, but only through housebreaking. Mother had only managed to buy a single ticket to the Opera on that night for the entire family, but she was determined to try and get us all in somehow.

So we arrived. My three sisters, my mother and myself. At the door of the theatre we found a vast, impatient crowd. This was just at the end of the war. The natural love innate in every Russian for music and ballet was made even stronger during those years by the fact that one was prepared to give anything in exchange for a little dream, a momentary escape from the nightmare of everyday life. The Russians' boundless spiritual resources, the profundity of their inner life—the sheer capacity that they have to cut themselves away from the sordidness of their daily struggles is for me perhaps the strongest explanation of the enormous success which almost any manifestation of art can command in the Soviet Union.

T.W.B.   G

The crowd was getting bigger and bigger every minute. It was pushing so strongly against the large doors of the Opera that suddenly they collapsed, the entrance was wide open and we were all literally propelled inside. Under cover of the general chaos, the five Nureyevs were in . . . in on one ticket.

I shall never forget a single detail of the scene that met my eyes: the theatre itself with its soft, beautiful lights and gleaming crystal chandeliers; small lanterns hanging everywhere; coloured windows; everywhere velvet . . . gold—another world; a place which, to my dazzled eyes, you could only hope to encounter in the most enchanted fairy-tale. That first visit to the theatre has left behind a unique memory, something illuminated within me in a quite special way, a very personal privilege. Something was happening to me which was taking me far from my sordid world and bearing me right up to the skies. From the moment I entered that magic place I felt I had really left the world, borne far away from everything I knew by a dream staged for me alone . . . I was speechless.

Even to-day I still feel the same sorcery whenever I enter a handsome theatre. The blue-and-silver Kirov, the red-and-gold Opera in Paris and London—they are for me among the most delightful visions I have ever known.

From that unforgettable day when I knew such rapt excitement I could think of nothing else; I was utterly possessed. From that day I can truthfully date my unwavering decision to become a ballet dancer. I felt "called". Watching the dancers that night, admiring their other-worldly ability to defy the laws of balance and gravity, I had the absolute certitude that I had been born to dance.

But how to leave that wretched existence in Ufa, how to leave the school? So many questions remained unanswered. Now the inner cry I had been living with had become deafening: "To Leningrad . . . to Leningrad . . ." I knew now how I wanted to live, but had no idea how to achieve it. It was then that I started a day-dream—an obsessive fantasy which even now stays with me. To escape from reality I imagined—and even convinced myself—that someday someone would come from the outside world, take me by the hand and point out the right road . . . the road to becoming an exceptional dancer. I still live with that hope. Although I may have made progress, I still wait for that person to come and show me what is really right.

So I waited for that miracle, for someone, who would say like all our friends and neighbours: "He is really good, he has so much talent he must go to Leningrad." But the dream remained a dream and there was nothing to do but go on with my Ufa life.

Our little folklore group had expanded some more. We had won various contests against other Bashkir schools. Occasionally, too, we had the chance of dancing before public audiences, and in the preparation for those simple performances I found a passionate delight. Since then I've always adored rehearsals. Even to-day my moments of highest pleasure often occur during the preliminary, solitary work of rehearsal when I feel I have brought some step, some harmonious new combination to a point of perfection—or as near to it as possible, at any rate.

These dancing successes as a child also gave me the illusion of a completely full life. I didn't share these joys with anyone—except my sister Rosa. She alone understood me. She was very musical and was studying to become a teacher of young children; she was doing a little dancing herself in order to demonstrate better to the children later how to hold themselves, how to participate fully in our folk dances. Rosa actively contributed to my initiation. She talked to me of the history of the dance, took me to lectures while still a child, and sometimes, to please me, she would bring home some ballet costumes. That, to me, was heaven. I would spread them out on the bed and gaze at them—gaze at them so intensively that I could feel myself actually inside them. I would fondle them for hours, smooth them and smell them. There is no other word to describe it—I was like a dope addict.

From the age of about eight I can truthfully say I was possessed. Just as a man consumed by a single passion becomes blind to the rest of the world, so I felt in me the urge, the blind need for dancing and for nothing else.

In school things went from bad to worse. From then on my marks were doomed to be an endless series of 2's and 3's (the top mark in Russia is 5). Besides dancing—or rather as a consequence of it—I had a strong urge to learn to play the piano. When I told this to my father he answered: "But Rudi, the piano is not really interesting. And it's very difficult to learn. You'd be much better off learning to play the accordion or a mouth-organ. An accordion is useful for making yourself popular at parties—and you take it

with you everywhere. But think of a piano . . . you can't carry it
on your back. Besides, not everybody likes a piano . . ."

True, not everybody liked it, but I adored it, and still do. I still
regret to-day I never could convince my father that music shouldn't
be limited to instruments you can carry on your back. But I haven't
given up the hope of learning to play some day. In 1960, with the
money I had made touring in East Germany, I bought a beautiful
piano and had it shipped to the apartment in Leningrad where
Rosa lives. That piano is still waiting for me there . . .

My craving for music is such that even without ever having
taken lessons I can sit at a piano for hours on end playing simple
airs from my favourite composers; I never get tired. If there is no
instrument to hand and I have no records with me (though nowadays I simply cannot bear to be without them, and always carry a
portable transistor record-player so I can listen to music whenever
I feel the need for it), I can get pleasure out of simply reading the
piano notes. I must confess I don't really enjoy what is known as
difficult music. But I can literally get drunk on Mozart, Prokofiev,
Chopin . . . their harmonies go straight to my heart. They can
make me forget anything I don't want to remember—and I've
often felt a need for that; to erase faces, events from my mind and
memory forever. Of all the composers I know, Scriabin is the one
I prefer by far. In my private hierarchy of artists I place him with
Dostoevsky and Van Gogh for the generosity and violence I feel
they share—they are my three favourite artists, anyway.

Of my third and fourth years at school I don't have much to say:
by then I was frankly a wretched pupil. Like any other child in
Russia I had become a Pioneer. Between ten and sixteen all Russian
children are incorporated into the Pioneers which, I suppose,
might be compared to the Scouts. There is nothing overtly political
about them—at least there was nothing political about them in
my mind when I joined them. Because nothing connected with
groups ever appealed to me I wasn't a very eager Pioneer, and I
can well imagine my group wasn't too fond of me either. All the
same, it's partially due to them that I made some decisive progress
in my dancing.

We had a dancing teacher in the Pioneers who adapted for us,
from Pioneer *Gazettes* edited in Moscow and Leningrad, dances
from all the Russian Republics. This was a very welcome change

since it enriched and enlarged our repertoire; at least I wasn't dancing exclusively Bashkir dances any more.

When I was eleven, thanks to a Pioneer-mistress who took me one day to the Ufa Scientists' Club, I met for the first time a woman —a very old woman—Udeltsova, who was *almost* a real ballet teacher. She had never really been a teacher but was extremely musical, highly cultivated and had danced, years and years ago, in the *corps de ballet* of Diaghilev's Ballets Russes de Monte-Carlo. I was to become extremely close to that remarkable woman of seventy who, every summer, took a trip to Leningrad to see what was new in the world of ballet. Thus it was that she had seen Japanese dancers and Indian dancers too, when they visited Leningrad; once back in Ufa she described everything to us, opening up our provincial eyes to a far wider scene.

It was Udeltsova who first talked to me of Anna Pavlova. She had probably met her in the Diaghilev Days. She told me what Pavlova brought to the world; how that greatest of ballerinas religiously trained to acquire her irreproachable technique but how, by the very atmosphere she distilled around her, she threw a veil over all outward manifestation of technique, creating an impression of utter spontaneity each time she danced. So much so that her audiences, under her spell, had the impression of watching a miracle in the making. This conception thrilled me. The art of hiding art: surely this was the key to greatness in an artist.

I know that there are people to-day who think that if Pavlova should come back now to dance she would not be interesting to us any longer. I know this is not so. All I saw of Pavlova during my first year of studies at the Leningrad Ballet School was an old, worn-out film, very primitively shot—she was dancing Anton Rubinstein's *The Night*, as a matter of fact. But I have never seen anything to match it: such gestures, such perfectly beautiful line; pure art. She spoke with her body, transposing Rubinstein's melodious music into sheer lyrical movement. I can find no words to describe such refinement of expression, such immaculate perfection; beauty which was beyond the human. And to think that this film had been made towards the end of her life. It was so moving you felt as if someone were very softly plucking feathers right out of your heart . . . a kind of exquisite pain . . .

In Leningrad, too, I saw another very old film shot a few

months before Pavlova died. She was dancing to some Chopin Preludes. She could no longer do very much and was limiting herself to a slight *pas de bourrée*, a few *ports de bras*, and the movements of her hands. There was almost nothing left of dancing yet, watching it, one couldn't refrain from weeping; it was so beautiful, so spiritual in its conception. One could see that her face was drawn together to a mask, yet that mattered not at all. One was looking at beauty. I've never been so moved as I was by those two old, primitive films.

I'm afraid the thought of Pavlova has side-tracked me out of my own story; it was, in fact, much later that I had this revelation of how great she was. But a Pavlova or a Nijinsky are not born every twenty years, and when the chance arises to defend their image from attack, I feel we should never postpone it.

But now back to Udeltsova. I was brought before her and told to dance a *gopak*, a *lezghinka* and various folk items with which I was absolutely familiar. I danced—and suddenly Udeltsova seemed absolutely stunned. When I stopped, she said that in fifty years of watching and teaching children how to dance this was the first time she could say with absolute conviction: "Child, you have a duty to yourself to learn classical dancing. With such an innate gift, you must join the students at the Maryinsky Theatre . . ." Udeltsova still called it by the name it bore in her younger days—the celebrated Imperial Maryinsky Theatre of Saint Petersburg. Later, while still retaining its historic traditions, it became known as the Leningrad Kirov, after a politician assassinated in Leningrad after the Revolution.

I blushed scarlet. But truthfully, I couldn't feel great surprise. I had already heard so much praise and "Go to Leningrad" had become such a familiar refrain. All the same, even a child of eleven could see there was a difference between a neighbour's predictions and those of a competent, informed woman such as Udeltsova. She offered to give me ballet lessons twice a week. One year later, having learned from her the correct five positions, my first *pliés*, my first *battements*, Udeltsova told me to continue with a friend of hers—an excellent teacher, Vaitovitch, who had been a soloist for years at the Kirov and had returned to Ufa as a professional teacher. Vaitovitch had a good technique and superb elevation—moreover, she could jump!

It is a rare gift. Chibukiani and Sergeyev, for instance, two of the greatest dancers of the last thirty years in Russia, have not got a big jump. But by *ballon* both succeed in creating an impression of jumping so perfectly that the illusion for the public is complete. It is all a question of stage mastery. Dudinskaya, for example, the unrivalled ballerina of the Kirov for some thirty years, seemed to us, as we watched her at work in the classroom, hardly to leave the floor. Nevertheless, she danced countless times the ballet *Laurencia* —a part whose variations called for powerful, man-size jumps. Thanks to *ballon*, and the technique of appearing to hang motionless in the air, once again illusion was perfect.

Anyway, Vaitovitch was born with that gift, and with her I started to make real progress. During the year that I was studying with her, I heard that a group of children was to be selected from throughout Bashkir, sent to Leningrad, and there be tested for possible entry into the Leningrad Ballet School. It felt as if my dream had come true. But the dream was destined to crash into a shattering disillusion, for the children left without me. I remember how I begged my father to come with me and make inquiries about how one set about joining the group. By then my father was already strongly opposed to my dancing and he advised me to forget about it. I pleaded with him, and finally, completely in the dark as we were, we approached the cashier of the Opera about how we should proceed for my inscription. But, of course, it was all in vain. I soon found out that the children had already left . . . left for Leningrad without me. It took me days to climb out of a state of black despair.

For a long time after this incident my father seemed embarrassed whenever he laid eyes on me. I never understood why, until a couple of years later when, having earned a little money, I took a three days' trip to Moscow. Then it all became clear to me: my father simply didn't have the necessary two hundred roubles—the price of the ticket from Ufa to Leningrad.

A DANCER'S LIFE

Elaine McDonald

Most of my childhood was spent in Scarborough on the North Sea coast, and it was there that I received my first ballet lessons. My sister and I attended classes once a week at a local ballet school, and besides ballet we learned tap, Modern, Greek and National dancing too. We found our lessons great fun, especially since we sometimes entered various Dance festivals, where we competed against other children for medals and trophies. Perhaps the best known of these is the nation-wide "Sunshine Festival", which is held every year and the proceeds go to help with the education of children in the Sunshine Homes for the Blind. The preliminary heats are held in regional centres all over Britain, and then the Finals are in London. I enjoyed learning all the dances, and meeting all the other children at these competitions, and I felt very lucky when we went to dance in London in the school holidays. During this time I was also working hard to pass the Royal Academy of Dancing Children's exams, and I found that I was beginning to enjoy my ballet lessons most of all.

My first serious step towards a career in ballet was taken when I was eleven. The Royal Academy of Dancing and *Girl* magazine were to give ballet scholarships to girls and boys aged between nine and eleven. These scholarships consisted of two free ballet classes a week at the nearest local centre which, in my case, was Leeds. My teacher suggested that I do the audition, and so, together with my mother and a friend, I travelled to Leeds. The audition was being held in a big church hall, and when we arrived it was full of children of my age, all displaying their *Girl* badges. We had been asked to wear swimming costumes instead of the usual white tunic, and my friend and I had both chosen red ones. As I got into mine I began to feel quite nervous, and it was then that I realised how much I wanted to win the scholarship. Soon my name was called and as I was going into the audition room my mother whispered, "Good

luck. You can only do your best, and I'll be praying for you both."
And sure enough, throughout the audition my mother sat and
prayed for us to do our best.

Once inside, we were all given numbers to pin on to our
costumes and we stood at the bars in numerical order. There were
lots of people watching, sitting behind tables at one end of the
room. We were to do an ordinary ballet class, and the person giving
the class was Miss Louise Browne. She came forward and told us
that we mustn't be nervous and we should try to enjoy ourselves.
To my surprise I found myself doing exactly that. The steps we
had to do were just like the ones we had been taught at our own
dancing school, and not too difficult. We were given some jumps
to do, and it was only when my head felt as though it had stayed
up in the air when I had landed that I realised I had a headache!

We finished the class and then certain numbers were called out,
mine and my friend's included. At first we thought we were to be
dismissed, but then we were told that we were being called for a
medical examination. This was to check on our physical condition,
the strength of our feet, our childhood illnesses, and so on. When
this was finished we were told that the results would be sent to us
by letter. Back at home, the seven days' wait seemed much longer,
particularly since all our friends kept asking us if we had had any
news. At last a letter came with an R.A.D. heading, to say that I
had been successful, and I felt very, very pleased. There were to
be ten other girls and three boys in the classes which would be held
on Saturdays and Mondays. The letter told us that we would have
to wear white tunics, pink belts and shoes for the classes. The boys
would wear black tights and white "T" shirts. The R.A.D. had
also notified my school that I had been awarded the scholarship,
and my headmistress gave her permission for me to do the classes.

So I began my journeys to Leeds. They were quite long,
Scarborough is seventy-five miles away, but I had great fun since
I had two companions from home who had also passed the
audition. We used to do our homework travelling back on the
train on Monday nights because, of course, our school work could
not be allowed to suffer in any way. I enjoyed the classes very much
and found that I worked hard in them. Each year there was a re-
test which took place in London and the examiners decided whether
or not to award your scholarship for another year. In my third year

the centre for the classes was moved to York, and this made things much easier, reducing our travelling time by half. In all, I spent four years as an R.A.D. scholar and I enjoyed the classes tremendously. I was also completing my education at school, which is very important to anyone who wants to continue with a ballet training. Some Education Authorities give grants for this, but you need to have G.C.E. "O" levels, and so, together with my other school friends, I did my "O" levels.

I now felt that I would like to try to make dancing my career, and Miss Browne suggested that I should write to the Royal Ballet School for an audition. This was held in London in the Royal Ballet School's famous Baylis Hall. There were five very nervous girls—including myself—doing the audition, which consisted of a normal ballet class. We began with work at the bar—*pliés, battements, ronds de jambe*—in fact, all the exercises which form the basis of classical ballet. Then we moved into the centre of the room and I began to relax a little, but it was difficult, especially with the Principal and some of the teachers of the Royal Ballet School watching! In the centre we were given a series of *enchaînements Enchaînements* is a French word—like many of the terms used in ballet—and it means several steps following one after the other and danced to a piece of music. The ballet mistress gave us the steps, then we were allowed to practise or "mark" them. After that the pianist played the music and we danced the *enchaînement* as well as we could. Full-length ballets are formed in this way. The choreographer, or person who composes the ballet, builds it up by adding on steps and movements until a whole story is told. In the audition we were asked to do *enchaînements* with balancing steps, turns— or pirouettes—and jumps. Afterwards there was a medical examination, and then—to my joy—I was informed that I had been accepted.

I started my training at the Royal Ballet School in the September after my fifteenth birthday. It was all very new and strange living in London and having classes every day. It was like a dream working in the same building as all the famous ballerinas and being taught by the same teachers. Besides our daily ballet class we had classes in which we learned the full-length ballets like *Swan Lake* and *Giselle*. I found this very absorbing and also very demanding— keeping in line when learning the *corps de ballet* work and attempting

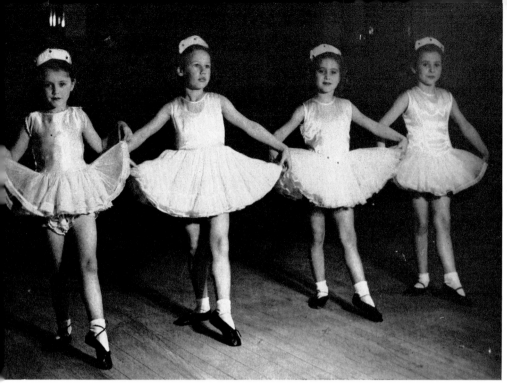

Elaine McDonald (on the left) in one of her earliest stage performances

Elaine McDonald at the age of nine

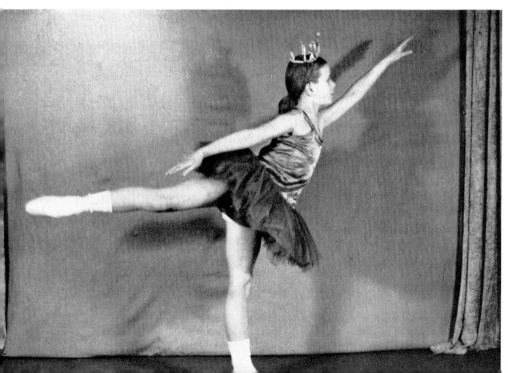

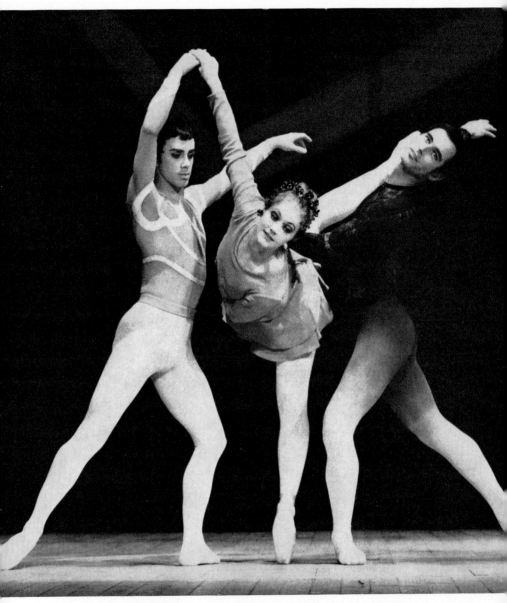

Elaine McDonald as a soloist of the Western Theatre Ballet in
Ephemeron with Ken Wells and Peter Cazalet

steps in solos which had seemed impossible when I had watched them on the stage. We were sometimes allowed to watch dress rehearsals at Covent Garden and encouraged to attend actual performances. This was a great treat for me, because in Scarborough it had been difficult to see live performances by a professional company.

I had been at the school nearly one and a half years when I decided it was time to gain some kind of stage experience. We had five weeks' holiday at Christmas and I auditioned successfully for a pantomime called *The Sleeping Princess*, which was being produced by Cyril Fletcher. It was to run for five weeks—just the length of our holidays. We did two weeks' rehearsals, working very hard all day, but the tiredness was forgotten on the first night in the excitement of performing before a live audience. One of the most interesting things in the pantomime for me was the variety of roles which we dancers had to perform. We were a different character each time we made our entry on the stage. We were "Puppets", then "Children", "Flowers" and also "Princesses". I felt glad of my training in tap-dancing, and all the other types of dancing, as it was very useful to me now.

After five weeks on the stage it was back to school, and I was determined to work even harder to improve my dancing and try to join a ballet company. Before the end of the summer term I heard that a new young company, the London Ballet, with Walter Gore as Artistic Director, were looking for dancers for the *corps de ballet*. Shortly afterwards an announcement to this effect was posted on the school notice board, giving the time and place of the audition. I went along and found that there were eighty girls there, auditioning for only ten places in the *corps de ballet*. The chances looked very slim. We were divided into three groups, each group to do an hour's class. Since I was in the last group, I had to go back in the afternoon. I did the class and was one of twenty girls asked to go back the next day. At the end of the class on the following day I was offered a contract as a student member of the company. Two friends of mine were also included in the ten girls chosen, and we were to begin work on the Monday of the following week. The contract was for an eighteen-week tour of Britain, preceded by five weeks' rehearsals.

The first day of my new life began with a ballet class of one and a half hours. Then we had a break of a quarter of an hour. This break was really quite astounding for me. One moment there was a rehearsal room full of dancers all working terribly hard in class. The next, it seemed to me as though chaos had broken out. Some dancers went into the little kitchen to make coffee; others had brought flasks and sat on the wooden stage at the end of the hall, chattering to their friends or discussing the new roles that they had to learn. Others began practising steps in the centre, then ran up to someone else in the room, saying: "Oh, could you tell me about the arms in this", or "What happened after that turn? I just can't remember." My friends and I sat and watched it all, and I wondered how anyone could practise anything in front of all those people! But it was not long before I realised the value of practising anywhere to get something right.

Lists had been posted giving details of the roles for each dancer, and after the break everyone settled down to the important task of learning and rehearsing these roles. *Giselle* was one of the ballets included and I was to be a stately court lady who accompanies Count Albrecht on his hunting expedition in Act One. Then I was to be one of the Wilis, or spirits of dead maidens, who dance with the spirit of Albrecht's dead love in Act Two. After another hour and a quarter's work we broke for lunch at one-thirty. Then back at two-thirty until six. I have since learned that this is the regular day for most ballet companies all over the world. It is rewarding but very hard work, and really necessary if one is to succeed as a dancer.

At the end of five weeks we had learned all the ballets which we were taking on tour. A notice had been posted giving lists of accommodation in the various towns included in our tour, together with the time of the train which took us to our first town on the Sunday. I had taken down some of the addresses and had written to ask for accommodation at the ones which seemed most reasonable. This comprised bed and breakfast and supper at the end of the performance. As the tour was to start in the autumn and finish at Christmas, it was quite a problem to decide what clothes to take. Finally I made my decision in favour of winter clothes rather than summer ones, as this tour was to include four towns in Scotland.

The accommodation in the first town was very good and the landlady offered tea when I arrived. I unpacked my things and decided to go and look at the theatre. The dressing-room list was on the notice board, and since I was a student member of the company I was sharing a dressing-room right at the top of the theatre. It was a very large theatre and there was plenty of room. The scenery for the ballets had already been unpacked and the wardrobe mistress and her assistant were busy ironing all the costumes. The whole theatre was alive and I felt butterflies in my stomach in anticipation of the following night's performance. Then it was time to unpack all my ballet clothes from the boxes we had been given, and put out my make-up. I had knitted some woollen tights and bought some coloured tops because there was no set uniform and we could wear what we liked for practice and rehearsals. The company provided us with point shoes for rehearsals and performances—we just had to sew on the satin ribbons and keep them clean.

The next day the morning class was held on stage at ten, and for a bar we used scenery and anything that was solid enough to support us. For the rehearsal that followed, those of us who were newcomers wore our costumes to make sure that everything was in order. What a difference to practice clothes! The long, heavy velvet dress for the court lady in *Giselle* certainly helped you to walk in a slow, stately manner. It was impossible to do anything else but walk slowly. In contrast, the Wili costumes for Act Two were made of white net, and though they were long, they were very light and floating—just right for the spirit of a dead maiden!

During the morning we also mapped out the stage so that we knew exactly where we had to stand to keep in line, and how much room there was to dance in. Then at two o'clock we were told that we had finished until the evening performance. This left enough time to check last minute details such as cleaning shoes, making sure that I had enough hairpins, and trying hair styles with headdresses to make sure I knew the best way to make them stay firmly fixed.

The time arrived to get ready. I had been taught about make-up at the Royal Ballet School, and I hoped I had remembered everything correctly as I put it on. The Tannoy radio relayed a message from the Stage Manager to all the dressing-rooms: "Good evening, Ladies and Gentlemen. This is your half-hour call. Half an hour, please." Half an hour before the curtain went up. I began to feel very nervous. By the time the quarter of an hour call came I was ready, and I decided to go down on stage to go over the ballet. I felt sure that I could not remember the steps at all, but when I met an older member of the company she told me that it was just a very natural form of nerves.

The performance went well and I didn't forget any steps. At the end, the ballet master came round and gave us dozens of notes about our dancing. I wondered how the performance could possibly have gone well with so many notes! Now I know that there are always lots of notes after any performance—this is the only way to achieve perfection. After the first night the week seemed to fly by, and before I knew it, it was time to pack up on Saturday.

The following weeks of the tour were very similar to the first. But no two weeks were ever quite alike. The towns we visited were so varied, so were the audiences who came to see our performances. The theatres were different. Sometimes the stages were enormous; sometimes they were so small that we wondered how we would all manage to dance on them. But with planning and careful rehearsal we succeeded. If we had a free afternoon we occasionally visited a cinema, or were taken out into the countryside.

Four weeks before the end of the tour we were told that the next contract was to start from the following February. We had to go and see the director individually to find out whether we were going to be offered a contract or not. All I could do was pray that I would be accepted again, and I felt as though my prayers had been answered when the director offered me a contract. And this time not as a student member—as a full-time member of the company.

The tour finished at Christmas, and we were all to begin rehearsing again in February. I wanted to find some work for the eight weeks in between and decided to try another pantomime. This lasted for five weeks and was just as enjoyable as before.

When the company reassembled in the spring, we found that we were taking lots of new ballets on a tour which was to last twenty weeks. One of the ballets was Les Sylphides, and five of us were to learn the Prelude. Eventually two would be chosen to perform it. This was a chance to dance a solo role for the first time and I was determined not to miss such an opportunity. I worked very hard to get to know the steps so well that I could make them look soft and easy when I danced them. *Les Sylphides* is a very flowing, romantic ballet. The day arrived when we had to dance the Prelude separately, to see who would dance the performance. When the time came, I felt that I had to dance as I had never danced before, and I must have succeeded for I was one of the two girls finally chosen. Now the work really began because besides the solo there were lots of small pieces to learn and, of course, all the *corps de ballet* work.

We went on tour and I danced the Prelude and enjoyed it very much, even the director seemed quite pleased with the performance. I also danced two other solo parts. Each time a performance finished I wished I could do it again and do it better. Some of the new ballets were not strictly classical and I began to be very interested in these and loved watching them. Towards the end of the twenty weeks we began to hear rumours that the company was in financial difficulties and might have to disband. Some of the rumours grew quite wild, and finally an official announcement was issued. It was true. The Directors did not think that there would be enough money to continue. This was a shock for all of us. The thought of not doing the ballets again and missing all our friends was awful. At the end of the tour we were told that we would be notified by letter within two weeks if the company was to re-assemble. I waited the two weeks, praying that they would find the money, but alas it was not so, and now I had to find a new job.

A friend of mine was working at the London Palladium and, as one of the girls in the group was ill, she asked me if I would like to audition, because I was the right height. I was accepted for the ballet group which opened the second half of the show. It was quite an experience being on the same bill as people like Frank Ifield and Susan Maughan. Life backstage was just as interesting. We met a lot of the other artistes, and it was fascinating to watch the tumblers doing a last minute warm-up in the corridor. The performances were mainly in the late afternoon and early evening, which left our days free, and plenty of time to do ballet classes at Cleo Nordis. I felt it was important to keep on trying to improve and usually did at least one—sometimes two classes a day—with this teacher, the best professional teacher I know.

I finished the show at the Palladium just before Christmas, and went for an audition with a company called The Western Theatre

Ballet. I did not know much about the company, but I had heard and read that it was young, vital and very forward-looking. There were only twelve dancers in it—six boys and six girls. After the audition I was asked to do a company class the following day. This class was even more of an ordeal than the audition, as the whole company were watching as well as the director. I knew that I must dance well in spite of this, and breathed very deeply before each exercise.

I was accepted and offered a contract for one year, which also included a two-week visit to Denmark in the spring. We were to go out on tour immediately, spending one night in each town, and I had to learn some of the ballets as we went along. Being one night in each town was a very new experience for me. The company travelled all together in a special bus, with the scenery and costumes stored at the back. As soon as we reached our destination, sometimes in the morning, sometimes in the afternoon, everybody unpacked and then did a class on stage. Whilst this was going on, the stage staff were mounting the scenery and setting the lighting. Sometimes there was just enough time to get ready for the performances when we had finished. The life was a very hectic one, and because of this we only did such tours for a limited period in the year. But the work was very rewarding. We visited halls, Institutes and schools as well as theatres, and always with capacity

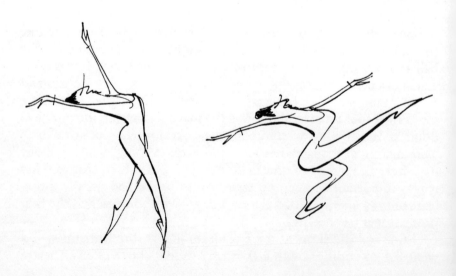

audiences. We enjoyed our school visits very much. Sometimes we went to lunch in the school hall, and the children used to ask us hundreds of questions. I wish that we could have been as lucky when we were at school!

When I joined the Western Theatre Ballet it was considered one of the most modern companies in Britain. Not because the basic steps were different—we still use the steps that I have known since I was a child. But because the stories which some of our ballets tell are stories of everyday life. Our repertoire is very varied. It includes *La Ventana*, one of the very first classical ballets to be performed; *Mods and Rockers '63*, danced to the music of The Beatles, with such tunes as "She Loves You". We have learned a new ballet choreographed by our Artistic Director, Peter Darrell, with the story written by Colin Graham and music specially commissioned for the occasion from Theo Musgrave. We performed this ballet at our last London Season at Sadler's Wells, when we danced under our new name, the Scottish Theatre Ballet, because the company is now the official National Ballet of Scotland. But the most important feature for me is the fact that the company never stands still. It is hard working and always experimenting with new ways to improve still more, as I have to be if I want to go on improving as a dancer.

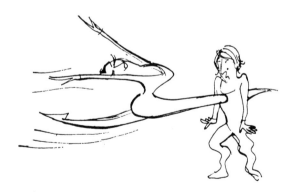

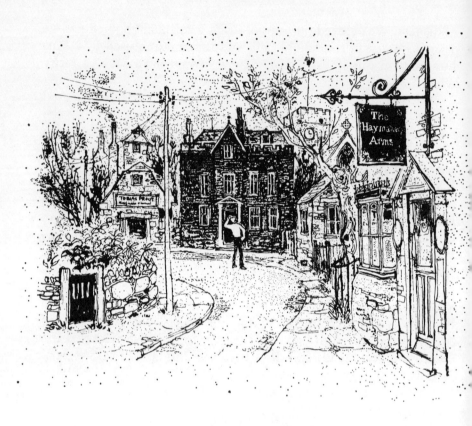

THE ROSE
OF PUDDLE FRATRUM

Joan Aiken

Right, then: imagine this little village, not far back from the sea,
in the chalk country, Puddle Fratrum is its name. One dusty,
narrow street, winding along from the Haymakers' Arms to Mrs.
Sherborne's Bed and Breakfast (with French marigolds and
bachelors' buttons in the front garden); half-way between these

two, at an acute bend, an old, old grey stone house, right on the pavement, but with a garden behind hidden from the prying eyes of strangers by a ten-foot wall. And the house itself—now here's a queer thing—the house itself covered all over *thick*, doors, windows, and all, by a great climbing rose, fingering its way up to the gutters and over the stone-slabbed roof, sending out tendrils this way and that, round corners, over sills, through crevices, till the place looks not so much like a house, more like a mound of vegetation, a great green thorny thicket.

In front of it a B.B.C. man, standing and scratching his head.

Presently the B.B.C. man, whose name was Rodney Cushing, walked along to the next building, which was a forge.

Tobias Prout, Blacksmith and Farrier, said the sign, and there he was, white-haired, leather-aproned, with a pony's bent knee gripped under his elbow, trying on a red-hot shoe for size.

Rodney waited until the fizzling and sizzling and smell of burnt coconut had died down, and then he asked,

"Can you tell me if that was the ballerina's house?"—pointing at the rose-covered clump.

B.B.C. men are used to anything, but Rodney was a bit startled when the blacksmith, never even answering, hurled the red-hot pony shoe at the stone wall of his forge (where it buckled into a figure-eight and sizzled some more), turned his back and stomped to an inner room where he began angrily working his bellows and blowing up his forge fire.

Rodney, seeing no good was to be had from the blacksmith, walked along to the Haymakers' Arms.

"Can you tell me," he said to Mr. Donn the landlord over a pint of old and mild, "can you tell me anything about that house with the rose growing over it?"

"Arr," said the landlord.

"Did it belong to a ballet dancer?"

"Maybe so."

"Famous thirty years back?"

"Arr."

"By name Rose Collard?"

"Arr," said the landlord. "The Rose of Puddle Fratrum, they did use to call her. And known as far afield as Axminster and Poole."

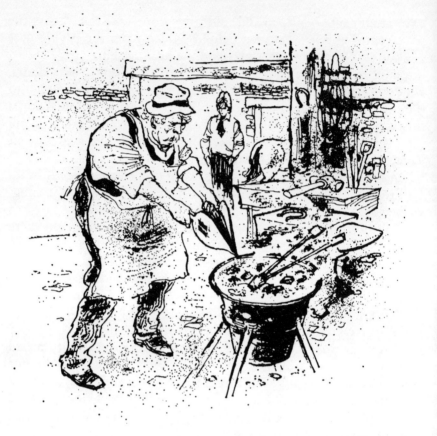

"She was known all over the world."

"That may be. I can only speak for these parts."

"I'm trying to make a film about her life, for the B.B.C. I dare say plenty of people in the village remember her?"

"Arr. Maybe."

"I was asking the blacksmith, but he didn't answer."

"Deaf. Deaf as an adder."

"He didn't seem deaf," Rodney said doubtfully.

"None so deaf as them what won't hear. All he hears is nightingales."

"Oh. How very curious. Which reminds me, can you put me up for the night?"

"Not I," said the landlord gladly. "Old Mrs. Sherborne's fule enough for that, though; she'll have ye."

Mrs. Sherborne, wrinkled and tart as a dried apricot, was slightly more prepared to be communicative about the Rose of Puddle Fratrum.

"My second cousin by marriage, poor thing," she said, clapping down a plate with a meagre slice of Spam, two lettuce leaves and half a tomato. "Slipped on a banana-peel, she did; ('twas said one o' the scene-shifters dropped it on the stage); mortification set in, they had to take her leg off, and she never danced again."

"Did she die? Did she retire? What happened to her?"

In his excitement and interest, Rodney swallowed Spam, lettuce, tomato and all at one gulp. Mrs. Sherborne pressed her lips together and carried away his plate.

"Came back home, went into a decline, never smiled again," she said, returning with two prunes and a dollop of junket so thickly powdered over with nutmeg that it looked like sandstone. "Let the rose grow all over the front of her house, wouldn't answer the door, wouldn't see anybody. Some say she died. Some say she went abroad. Some say she's still there and the nightingales fetch her food. (Wonderful lot of nightingales we do have hereabouts, all the year round). But one thing they're all agreed on."

"What's that?" The prunes and junket had gone the way of the Spam in one mouthful; shaking her head, Mrs. Sherborne replaced them with two dry biscuits and a square centimetre of processed cheese wrapped in a seamless piece of foil that defied opening.

"When she hurt her leg she was a-dancing in a ballet that was writ for her special. About a rose and a nightingale, it was. They say that for one scene they had to have the stage knee-deep in rose-petals—fresh every night, too! Dear, dear! Think of the cost?"

Mrs. Sherborne looked sadly at the mangled remains of the cheese (Rodney had managed to haggle his way through the foil somehow) and carried it away.

"Well, and so?" Rodney asked, when she came back into the dark, damp little parlour with a small cup of warm water into which a minute quantity of Dark Tan shoe-polish had almost certainly been dissolved. "What about this ballet?"

" 'Twas under all the rose-petals the banana-peel had been dropped. That was how she came to slip on it. So when Rose Collard retired she laid a curse on the ballet—she came of a witch family, there's always been a-plenty witches in these parts, as well as nightingales," Mrs. Sherborne said, nodding dourly, and Rodney thought she might easily qualify for membership of the Puddle Fratrum and District Witches' Institute herself—"laid a curse on the ballet. 'Let no management ever put it on again,' says she, a-sitting in her bathchair, 'or, sure as I sit here—' "

"Sure as I sit here, what?" asked Rodney eagerly.

"I disremember exactly. The dancer as took Rose's part would break her leg, or the stage'd collapse, or there'd be some other desprat mischance. Anyway, from that day to this, no one's ever dared to do that ballet, not nowhere in the world."

Rodney nodded gloomily. He already knew this. It had been extremely difficult even to get hold of a copy of the score and choreographic script. *The Nightingale and the Rose* had been based on a version of a story by Oscar Wilde. Music had been specially written by Augustus Irish, choreography by Danny Pashkinski, costumes and scenery designed by Rory el Moro. The original costumes were still laid away in mothballs in the Royal Museum of Ballet. Rodney was having nylon copies made for his film.

"Well, you won't be wanting nothing *more*, I don't suppose," Mrs. Sherborne said, as if Rodney were likely to ask for steak tartare and praline ice. "Here's the bath plug, I dare say you wish to retire as the TV's out of order. Put the plug back in the kitchen after you've had your bath."

This was presumably to discourage Rodney from the sin of taking two baths in quick succession, but he had no wish to do so. The water was no more than lukewarm. When he ran it into the tiny bath, a sideways trickle from the base of the tap flowed on to the floor, alarming an enormous spider so much that all the time Rodney was in the bath he could hear it scurrying agitatedly about the linoleum. A notice beside a huge canister of scouring powder said PLEASE LEAVE THIS BATH CLEAN, after which some guest with spirit still unbroken had added WHY USE IT OTHERWISE?

Shivering, Rodney dropped the bath plug in the kitchen sink and went to his room. But the bed had only one thin, damp blanket; he got dressed again, and leaned out of the window. Some nightingales were beginning to tune up in the distance. The summer night was cool and misty, with a great vague moon sailing over the dim silvered roofs of Puddle Fratrum. Due to the extreme curve in the village street, the corner of Mrs. Sherborne's back garden touched another, enclosed by a high wall, which Rod was almost sure must be that of the legendary Rose Collard.

He began to ponder. He scratched his head.

Then, going to his suitcase, he extracted a smallish piece of machinery, unfolded it and set it up. It stood on one leg, with a tripod foot.

Rodney pulled out a kind of drawer on one side of this gadget, revealing a bank of lettered keys. On these he typed the message, "Hullo, Fred."

The machine clicked, rumbled, let out one or two long experimental rasping chirrs, not at all unlike the nightingales warming up, and then replied in a loud creaking voice,

"Friday evening June twelve nineteen seventy eight-thirty p.m. Good evening, Rodney."

The door shot open. Mrs. Sherborne came boiling in.

"What's this?" she cried indignantly. "I let the room to *one*, no more. Entertaining visitors in bedrooms is strictly against the—" She stopped, her mouth open. "What's *that*?"

"My travelling computer," Rodney replied.

Mrs. Sherborne gave the computer a long, doubtful, suspicious glare. But at last she retired, saying, "Well, all right. But if there's any noise or bangs, mind, or if neighbours complain, you'll have to leave, immediate!"

"I have problems, Fred," Rodney typed rapidly as soon as the door closed. "Data up to the present about Rose Collard are as follows:" and he added a summary of all that he had learned, adding, "People in the village are unhelpful. What do you advise?"

Fred brooded, digesting the information that had been fed in.

"You should climb over the garden wall," he said at length.

"I was afraid you'd suggest that," Rodney typed resignedly. Then he closed Fred's drawer and folded his leg, took a length of rope from a small canvas holdall, and went downstairs. Mrs. Sherborne poked her head out of the kitchen when she heard Rodney open the front door.

"I lock up at ten sharp," she snapped.

"I hope you have fun," Rodney said amiably, and went out.

He walked a short way, found a narrow alley to his left and turned down it, finding, as he had hoped, that it circled round behind the walled garden of the rose-covered house. The wall, too, was covered by a climbing rose, very prickly, and although there was a door at the back it was locked, and plainly had not been opened for many years.

Rodney tossed up one end of his rope, which had a grappling hook attached, and flicked it about until it gripped fast among the gnarled knuckles of the roses.

Inside the wall half a dozen nightingales were singing at the tops of their voices.

The place sounds like a clock factory, Rodney thought, pulling himself up and getting badly scratched. Squatting on top of the wall, he noticed that all the nightingales had fallen silent. He presumed they were staring at him but he could not see them; the garden was full of rose-bushes run riot into twenty-foot clumps; no doubt the nightingales were sitting in these. But between the rose thickets were stretches of silvery grass; first freeing and winding up his rope, Rodney jumped down and began to wander quietly about. The nightingales started tuning up once more.

Rodney had not gone very far when something tapped him on the shoulder.

He almost fell over, so quickly did he spin round.

He had heard nothing, but there was a person behind him, sitting in a wheelchair. Uncommon sight she was, to be sure, the whole of her bundled up in a shawl, with a great bush of moon-silvered white hair (he could see the drops of mist on it) and a long thin black stick (which was what she had tapped him with), ash-white face, thinner than the prow of a viking ship, and a pair of eyes as dark as holes, steadily regarding him.

"And what do *you* want?" she said coldly.

"I—I'm sorry, miss—ma'am," Rodney stammered. "I did knock, but nobody answered the door. Are you—could you be—Miss Rose Collard?"

"If I am," said she, "I don't see *that's* a cause for any ex-Boy Scout with a rope and an extra share of impertinence to come climbing into my garden."

"I'm from the B.B.C. I—we did write—care of Covent Garden. The letter was returned."

"Well? I never answer letters. Now you *are* here, what do you want?"

"We are making a film about your life. Childhood in Puddle

Fratrum. Career. And scenes from the ballet that was written for you."

"So?"

"Well, Miss Collard, it's this curse you laid on it. I—" he hesitated, jabbed his foot into a dew-sodden silvery tussock of grass, and at last said persuasively, "I don't suppose you could see your way to taking the curse *off* again?"

"Why?" she asked with interest. "Is it working?"

"*Working!* We've had one electricians' strike, two by the musicians' union, three studio fires, four cameras exploding, and five dancers with sprained ankles. It's getting to be almost impossible to find anyone to take the part now."

"*My* part? Who have you got at present?"

"A young dancer called Tessa Porutska. She's pretty inexperienced but—well, no one else would volunteer."

Rose Collard smiled.

"So—well—couldn't you take the curse off? Please? It's such a long time since it all happened."

"Why should I take it off? What do I care about your studio fires? Or your sprained ankles?"

"If I brought Tess to see you? She's so keen to dance the part."

"So was I keen, once," Rose Collard said, and she quoted dreamily, " 'One red rose is all I want, cried the Nightingale.' "

"It's such a beautiful ballet," pleaded Rodney. "I mean—it *would* be, if only the stage didn't keep collapsing, and the props going astray, and the clarinettist getting hiccups—"

"Really? Did all these things happen? I never thought it would work so well," Rose Collard said wistfully, as if she rather hoped he would ask her to a rehearsal.

"What exactly were the terms of the curse?"

"Oh, just that some doom or misfortune should prevent the ballet ever being performed right through until Puddle church clock ran backwards, and the man who dropped the banana-peel said he was sorry, and somebody put on the ballet with a company of one-legged dancers."

Rodney, who had looked moderately hopeful at the beginning of this sentence, let out a yelp of despair.

"We could probably fix the church clock. And surely we could get the chap to say he was sorry—where is he, by the way?"

"How should I know?"

"But *one-legged* dancers! Have a heart, Miss Collard!"

"I've only got one leg!" she snapped. "And I get along. Anyway, it's not so simple to take off a curse."

"But wouldn't you *like* to?" he urged her. "Wouldn't you enjoy seeing the ballet? Doesn't it get a bit boring, sitting in this garden year after year, listening to all these jabbering nightingales?"

There was an indignant silence for a moment, then a chorus of loud, rude jug-jugs.

"Well—" she said, looking half convinced, "I'll think about it. Won't promise anything. At least—I tell you what. I'll make a bargain. You fix about the church clock and the apology, I'll see what I can do about remitting the last bit of the curse."

"Miss Collard," said Rodney, "you're a prime gun!" and he was so pleased that he gave her a hug. The wheelchair shot backwards, Miss Collard looked very much surprised, and the nightingales all exclaimed,

"Phyooo—jug-jug-jug-jug-jug!"

Rodney climbed back over the wall with the aid of his rope. Mrs. Sherborne had locked him out, so he spent the night more comfortably than he would have in her guest room, curled up on a bed of hassocks in the church. The clock woke him by striking every quarter, so he rose at six-forty-five and spent an hour and a half tinkering with the works, which hung down like a sporran inside the bell tower and could be reached by means of his rope.

"No breakfasts served after eight-fifteen!" snapped Mrs. Sherborne, when Rodney appeared in her chilly parlour. Outside the windows mist lay thick as old-man's-beard.

"It's only quarter-to," he pointed out mildly. "Hark!"

"That's funny," she said, listening to the clock chime. "Has that thing gone bewitched, or have I?"

Rodney sat down quietly and ate his dollop of cold porridge, bantam's egg, shred of marmalade and thimble full of tea. Then he went off to the call-box to telephone his fiancée Miss Tessa Prout (Porutska for professional purposes) who was staying at the White Lion Hotel in Bridport along with some other dancers and a camera team.

"Things aren't going too badly, love," he told her. "I think it might be worth your while to come over to Puddle. Tell the others."

So presently in Puddle High Street, where the natives were all scratching their heads and wondering what ailed the church clock, two large trucks pulled up and let loose a company of cameramen, prop hands, ballet chorus, and four dancers who were respectively to take the parts of the Student, the Girl, the Nightingale and the Rose. Miss Tessa Porutska (*née* Prout), who was dancing the Rose, left her friends doing *battements* against the church wall and strolled along to Mrs. Sherborne's, where she found Rodney having a conversation with Fred.

"But Fred," he was typing, "I have passed on to you every fact in my possession. Surely from what you have had you ought to be able to locate this banana-peel dropper?"

"Very sorry," creaked Fred, "the programming is inadequate," and he retired into an affronted silence.

"What's this about banana-peel?" asked Tess, who was a very pretty girl, thin as a ribbon, with her brown hair tied in a knot.

Rodney explained that they needed to find a stage-hand who had dropped a banana-peel on the stage at Covent Garden thirty years before.

"We'll have to advertise," he said gloomily, "and it may take months. It's not going to be as simple as I'd hoped."

"Simple as pie," corrected Tess. "That'll be my Great-Uncle Toby. It was on account of him going on all the time about ballet when I was little that I took to a dancer's career."

"Where does your Uncle Toby live?"

"Just up the street."

Grabbing Rodney's hand, she whisked him along the street to the forge where the surly Mr. Prout, ignoring the ballet chorus who were rehearsing a Dorset schottische in the road just outside his forge and holding up the traffic to an uncommon degree, was fettling a set of shoes the size of barrel-hoops for a brewer's dray-horse.

"Uncle Toby!" she said, and planted a kiss among his white whiskers.

"Well, Tess! What brings you back to Puddle, so grand and upstage as you are these days?"

"Uncle Toby, weren't you sorry about the banana-peel you dropped that was the cause of poor Rose Collard breaking her leg?"

"Sorry?" he growled. "Sorry? Dang it, o' *course* I was sorry. Sorrier about that than anything else I did in my whole life! Followed her up to London parts, I did, seeing she was sot to be a dancer; got a job shifting scenery so's to be near her; ate nowt but a banana for me dinner every day, so's not to miss watching her rehearse; and then the drabbited peel had to goo and fall out through a strent in me britches pocket when we was unloading all they unket rose-leaves on the stage, and the poor mawther had to go and tread on it and bust her leg. Worst day's job I ever did, that were. Never had the heart to get wed, on account o' that gal, I didn't."

"Well, but, Uncle Toby, did you ever tell her how sorry you were?"

"How could I, when she shut herself up a-grieving and a-laying curses right, left, and rat's ramble?"

"You could have written her a letter?"

"Can't write. Never got no schooling," said Mr. Prout, and slammed down with his hammer on the horseshoe, scattering sparks all over.

"Here, leave that shoe, Uncle Toby, *do*, for goodness' sake, and come next door."

Very unwilling and suspicious, Mr. Prout allowed himself to be dragged, hammer and all, to the back of Rose Collard's garden wall. Here he flatly refused to climb over on Rodney's rope.

"Dang me if I go over that willocky way," he objected. "I'll goo through the door, fittingly, or not at all."

"But the door's stuck fast; hasn't been opened for thirty years."

"Hammer'll soon take care o' that," said Uncle Toby, and burst it open with one powerful thump.

Inside the garden the nightingales were all asleep; sea-mist and silence lay among the thickets. But Uncle Toby soon broke the silence.

"Rose!" he bawled. "Rosie! I be come to say I'm sorry."

No answer.

"Rose! Are you in here, gal?"

Rodney and Tess looked at one another doubtfully. She held

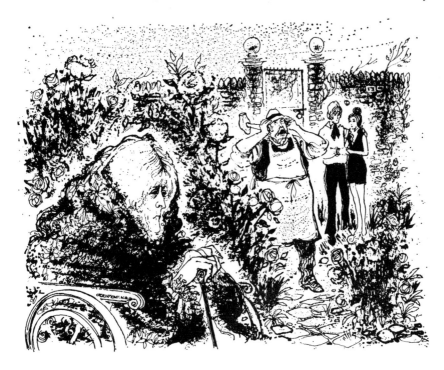

up a hand. Not far off, among the thickets, they heard a faint sound; it could have been somebody crying.

"Rosie!" shouted Uncle Toby. "Said I was sorry, didn't I? Can't do no more'n that, can I?"

Silence.

"*Rosie?* Confound it, gal, where are you?" And Uncle Toby stumped purposefully off among the thickets.

"Suppose we go and wait at the pub?" suggested Tess. "Look, the sun's coming out."

An hour later Mr. Prout came pushing Miss Collard's wheel-chair along Puddle Fratrum's main street.

"We're a-going to get wed," he told Rodney and Tess, who were drinking cider in the little front garden of the Haymakers' Arms. (It was not yet opening hours, but since the church clock now registered five a.m. and nobody could be sure of the correct time there had been a general agreement to waive all such fiddling rules for the moment.) "A-going to get wed we are, Saturday's a fortnight. And now we're a-going to celebrate in cowslip wine and huckle-my-buff, and then my intended would like to watch a rehearsal."

"What's huckle-my-buff?"

Huckle-my-buff, it seemed, was beer, eggs and brandy, all beaten together; Tess helped Mr. Donn (who was another uncle) to prepare it.

The rehearsal was not so easily managed. When the chorus of village maidens and haymakers were half-way through their schottische, a runaway hay-truck, suffering from brake-fade, came careering down the steep hill from Puddle Porcorum and ran slap against the post office, spilling its load all up the village street. The dancers only escaped being buried in hay because of their uncommon agility, leaping out of the way by means of a variety of *jetés, caprioles* and *pas-de-chamois*, and it was plain that no filming would be possible that day, until the hay had somehow been swept, dusted or vacuumed away from the cobbles, front gardens, door-steps and window-sills.

"Perhaps we could do a bit of filming in your garden, Miss Collard?" Rodney suggested hopefully. "That would make a wonderful setting for the scene where the Nightingale sings all night with the thorn against her heart, while the Rose slowly becomes crimson."

"I don't wish to seem disobliging," said Miss Collard (who had watched the episode of the hay-truck with considerable interest and not a little pride; "*Well*," she had murmured to her fiancé, "just fancy my curse working as well as that, after all this time!"), "but I should be really upset if anything—well, anything troublesome was to happen in my garden."

"But surely in that case—couldn't you just be so kind as to remove the curse?"

"Oh," said Rose Collard. "I'm afraid there's a bit of difficulty there."

"What's that, Auntie Rose?" said Tess.

"As soon as you get engaged to be married you stop being a witch. Soon as you stop being a witch you lose the power to lift a curse."

They gawped at her.

"That's a bit awkward," said Rodney at length. He turned to

Tess. "I don't suppose *you* have any talents in the witchcraft line, have you, lovey, by any chance?"

"Well, I did just have the rudiments," she said sadly, "but of course I lost them the minute I got engaged to you. How about Mrs. Sherborne?"

"The curse has to be taken off by the one who put it on," said Rose.

"Oh." There was another long silence. "Well," said Rodney at last, "maybe Fred will have some suggestion as to what's the best way to put on a ballet with a company of one-legged dancers."

They drank down the last of their huckle-my-buff and went along to Mrs. Sherborne's.

"Hullo, Fred. Are you paying attention? We have a little problem for you."

*   *   *

And that is why, when *The Nightingale and the Rose* ballet was revived last year, it ran for a very successful season at Covent Garden, danced by a company of one-legged computers, with Fred taking the part of the Nightingale.

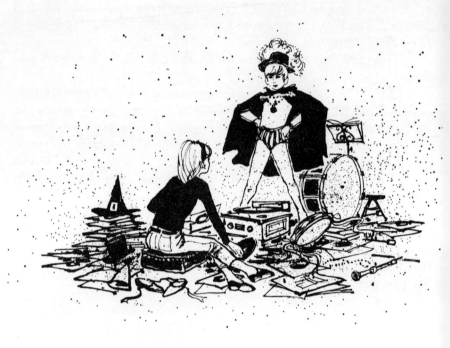

BALLET YOU CAN MAKE

Robina Beckles Willson

Sometimes, when you have to wait nearly a week until your next ballet lesson, when you have completed any suggested exercises for that day, when you have swallowed all the information you can digest, you may wonder: "What can I do, here at home?" Why not try to create your own ballets, with music? It will be as if you are hearing your own dancing.

This article is not a technical one: it is concerned more with the fun and games side of ballet, even though I realise that you will take your dancing seriously. And, while ballet is a demanding art, it is also an overflowing and rich one, which can spill into odd corners of our lives, so that you may eventually wonder what you *did* before you thought of making ballet for yourself.

First, then, I suggest, you can learn to listen. Margot Fonteyn has said: "I take all my guidance from the music." I am sure that is one of the reasons for the success of her brilliant career. It is a matter of teaching yourself to concentrate, to listen to sounds so hard that no detail escapes you. For instance, you may want to use a flutter on the flute for a frilly movement of your fingers. If you do not bother to hear it and place it, how can you match your movements to a few notes?

People complain to-day, with some reason, that there is too much music. It is even blaring in stations or whining in shops, a constant background, rightly given an ugly name, MUSAK, which reduces music to an annoying noise. But we can take a more positive attitude. We can put to use all the modern aids of recording and reproduction to improve our grasp of music; we can learn to know by ear just "what happens next" in familiar pieces of ballet music.

In your home it is very likely that you have either radio, or a television, and possibly a record-player. Perhaps you have all three. Then you are really lucky, because you can probably retreat by yourself and listen without distractions to a piece of music you like or want to know. You might start with ballet scores, like Tchaikovsky's *Swan Lake* or *Nutcracker*. But you won't need me to tell you that in this century all kinds of music have been used for ballet. And we want to be able to take in any music, and see if we can "hear" it for dancing.

At your next dancing class, when you are resting, watch the others closely. Are they really listening to the music? Or are they thumping away, only thinking of their aching feet, or lazy backs? Are they really *hearing* the beat? Are they then dancing to the music, or merely alongside it, as a convenient noise to drown any heavy thuds? It sounds obvious, but do they, and do you, really hear the rhythm, and convey it by exact timing? It is the dancer's response to the music which makes ballet an art, rather than a series of carefully plotted movements, with excellent muscular control, like graceful "physical jerks".

T.W.B.   I

Then there is the way you use the music. Beryl Grey reported that, when she rehearsed with the Bolshoi Ballet in Moscow, dancing to counts of the beat was unheard of: it was just not allowed. Always new choreography was taught by the music, piano or orchestra. And any repetition of a sequence, however short, also had the music as accompaniment. This is an ideal, of course, but I think it has the right emphasis.

Now that you are teaching yourself to listen hard to music, watching out for radio programmes, begging and borrowing records, what happens next? You find that you have favourites. Start with short pieces and repeat them often, listening hard all the time. Give yourself, and your long-suffering family, breaks! And you find that the music will play on in your mind. You will get a tune "on the brain".

That is the time to let our imaginations start to work, by imagining the actual dancing. Some people close their eyes when listening to music. We can take this a stage further, and when we listen to music we can begin to see movement and dance. Or maybe you will prefer to start moving as soon as the music gives your imagination ideas. This is the beginning of your own inter-pretation. Your "tools" are your body, your limbs, your face; your aids are the rhythm you hear, and your imagination.

I take it for granted that you have watched live, on television or film, all the ballet you can. But to create something of your own you will obviously not make your first attempt a story in three acts! You will be thinking of an episode, a ballet in miniature. Supposing you choose two contrasting pieces that you like. You may know Ravel's short "Pavane for a Dead Infanta", which has, in fact, been used for ballet. But you can approach it freshly, and invent your own dance to the haunting, dreamy music. Will you be a sorrowing mother, grieving and remembering, hugging your grief to your bowed body, and unable to rest? The Pavane, always a dignified and solemn dance, was first of all for Kings, Queens, Princes and Princesses. Perhaps this inspires you to become a royal mourner, and to dance with restraint, as if in a state procession, representing a nation's sorrow, and keeping your own feelings private? You will think then of your heavy robes weighing you down as a symbol of heavy mourning.

I hardly expect that you have your own dance studio, with

mirrors on every wall, to watch and correct your positions, so that your body, arms, legs and feet do what you *mean* them to do, and don't poke in gawky angles, unless you intend it so. You can use a bedroom mirror, perhaps, but your dance is likely to be a prinking fidget on the spot if you use that alone. So now is the time to enlist a good friend or relation, who will not laugh if you lose balance or trip over your own feet.

When you choose a partner, the ideal choice would be a friend who dances and, of course, this is easier at a ballet school. Then you can both prepare your own dances to the Ravel "Pavane", and perform to each other. This is important, because, once you have an audience, you meet the challenge which faces any creative person. Does your miniature ballet "say what you mean" about the music? Would your audience know you were sad? Or wonder if you were ill? Would they guess you were mourning in a state procession, or would they think you were captive in a nightmare, sleepwalking?

If your friend is both honest and sympathetic, she may help you; and if you can swallow friendly criticism, you will learn from her. Next you might try to combine the best of your ideas into one dance. Before you leave the "Pavane", it is worth experimenting with clothes. In classes, dancers wear their leotards and tights for freedom, and uncluttered views in the mirrors, but, occasionally, they will practise with robes and head-dresses, and you could allow yourselves this luxury and great pleasure.

Dressing-up is an enormous help. It is so much easier to feel a Queen if you have a long flowing cloak, even if it is only a bedspread. Different everyday clothes make us feel different: a uniform seems ordinary; a party dress gay; sweater and jeans relaxed, but ready to be active, certainly free and easy to wear. And it is the same with costume. The clothes and props help us to assume a character, particularly if it is one far from our own.

So, in spite of protests, let nothing that will come in for dressing-up be thrown away in your house. Attend local jumble sales, then assure your mother that you *will* wash what you bring home. Stow it away in your box, which is an essential possession, even if it is only a cardboard carton from the shop around the corner. Look out for old hats, from everyone who still wears them, or persuade them to give up wearing them, in your favour. Men's hats help particularly when you want to take a male part. Wigs are so expensive they are unlikely to be thrown away, but, if you feel painstaking, they can be made with wool, brushed out or not, with teased-out string, even with raffia. Long nighties or evening dresses are invaluable. Net curtains make magnificent veils and draperies. Keep them all. And speak kind words to dressmakers, who may spare you a luscious remnant for decoration, or even short cloaks to whisk round your shoulders.

You are ready now to form a group with some friends. Dressing-up is better shared, and you can jointly make a selection of clothes to keep with one of the mothers, who might even supply a junk cupboard as the collection grows. If you form a group from your dancing class you might persuade any boy dancers to join you. So often they are in the minority and might be glad of meetings with fellow enthusiasts. You need not limit yourselves to dancers either. Elder or younger sisters might help with the clothes, or arrange refreshments, because, after their exertions, dancers always seem to be ravenous.

Now supposing you have brought the group together. You may take it in turns to be host or hostess, or go where there is most space available. At your first meeting you could take another short piece, for piano, Debussy's "Golliwog's Cake-walk", from his "Children's Corner Suite".

I suggest this as the contrasting piece to the "Pavane", which, if you have the nerve, you might perform first. Then invite each of the group to improvise a dance to the "Cake-walk", which is marvellously gay and syncopated. Vote on which has the best steps and interpretation of the mood of the piece. Then the winner can teach the others, in a follow-my-leader way, just as you do in class. If you are the leader, you may spot here someone who is good at being a "clown". He or she may be loose-limbed and floppy while playing the fool, able to keep a completely "straight" face. If this is so, make a note that this talent can be used when you make a story. And look for strength in supporting, and bounce in jumping in any boys.

From these small beginnings you can enlarge your efforts. And when you think that you are all capable of really listening, and "obeying" music, you can banish it for a while and turn to acting.

You might begin by further practice in miming, beyond what you do in class. Take it in turn to mime a mood, and see if the others can guess correctly when you are being happy, angry, frightened, violent, guilty, thoughtful, jealous, cunning, greedy, hungry. Or you might each write a mood on a piece of paper, then draw lots, so that you have no choice; and you might have something difficult to convey, like "bullying".

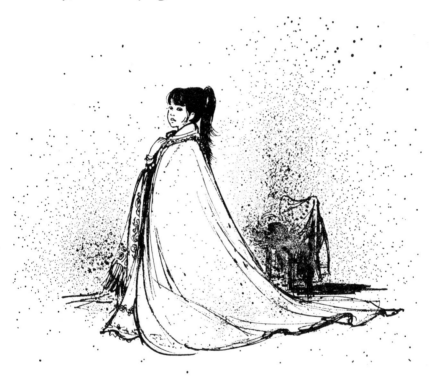

Then you could go on to act situations: a farewell; a reunion; a quarrel and its reconciliation. You could practise actions: digging, lifting, carrying various objects; again given a choice, say, a baby, or a bag of potatoes, a vase of flowers, or a bag for the launderette. And you could try keeping absolutely still, perhaps the hardest of all for someone young and energetic.

How can you improve your miming and acting, if it does not come easily to you to become a weary old woman, then a fretful child, then a taunting devil, using just your own face and your own body? I suggest that your best aid is observation. Use your eyes. You won't, I hope, meet devils sauntering down the High Street, but you may see ill temper on someone's face, see an angry movement, or a spiteful slap. Watch how people move when they are tired, when they are in a long queue. Do they drag their feet or hang their heads, or scowl? Do you? The more you notice, the more material you have for copying. The more exactly you can mirror life, the easier it will be for other people to recognise. And, of course, you will be rewarded by much amusement from observing so carefully. Even your walk to school, the bus or train, will be a great deal more entertaining.

By now your group will have gained a shrewd idea of the talents of its members. And this is an enduring hobby of dancers, watching other people and learning by their mistakes. We come to know who can be funny, who giggles at the wrong moment, who has the best ideas, and who is best at carrying them out; who can be flexible and fit in with other dancers' ideas or movements, without sulks or collisions.

Now you are ready to move on to stories. If you find it easy, you can invent one. If not, you can use or adapt one you like, perhaps an old fairy or traditional story, even a detective story with a clear plot. But, as you choose, look round the group and try to make your story fit their talents. You might have an ideal fierce villain, with piercing eyes and claw-like hands, an acrobatic jester, an exquisitely light dancer ideal for a fairy, or a ghost; or a pair of dancers who complement each other, and seem to be made to be twins, or shadows.

Next you return to music, and you will be glad of all the listening you have done, because you will want to be able to choose something to match your ideas. You can use an extract from a long piece; perhaps the war-like "Mars" from Holst's "Planets" Suite; or a piece from a Bach Brandenburg Concerto; some jazz by Johnny Dankworth; a Beatles' song; a piece from a Benjamin Britten Opera; a folk song, which might tell its own story. What matters is that *you* should see a connection between the music and your story. Then you can begin to knit them together with steps and movements, perhaps plotting first on paper with stars and arrows for direction, or using toy soldiers to be your puppets as you imagine a tiny ballet. Or work it out by dancing to yourself first, back in your bedroom.

In a small way, you are becoming a choreographer, and if this develops into your chief talent, you will be valuable. Good choreographers are always needed. Also I think you will appreciate how much more difficult it is to design ballets than it appears to be. Perhaps in a group you can't all manage this, but, when several of you have set small stories to music, you are ready to look for an audience.

As for a performance, choose the next birthday, or Christmas, and work towards a date, so that you have a reason for trying to complete a work worth being seen by a few friends, or the families, or your teacher. Explain what you have been doing. You might even collect for a charity if you have enough material to make a performance, but, as an introduction, you could easily entertain at a younger children's party, when the mother will be glad for them to sit down quietly for a few minutes after gigantic teas. As they will probably be more admiring than critical, that would be encouraging. You may not have much room, so you will have to clear as much as possible, unless you are lucky enough to use a lawn on a summer's day.

It is from these experiments, undertaken for pleasure, that we incidentally learn quite a lot. The group will keep going if you welcome new members and their new ideas, limit your meetings so that you don't get stale, and, above all, *experiment*.

Nobody will expect polished professional performances from you. They can get those elsewhere. But they will, if they know you, enjoy seeing what you can do with hard work and enthusiasm, just as you enjoy watching each other.

We are living in an age of experiment. Ballets are being danced to electronic music, to silence, to jazz, to medieval music. We see men dancing attached to kites which pattern the air as they dance; others float beneath sheets and gauzes, under flashing, rotating lights, against films. There are hundreds of other novelties and ideas, some brilliant and some almost ridiculous, which are bringing new life to ballet. I even read of a dancer dancing to jazz with a gas-filled balloon tied to one toe, if you want to try something really tricky!

From all these experiments will come new forms and exciting

opportunities for the dancers of the future. Eventually you may join those who are versatile, who also may have begun to experiment in their own gardens and bedrooms, and who now are eager to use their ears, their bodies, limbs, intelligence and imagination to "speak" the international language of dancing all over the world.

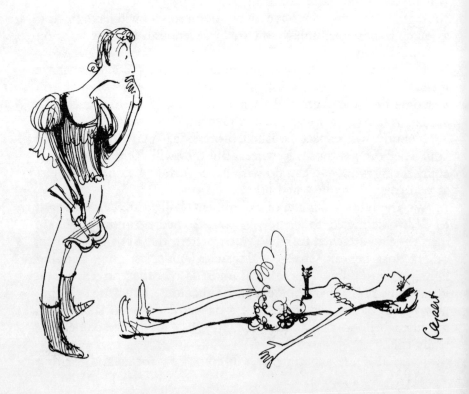

MAKE-UP FOR BALLET

Richard Blore of Leichner Creative Studios

There is a lot of fun to be had from dancing. It makes you feel good, look good, and be more attractive in every way. But there is also a lot of hard work and study involved if you are going to appear as enchanting as you feel to the audience. Apart from your technical ability in dancing, you have to be able to project your personality, have a flair for wearing costume and, very important, know how to apply a clean, professional make-up that is in character with the role you are dancing. Don't forget that in one show you may be dancing as a young romantic character, in the next you may have to appear as a witch.

Why is make-up necessary? First because you will be appearing under stage lighting which is far more powerful and intense than the light you have at home. The effect of this is to drain colour from your skin and also to make your face look flat. Not only has colour to be replaced with make-up, but flat features have to be remoulded with highlight and shadow. There is also another problem with light. In order to create interest and atmosphere in the ballet, as well as to establish the time of day, colour filters are used in front of the spotlights. If the scene is set at night, a steel-blue filter might be used to suggest moonlight. If the scene is set during the day, a pink or light amber filter might be used to give the impression of sunlight. All these filters have a different effect on the colour of make-up which has to be carefully selected to counteract any adverse effect. For instance, under primary red lighting cheek and lip colours will look very pale and darker red lipstick would have to be used, under blue lighting cheeks and lips would appear rather purplish, and lighter reds would be necessary.

Ballet is often performed in large halls and theatres and the make-up used, especially the eye make-up, is sometimes made a little bolder and more exaggerated so that the correct appearance can be seen as far back as possible, without appearing overdone to the people who sit in the front rows. And finally, you have to select and apply your make-up carefully to appear in character—remember, if you are dancing the role of a witch, you have to look like one.

Greasepaint is the popular form of make-up used in the theatre because it can spread easily and quickly across the skin, and the various colours used can be blended off into each other so smoothly. Leichner Greasepaints are made in a wide range of shades, but a beginner's box would include Numbers 5 and 9 because they have many uses. They can be blended together in various proportions to make a very wide range of flesh tints for both girls and boys, the No. 5 (Ivory) by itself is used for highlighting and the No. 9 (Brick Red) is often used for cheeks and lips. For shading No. 16 (Dark Brown) mixed with No. 25 (Crimson Lake Liner) is excellent. This shading may also be used on the eyelids of boys, who would use the No. 9 greasepaint on the lips, while girls may use No. 326 (Medium Blue) or Green 2 on the eyelids and the Carmine 1 Liner on the lips. The eyes should be lined along the base of the eyelashes with the No. 78 Spot-Lite Pencil in either Brown or Black. The beginner's outfit would also include Rose Blending Powder for setting the make-up and removing the shininess, and also Removing Cream.

How can you acquire skill in the application of make-up? Mainly by observation and practice. Study the features of other people and study your own face. Then try a simple straightforward make-up and go on trying until you are satisfied with the result.

You may wish to follow this routine, remembering that greasepaint should be applied to a clean skin which has no greasiness on it, and therefore all you need do to start is to wash with soap and water. Rub the greasepaint stick across the palm of one hand, rub the hands together vigorously, and then apply with a washing movement across the face until the skin, including that over the neck and ears, is covered with a light film, and finally pat with the finger-tips to a smooth even surface. Blot with tissue to remove any excess. Next apply colour to the cheeks and lips and use shadows and highlights to mould the contours of the face. As a rule, shadows are used to tone down over-prominent features, and highlights to bring features into prominence. When applying lip colour first dry the lips thoroughly with a tissue, paint to the shape required either directly with the liner or with a lip brush, blot by biting on a tissue to remove surplus, powder with Rose Blending Powder, and finally dab with cold water to set. The eyes are, of course, the most expressive feature, and make-up for them should be carefully selected and applied to enhance their colour and to make them appear bigger. Simply apply the eyeshadow to the upper lids, fading gradually away outwards about half an inch from the outer corners and then line along the base of the lashes with the Spot-Lite Pencil, which does not smudge. Add a touch of No. 9 to the eye-hollow (the area between the eyelids and the eyebrows) and apply Mascara to the eyelashes. Powder the make-up with Rose Blending Powder, pressing the powder firmly in to the make-up, brush away any surplus with a complexion brush or with cotton-wool, and then dab over the skin with cold water.

When you are satisfied that you can do this simple make-up satisfactorily, try experimenting with simple facial alterations. A simple one is making a rather round face look thinner (which, for instance, you might have to do if you were dancing in *Swan Lake*). Place a little No. 9 or Carmine 1 on the cheeks, fading gently up-wards and outwards over the cheekbone, and let this also fade into a highlight of No. 5 on the top part of the bone. Immediately underneath the cheekbone place a shadow, fading out towards the jawbone. Incidentally, if the No. 9 is placed on the roundness of the cheek, and taken almost horizontally towards the side of the face, the thin face will appear to be plumper. Narrow foreheads can be widened by merging No. 5 into the foundation shade at both sides, and similarly a very wide forehead can be adjusted by placing shadows at the sides. A prominent chin can be toned down by placing a shadow lightly over the foundation covering the pro-truding area, and if the chin is not very prominent, a highlight over the area will appear to make it stand out. Many exciting alterations can be made to the nose. A shadow on each side of the nose, starting from the top of the nose and running straight down to the tip and carried high up the sides of the nose, will make a broad nose look thin. If the nose is too long, a shadow placed below the tip will make it look shorter, whereas a highlight carried under the tip will make a short nose look longer. If the shadows at the sides of the nose are angled slightly the nose will appear to be bent.

When grotesque noses are required, as for an Ugly Sister or Witch in ballet, Nose Putty is used. This is supplied in stick form

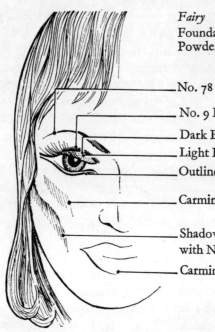

Fairy
Foundation: Peach Dark
Powder: Rose Blending Powder

No. 78 Brown Spot-Lite Pencil

No. 9 Lightly on eyehollow

Dark Blue Liner on crease

Light Blue on lid

Outline with Brown Spot-Lite Pencil

Carmine 1

Shadow under bone of No. 16 mixed
with No. 25 Crimson Lake Liner

Carmine 1

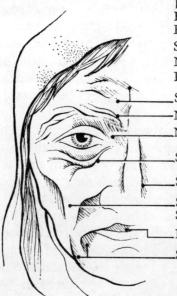

Witch
Foundation: No. 6
Highlights: No. 5
Shading: No. 16 mixed with
No. 25 Crimson Lake
Powder: Rose Blending Powder

Shadows with highlights above

No. 22 White Liner

No. 25 Crimson Lake   No. 5 on eyelids

Shadows with highlights between

Shade Sides of Nose

Shade under cheekbone
Shadow with highlight above

No. 25 Crimson Lake on lips

Shadows with highlights above

and the method of application is to break a piece from the stick and knead between the fingers until it is soft and pliable. It is then roughly shaped as required, pressed firmly on to the nose, and the edges smoothed out into the skin. Greasepaint is used over the Nose Putty to give it the correct colour.

A witch would have to look considerably older, and you can have really enjoyable make-up sessions if you practise ageing. It's always great fun to surprise your parents and your friends by looking as you probably will do in about eighty years' time. Ageing with make-up is normally achieved by trying to simulate the ageing folds of tissue with highlights and shadows. The chart for the witch illustrates the method.

Leichner have a series of helpful make-up charts covering straight, middle-aged and elderly characters as well as racial types, and also a book on make-up called *Stage Make-Up*. The Leichner Creative Studios, 44a Cranbourn Street, London, W.C.2, is open every week-day for the purpose of advising on all problems of make-up. Do not hesitate to ring for an appointment (Tel.: 01-734 7166) if you would care to call for advice and a demonstration of the application of make-up.

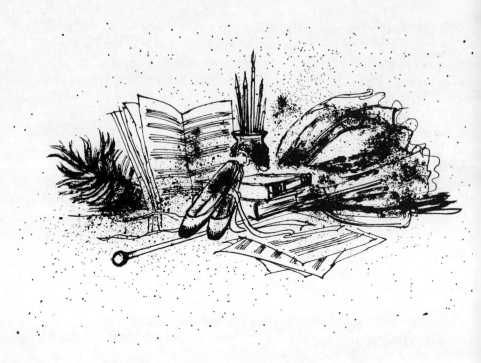

CHOREOGRAPHY

Elizabeth Malcolm

When you went to your first performance of a ballet, did you think that the dancers were just floating around the stage, allowing the music to tell them what to do? Or did you realise that the graceful shapes and patterns made by the soloists and *corps de ballet* were, in fact, very carefully rehearsed, practised and composed to suit the music, the story and style of the particular piece?

Ballet is one of the most complete ways of expressing ideas and stories yet devised for the theatre. The bodies and faces of the dancers "speak" just as actors say their lines in a play, or members of an orchestra play their part in a symphony or concerto. Yet in ballet there is more, for the music, scenery and costumes are also a vital part of the work.

What is choreography? The actual word comes from the Greek *choreos*, dance, and *grapho*, to record, "choreography" meaning the art of dance or ballet composition. Nowadays this is understood to mean the composition of a series of movements, either telling a story or expressing an idea. A composer of a piece of music or the author of a play is similar to a choreographer. The choreographer will choose his theme and music and will then arrange the steps, gestures and the mime as he wishes. He will also make sure that the complicated patterns that you see on the stage, performed by the *corps de ballet* and soloists, are exactly what he wants. Different seats in a theatre make quite a difference to what you see; from high up in the gallery you would see more of the patterns made on the stage, but from the front seats (the stalls) you would see more of the expressions and details of each dancer's performance.

There have been many different forms of choreography in the past, but not until the Italian Renaissance in the fifteenth century did the idea of composing purely for dancers become popular. The Italian nobles began to combine music and movement in the elaborate courts and palaces of the Renaissance. All the courtiers learnt dancing and performed complicated dances together at the court functions and parties, moving in and out of circles, and holding, then dropping their hands. They developed a style of "ballet" which had graceful movements of the head, arms and top of the body with small, delicate leg movements creating elaborate floor patterns and rhythms. They were limited by their clothes to movements that did not involve jumps and restricted the legs. (If you look at some of the famous Italian paintings of that time, you will be able to see for yourself the sort of movements that the Italians liked.) For these more complicated dances, a choreographer was employed by the court, and fairly soon a technique of ballet was evolved. Important visitors to the Italian courts were welcomed and entertained with festivals which often included dancing, poetry, songs and even choreography on horseback! Milan became the centre of ballet, and in 1564 the future King of France, Henri III, saw an Italian "ballet" and afterwards met the choreographer. He was so impressed that he employed Italian dancing masters and choreographers in the French capital. Louis XIV of France was the first monarch to dance himself. When he became too fat to perform, he followed the suggestion of his dancing master and engaged professional dancers. This is the first time that dancers were encouraged to become professional, and a ballet school, part of the Paris Opéra, was started and exists to this day. Girls started to train to become dancers, and in 1669, when the French court ceased dancing completely, ballet became a public and professional form of entertainment.

Dancing masters were also the choreographers and quite often had to play the violin as well whilst they were teaching! Ballet in Italy went through many stages, using masks and stylised movements, and then, under the influence of the Frenchman Noverre, returning to the use of mime and facial expression. It was also Noverre who arranged ballets in conjunction with composers such as Mozart and Glück. His experiences as a ballet teacher are preserved in a book, *Lettres sur la Danse*, in which he laid down the basic principles of ballet, principles which still apply to this day.

Noverre was very important as a teacher, and it was during his time that many individual "stars" were launched and acclaimed as ballerinas. Marie Sallé managed to become famous by using her own ideas. She scandalised the English by discarding the stiff courtly costumes and wearing flowing veils and loose hair! Another great ballerina, Marie Taglioni, created an everlasting fashion by dancing on her "pointes" (or the tips of her toes) for the first time in 1832.

During the mid-nineteenth century the first great "romantic" ballets were choreographed, ballets such as *Les Sylphides* and *Giselle*, and at the same time the male dancer's role became one of supporting the ballerina. These famous dancers of the Romantic period inspired many choreographers to compose ballets which, alas, have mostly been lost and forgotten. But if you have seen either *Les Sylphides* or *Giselle*, you will be able to recognise the features of this period. There are very few male dancers in the cast, and often the *corps de ballet* become mysterious spirits who float across the stage in beautiful and complicated patterns. Taglioni's father was the choreographer of *Les Sylphides*, but *Giselle* was created for another famous Italian ballerina of the Romantic period, Carlotta Grisí. Italians were still influencing the ballet world, and in Milan another teacher, Carlo Blasis, trained dancers to jump, requiring his students to practise daily. His book of exercises (called *The Code of Terpsi-chore*) is still the basis of classical training to-day.

Although France and Italy were the centres of ballet until the beginning of this century, other European countries also enjoyed watching ballet. In Denmark, Auguste Bournonville established the Danish style of dancing in the nineteenth century. This special-ises in quick, brilliant footwork, for which the Danes are famous to this day. Bournonville has left us several ballets, for example, *Napoli* and *Flower Festival at Genzano*, both of which are marvellous examples of this style. English audiences were also very appre-ciative of ballet, and although the English theatre was mainly devoted to plays, ballet dancers who visited London were received enthusiastically.

We are unable to study the choreography that was fashionable until we reach the Romantic period. Why is this? The answer is simple. The early choreographers would devise a ballet, or an entertainment, for a special purpose, either a public performance or a court function. Once the courtiers had performed this work it would be forgotten and another would be arranged. There was no means of writing down the choreography, although many people tried to invent a system which would do this. Our idea of these early choreographic works is based on paintings and drawings, and on the few diagrams and descriptions which were written. Some of the more popular court dances, such as the gavotte, pavane and minuet, were developed and performed so much and for so many years that they *have* been passed down to us. But the original choreography for the court ballet was lost once it had been performed. It was only when individual ballerinas became popular that the ballets were preserved. Dancers, such as Taglioni, would perform a role not just once or twice, but many times, travelling throughout Europe and performing in different countries. These dancers would also teach their roles to favourite pupils so that when they died the ballets lived on.

During the Romantic period, dancers and choreographers started going to Russia. Marius Petipa left France and went to the Imperial Theatre in St. Petersburg (now Leningrad), where he became premier danseur. There he met Jules Perrot, a French dancer and choreographer who was the theatre's ballet-master. Together they tried hard to develop Russian dancers to take over from the Italian and French stars, but it was some years before the Russian audiences would accept and acclaim dancers of Russian origin. The Russians were, however, natural dancers, and Petipa succeeded in establishing the tradition of ballet there. The famous Russian style of ballet was born, a style which was, and still is, admired throughout the world.

Petipa succeeded in creating many beautiful ballets. He worked very closely with both soloists and composers, drawing some of his themes from traditional fairy-tales. It was with the music of Igor Tchaikovsky that Petipa created his most famous ballets, *Swan Lake*, *The Sleeping Beauty* and *The Nutcracker*, all produced between the years 1890 and 1902. These can be seen all over the world to-day and have become ballet classics. All three tell a story but also include important dances for the *corps de ballet*, many brilliant solo parts and very taxing roles for the ballerina. The part of the principal male dancer is very largely one of supporting the ballerina, although he has several important solos in each ballet. The ballets also include some wonderful character parts, such as the witch in *The Sleeping Beauty*.

With the close of the nineteenth century came the end of the popularity of classical ballets. Everywhere the artistic scene was undergoing immense changes. The Impressionist painters heralded a breakthrough in style, and painters, authors and composers were abandoning what they considered the old-fashioned ideas of their predecessors and creating works of art which seemed quite different. So it was with ballet. Petipa's popularity declined, and in St. Petersburg two of his pupils, Gorsky and Fokine, were experimenting with a new style of ballet which made use of male dancers as dancers in their own right and not just a support for the ballerinas. These new, modern ballets were watched with curiosity at first, then with passionate interest and devotion. In 1909 Serge Diaghilev formed a company in Russia and came to Paris; this is the year in which modern ballet was born. By this time the Russian dancers had established themselves as supreme, and Diaghilev employed some of the greatest for his company.

Diaghilev himself was neither a dancer nor a choreographer and yet, by being an extraordinarily intelligent and artistic man, he was able to involve the most important artists of every field in his new company. Painters such as Picasso, Bakst and Benois, com-

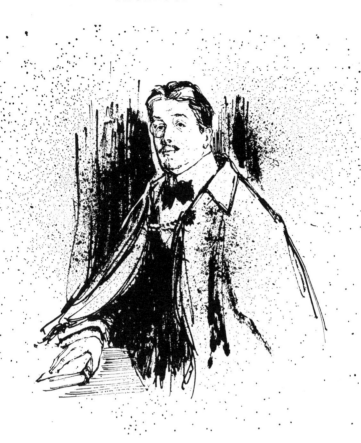

posers such as Stravinsky and Borodin, and dancers like Tamara Karsavina, Vaslav Nijinsky and Anna Pavlova, combined to form a magical company inspired by Diaghilev. From his group of dancers, choreographers of enormous importance emerged. The most famous of these are probably Mikhail Fokine, Vaslav Nijinsky (and later his sister, Bronislava Nijinska), Léonide Massine and George Balanchine. Their choreography is still an important part of the ballet repertoire to-day. Diaghilev toured the world with his company, astonishing and enthralling audiences everywhere. For the first time English dancers were to become famous, for Diaghilev engaged several for his company. At first they adopted Russian names (for instance, Alice Marks became Alicia Markova), but eventually, after English dancers became established, future dancers were able to keep their English names. After the Russian Revolution, the dancers and choreographers of Diaghilev's company settled in either Europe or the United States, thus spreading the ideas and style of Diaghilev and his company throughout the world.

Diaghilev's company broke away from traditional ideas and launched outstanding new forms of choreography. Fokine created *Les Sylphides* in a classical style, but followed it with *The Firebird*, with music by Stravinsky, and *Scheherazade*. Both these ballets are exotic and dramatic works, very different from the graceful choreography of *Les Sylphides*. In 1911 Fokine choreographed *Petrouchka*, again to music by Stravinsky. This great ballet combines the gaiety of a fairground with tenderness and poetry as three puppets come to life and dance and mime. It was for this same company that Nijinsky composed *L'Après-Midi d'un Faun*, another important work with himself as the mainspring of the ballet, dancing a series of beautiful movements based on the Greek vases. This ballet shocked the Parisian audience, mainly because Nijinsky wore a very scanty costume! Nevertheless, it is a very important step in the development of modern ballet.

For his first major work for Diaghilev, Léonide Massine drew his inspiration from quite a different source. After many visits to Spain he produced *The Three-Cornered Hat*, with music by a Spanish composer, de Falla. This is a rich and colourful ballet, very much influenced by the exciting flamenco dancing of Spain. Massine followed this with the successful *La Boutique Fantasque*, with beautiful choreography, humour and frenzied rhythms. After Massine left the company, Diaghilev asked Nijinsky's sister, Bronislava, to create some ballets, and she scored great triumphs with her Surrealist and Futurist ballets such as *Les Noces* and *Les Biches*. Throughout the 1920s the company continued to give birth to some exciting new styles in choreography. It was during this latter period that George Balanchine joined the company and began his meteoric career as a choreographer. In 1929, when Diaghilev died, the company was disbanded, and its dancers and choreographers joined or formed various companies throughout the world.

So ballet choreography developed from stylised court dancing, through the graceful Romantic period to the exciting years of Diaghilev, progressing further with choreographers such as Sir Frederick Ashton, Kenneth MacMillan and Norman Morrice. But

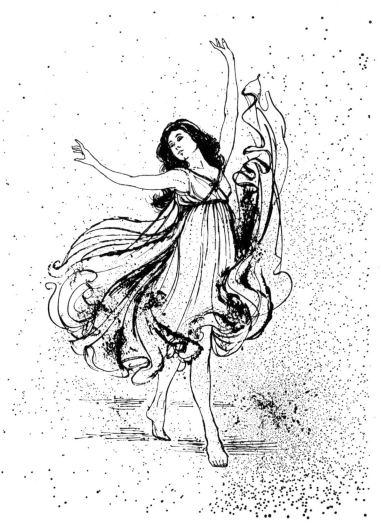

while companies in Europe at the beginning of this century were trying new styles of choreography, dancers in the United States were becoming dissatisfied with the technique of ballet. They complained that its rules made ballet stiff and unnatural, that it was now impossible to express real inspiration because the dancers were too concerned with accuracy in their technique. One woman, in particular, moved right away from the classical technique and used her body to just express her feelings. She ran, skipped and jumped, wearing flowing costumes and making wide movements with her arms. Her name was Isadora Duncan. Really, she was not a choreographer as she relied on her moods to express herself. She did, however, influence many dancers to try freer expression, and she had enormous personal successes on her tours in America and Europe.

Following Isadora Duncan, other choreographers started to explore movement without limiting themselves to the strict techniques of ballet. Martha Graham began to create works in which, at first, her movements were strong and sharp, and very dramatic. Gradually she started to combine these strong movements with flowing and soft ones. Her style is based on different positions and movements from classical ballet, but is, nevertheless, founded on a definite system, unlike Isadora's style which was based on her own emotions and feelings.

It was also in the United States that Jazz Ballet came into being, mainly through the talent of Jerome Robbins. He borrowed steps from jazz dancing and tap-dancing and composed exciting ballets to jazz rhythms. You have probably seen some of his most famous work, for it was Jerome Robbins who composed the dance sequences in *West Side Story*, which are so exciting and fast-moving.

Just like Petipa at the Maryinsky Theatre in St. Petersburg, choreographers nowadays are generally appointed to be a resident choreographer to a company. In this way they are able to rehearse the dancers, compose the ballets and discuss the scenery, costumes and probably the lighting with the people concerned with these specialised sides of a production. Sometimes the director of a ballet company is the resident choreographer as well, as in the case of Sir Frederick Ashton with the Royal Ballet.

Ballet relies entirely on movement, music, scenery and costumes so that there are no barriers of language. But it is unfortunate that there has been no universally established means of writing down new works. This sad state of affairs is changing now; to-day there are two different dance notations in existence for the recording of both ballet and general movement. One of these, the Benesh system of movement notation, has been adopted by many companies throughout the world, including the Royal Ballet. This system is able to record the finest details of movement. A library of ballet scores is being built up so that in future it will be possible to study, reproduce and compare with later works the choreography that is being created now. Ultimately, too, it is to be hoped that the dancers will learn their new roles in the same way as actors can study their parts and singers theirs.

A choreographer generally starts his career as a dancer; gradually he develops his choreographic talent whilst still dancing. Frederick Ashton and Kenneth MacMillan both became choreographers after they had danced with the Vic-Wells Company (later renamed the Sadler's Wells Company and later still the Royal Ballet). Dame Ninette de Valois founded the Sadler's Wells Company, and later the Ballet School, and choreographed many works for them, developing her style of choreography at the same time as the company were developing their style of performance and technique. We still enjoy works like *Checkmate* and *The Rake's Progress*, which she produced in the early days of the Vic-Wells Company.

And so, in this century, two completely different ways of seeking expression with movement were developed. Serge Diaghilev used the most brilliant choreographers, artists and composers to further classical ballet, and Isadora Duncan relied on emotions and free movement. Many modern choreographers produce both "abstract" ballets (without a story) and those which do tell a story. Frederick Ashton's *Symphonic Variations* (1946) is an example of an abstract ballet; beautiful, uncluttered and classical, it is a perfect example of pure ballet. His *La Fille Mal Gardée* is an excellent example of a story-ballet describing the love affair between a young country girl, Lise, and Colas, a country boy. This ballet is full of fun and laughter but also contains some beautiful *pas de deux* and solos for the two principals.

Since the Second World War many companies in Europe, the United States and Russia have produced new choreographic styles. Balanchine, in the United States, creates mainly abstract works with an almost purely musical approach. He has used classical and romantic scores by composers such as Brahms, Mendelssohn and Mozart, choreographing movement which is elegant and refined for classical music and full and flowing for romantic scores. He has also created works for contemporary music, and for these ballets he chooses spasmodic and disconnected phrases, sparse and concentrated to complement the twelve-tone score of modern music.

In the United States there is far more variety on the scene of modern dance than there is in ballet. Martha Graham has founded a school so that both her dance company and the school can continue her style of choreography. Two male dancers formerly with Graham's company have each developed their own style of choreography. One is Merce Cunningham, who believes that the main subject of dance is *dancing* and so he removes logical order from his choreography and leaves movements and placing to chance. By doing this, he has escaped clinging to a rigid technique and feels the results are more interesting than deliberate and contrived choreography.

Another former Graham dancer, Paul Taylor, has experimented with various styles. Once he stood absolutely still on the stage whilst a piece of electronic music was played through, and then danced wild and frantic movements. He continues to experiment with different styles and music, as does Alwin Nikolais. This choreographer, however, uses his props and dancers like pieces of sculpture, for example, once he covered the performers with pieces of material and plastic in order to create weird and wonderful shapes. This type of composition is mysteriously effective, depending a great deal on the stage lighting to change the shapes and shadows seen by the audience.

In Europe there are several important modern companies. The English Ballet Rambert, at first a classical ballet company, now has Norman Morrice as its director. This company is the home of modern ballet in England, and is brave and adventurous in its productions. Besides using choreography by Morrice, it commissions works by other modern choreographers. The Netherlands Dance Theatre, in Holland, has also established itself as a leader of modern styles of dance, and in Israel the Batsheva Company is breaking new ground.

Frederick Ashton, Kenneth MacMillan and John Cranko, to mention only three, are creating ballets for various European companies. Ashton has recently produced a short ballet in jazz style for the Royal Ballet, called *Jazz Calendar*. This was the first time the Royal Ballet had danced to a jazz score and it proved a great success. Ashton has also created a really exquisite short, abstract ballet, called *Monotones*. This is pure movement and is in two halves, using only three dancers for each half. Subtle lighting and simple sets and costumes help to make this ballet a real jewel in the company's repertoire. The dancers perform a *pas de trois* of quite outstanding poetry and grace.

MacMillan created a three-act ballet of *Romeo and Juliet*, also for the Royal Ballet. This tells the Shakespearian tragedy with great clarity, is full of beautiful choreography, exciting crowd scenes and contains a really memorable sword-fight. The last scene, where Romeo discovers Juliet in the tomb and thinks she is dead, gave MacMillan the opportunity to choreograph a very lovely *pas de deux*; Romeo takes Juliet's lifeless body in his arms and dances a very sad and touching series of movements. Another notable creation by MacMillan is *Song of the Earth*, which accompanies a song cycle by Gustav Mahler. The two singers sing each song as the dancers portray the ideas and moods behind the words.

For his present company in Stüttgart, Germany, where he is now working, John Cranko has been very active in choreography. He loves using complicated music (for instance, he composed a ballet to two of Bach's Brandenburg Concertos, called Brandenburg 2 and 4) and meticulously follows the different orchestral voices with his choreography.

The Russians have continued their great traditions in ballet. To-day their choreography does not aim to create beautiful but meaningless movements, and seeks to arouse the emotions of the audience. On the whole, the Russian choreographers tend to avoid abstract and symbolic ideas and instead create works which are clear, simple, dramatic and historically accurate. *Spartacus*, for example, is a faithful account of the hero of this name, and *Flames of Paris* relates, in a dramatic and accurate way, an episode in the history of the French Revolution. The stage in Moscow is so huge that an enormous cast can be used in which complicated and elaborate sets and scenery do not hamper the choreography. The style of Russian ballet suits this style of choreography perfectly, as the dancers are dramatic, acrobatic and athletic, and it has a wonderful tradition of male dancers. Great use is made of traditional dances in character ballet, and it is from Russia that many exciting new lifts and movements for *pas de deux* have emerged.

Each choreographer works in a different way. Some study the music for a long time, making very detailed notes and planning each phrase of movement exactly. This type of choreographer will decide what each dancer has to do on each phrase of music. When he has planned the ballet very thoroughly, he will then call the dancers together and demonstrate the movements. Perhaps he will then alter his original plan considerably as he sees how the movements suit the dancers and his ideas, or perhaps he will leave his original ideas, the dancers' ideas and his own together, until they achieve the effects they want. Again, many dancers themselves inspire choreographers to create ballets especially for them. Ashton has created several ballets for Margot Fonteyn. *Ondine* is, possibly, one of her most perfect roles, specially designed to make the most of her wonderful talents. It tells the story of a water-sprite who falls in love with a traveller on a ship. One of the most beautiful sections of the choreography is when the sprite sees her shadow and plays games with it, quite entranced to see how the shadow copies her every movement. Another great Ashton favourite is *Marguerite and Armand*, which he created for Margot Fonteyn and Rudolf Nureyev. This is a short ballet, depicting the tragic love-story between Armand and the dying Marguerite. It is a ballet of great tenderness and has some very moving choreography and mime.

It is difficult to give you an idea of how a choreographer creates a ballet as there are so many different ways of obtaining themes and ideas and the task of composing a new work is approached anew each time. Some ballets are composed to celebrate a special occasion, so that the basis of the ballet is chosen to suit the particular occasion. In 1964, the 400th anniversary of Shakespeare's birth, Ashton and MacMillan each composed a short ballet to celebrate the event. MacMillan chose some Shakespearian poems, each concerned with love, and built up a series of dance episodes to illustrate each poem. Ashton chose to make a ballet from the play *A Midsummer Night's Dream*, so that his ballet is a story-ballet, whilst MacMillan's is more abstract.

Sometimes a choreographer discovers a piece of music and feels he *must* create a ballet to this music. He will, of course, study and listen to the score many times, getting to know it very thoroughly. Then he will start deciding which parts of the music should be for solos, which for men and which for women, and so on. He will work, probably on his own, thinking of shapes that he would like to create, effects that he wants to produce, the type of movement (sharp and exciting, soft and flowing, simple or complicated) for each phrase. He will try out some of the steps, possibly using a mirror, which is one of the greatest aids to dancers and choreographers alike.

Perhaps a choreographer will "see" an idea for a ballet as he is walking along a street; a girl running to meet her boy-friend in a certain way may suggest a series of movements to him. Or a story he has read, or even an incident from a newspaper, may give him an idea for a ballet. Then he will think about the idea and search, sometimes for a long time, to find a piece of music to fit the idea. Early rehearsals almost always rely on a pianist to provide the music; the orchestra is only called in at the last few rehearsals. Of course, there are ballets created to electronic music too, so that then a tape-recorder or gramophone will be used.

Let's pretend that we are watching an early rehearsal of a ballet. The choreographer is called Henry, and he first tells his two soloists the ideas behind his ballet and what its moods are, how he wants them to interpret the music, what the other dancers are doing, and so on. Together they listen to the score while he explains and demonstrates.

HENRY: "Now, Ann and Paul, let's try this bit. Ann, I want you to be waiting for Paul over here. Your mother has told you that you cannot see him again, and you have to tell him. Try this . . . yes, an arabesque followed by a chassée and kneel, but leaning right forward like this . . . No, I want your hands to be full of resignation so they must be soft . . . Yes! that's better . . . and now you hear Paul coming in. Paul, you are happy and excited . . . can we have that phrase of music again, please? *That's* when you enter, Paul, on that high note. O.K? All right, I want you to come in and run towards Ann . . . That's it. And then what do you see? You see Ann, full of misery . . . so let's take that phrase again.
ANN: When I hear Paul's footsteps, do I jump up?
HENRY: No! No! You gradually rise . . . look, like this.
ANN: I see . . . with a sort of swirl round, on those chords.
HENRY: That's it.
PAUL: And you want me to be poised mid-flight when Ann turns?
HENRY: Yes . . . that's about it. Slowly I want you to realise that there is something wrong. You must look questioning, so that I want your hands to go out slowly like this. O.K. Once more with the music . . . good! That's just it! Now, Ann, having shown Paul how beastly

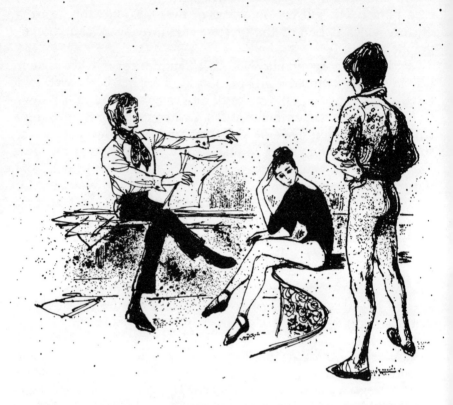

everything is, I want you to do a dejected little run and then jump into
his arms for comfort. Just listen to that piece . . . there! *That* note is
where you jump.

PAUL: So in fact I have to take a step or two to meet her?

HENRY: Yes. Look, this is how you must take her, Paul. Try it with me,
Ann . . . Good, do you see, Paul? I want you to take her in your arms
like this, and then on that next phrase of music to rock gently, twisting
round a little. Try again.

ANN: Here goes . . .

HENRY: No! No! Ann, try and make your run more like this . . . yes,
that's better. Like a wounded animal . . . yes, good! that's great . . .
and now, Paul, walk with her through the next phrase . . . can we hear
the next phrase, please? Right . . . and here, when you are right down-
stage, you, Ann, move into a sort of arabesque like this . . . yes, but I
think we will try it with your head down instead . . . as low as possible
. . . and bend your raised leg even more . . ."

And so it goes on. In fact, there is a good deal more demonstrating than talking usually, and always a great deal of waiting to be done before these early rehearsals. The choreographer tries to rehearse only the dancers that are required for each scene, but even so, most of the time the dancers will be sitting on the floor, watching the other dancers trying again and again, or they may be trying out their own steps, lifts and patterns at the back of the rehearsal room. Gradually the ballet begins to take shape, and the cast start projecting personality and character into their parts or, in the case of an abstract ballet, they start capturing the right moods and conquering the more difficult movements. They will start to see the patterns of the *corps de ballet* emerge, and so will the choreographer. He may decide to change something, or add something, or cut a piece of the music. *His* idea of a character may be influenced by the dancer who is portraying that particular character so that he may suggest a different type of movement. Thus the ballet will be taught, adapted, developed and practised and practised.

There are no laws to be followed in the creation of a ballet, just as there are none to follow in the writing of a book or the composing of music. Once the idea has been born and the music chosen, the choreographer can arrange his ballet and dancers as he pleases. There are no longer any restrictions about what he may or may not do, unlike the ballets created a century ago. Of course, the question of the cost of mounting a new production has to be considered, but a choreographer is not hampered by tradition or restrictive costumes any longer. Ballet to-day has become such an important and popular form of the theatre that each day new companies are being founded, or new works created and new dancers discovered. It is enough to say that ballet will continue to develop and will undergo further transformations, for ever being influenced by new ideas in other artistic fields, and yet never rejecting its rich heritage from the past.

CHOREOGRAPHER
IN HIS ELEMENT

from "Balanchine" by Bernard Taper

The rehearsal studio of a ballet company is something of a cross between a convent and a prizefight gym. Before the dancers go into action they paw a resin box in a corner, like fighters, and when they make their way about the room between classes or rehearsal sessions they are apt—even the most petite of ballerinas—to walk with a pugilist's flat-footed but springy gait, shoulders swaying with a bit of swagger, arms hanging loosely. There is the acrid sweat smell of the gym, and the same formidable presence of lithe, steel-muscled, incredibly trim and capable bodies ruthlessly forcing themselves to become even trimmer and more capable. But there is also an aura of asceticism, of spirituality—a spirituality achieved paradoxically, by means of single-minded concentration on the body. The mirror covering one whole wall from ceiling to floor would seem to speak of gross vanity, but the dancers, though they may have embarked on their careers from vain motives, have learned to rid themselves of conceit when they work. They use the mirror dispassionately, measuring their reflected selves with almost inhuman objectivity against the conception of an ideal to which they have dedicated their lives. The ideal, of course, is that of a particular kind of beauty, a centuries-old, thoroughly artificial way of moving which, when shaped into ballets by a choreographer, becomes art of a special sort—an elusive, evanescent art, as fleeting as fireworks or soap bubbles, that nevertheless has the power not only to entrance beholders but even, in some mysterious manner, to convey an experience of lasting significance.

To see George Balanchine in such an environment, rehearsing his New York City Ballet Company or, better yet, creating one of the new ballets he brings forth bountifully, season after season, is to have a rare pleasure—the pleasure of seeing someone who appears completely attuned to his world. In his person, Balanchine suggests the quintessence of the ballet studio's paradoxical combination of qualities. A noble-looking man, with a proud, elegant bearing—"a grand seigneur", Cecil Beaton has called him—Balanchine does not hesitate to throw himself on the studio floor in the course of demonstrating to his dancers some movement in one of his ballets, and he will often work himself into a dray-horse lather of perspiration during a rehearsal or choreographic session. In him, an intense, dedicated vision of a perfection of grace merges with an unquestioning willingness to submit to the arduous discipline, the specific physical efforts, required to attain—or, at any rate approach—this vision. "First comes the sweat," Balanchine says, speaking in a low, agreeable voice, tinged with the accents of his native Russia. "Then comes the beauty—if you're *vairy* lucky and have said your prayers." Someone once observed of ballet that it is "a science on top of which an art is precariously balanced". Balanchine would agree, although he would prefer to substitute the word "craft" for the more resounding "science".

In the half-century since his introduction to this craft, at the age of ten, in the Imperial School of Ballet in St. Petersburg, he has knocked about in many parts of the world, but wherever, in the course of his wanderings, he has been able to find a ballet studio, with a complement of dancers in need of something new to dance, there he has been at home and in his element. The ballet studio—whether it be in Russia, France, Denmark, Italy, Monaco, Argentina, England or the United States—is his true native heath. It is much more to him than just the setting in which he works; it provides the vital stimulus to his creativity—the rare and indefinable kind of creativity that has made him the most esteemed and prolific inventor of ballets in our time, whose works are to be found in the repertory of every major ballet company in the West. "I'm not one of those people who can create in the abstract, in some nice quiet room at home," he says. "If I didn't have a studio to go to, with dancers waiting for me to give them something to do, I would forget I was a choreographer. I need to have real, living bodies to look at. I see how this one can stretch and that one can jump and another one can turn, and then I begin to get a few ideas."

As a man, aside from ballet, the impression Balanchine makes is of someone who is pleasant, mercurial, authoritative and fundamentally enigmatic. In tastes and interests he falls into no category; he is highbrow, lowbrow and middlebrow all mixed up together in a blend of his own. He likes Braque, Pushkin, Eisenhower, Stravinsky, Jack Benny, Piero della Francesca, science fiction, TV Westerns, French sauces and American ice-creams. A communicant of the Greek Orthodox Church, he is deeply religious. He patronises only the best and costliest tailors, but the clothes he wears are a sort of Russianised version of a Wild West dude's garb—bright, pearl-buttoned shirts, black string tie, gambler's plaid vest, frontier pants. On him, these surprising outfits appear natural and elegant. After some three decades in America, he is still enthusiastic about the country. He says he loves the way it looks, sounds and smells; and on occasion, sometimes to the surprise of his auditors, he can be heard to remark what a pleasure it is to pay taxes to support a country it is such a pleasure to live in. Most of the time he would rather talk about politics, or almost anything else, than about ballet—ballet, he feels, being something you do, not discuss. He relishes luxury but does not give a hang for money. Gay, witty, and often playful, he is, however, fundamentally reserved about himself. Most people who have anything to do with him speak of him with great devotion and affection, but they also say that while he is a very easy person to be with, he is not an easy person to know.

Those who admire Balanchine's work are apt to rank him very high among the creative artists of the world. The word "genius" is used freely in referring to him. The poet W. H. Auden has been heard to remark that if he has ever known anyone who could be called a genius, it is Balanchine. The painter and stage designer Eugene Berman, in a memoir published in the *Saturday Review* in 1957, wrote that one of the privileges of his life had been the opportunity to work with Balanchine, whom he called "not only the greatest living choreographer, but in my view the greatest of all time, the Mozart of choreographers". The music critic B. H. Haggin wrote a few years ago that Balanchine was for him "an artist of the same magnitude as Picasso, and the only one I can think of now working in any of the arts", adding, "he is, it seems to me, even more disciplined in the exercise of his powers than

Picasso: the originality, no matter how astounding, always remains part of the continuous development".

It is one of Balanchine's most pleasing traits, to those who know him, that he can never be heard speaking in such terms of himself or his work. He can seldom ever be trapped into speaking of ballet as an art or himself as an artist. He prefers to view himself as an artisan, a professional maker of dances. When he talks of what he does, he often compares himself to a chef (he is, incidentally, a superb cook), whose job it is to prepare for an exacting clientele a variety of attractive dishes that will delight and surprise their palates, or to a carpenter, a good carpenter, with pride in his craft— a cabinetmaker, say. Balanchine does not keep scrapbooks, pro- grammes or reviews of his work; in fact, he almost never bothers to read what critics and admirers write about him or about the ballet. If someone happens to tell him about an article propounding a theory in regard to his ballets, he is perfectly willing to listen politely. Then he will make his standard comment: "Too fancy!" He does not particularly blame writers for going on at length about ballet, if that is how they want to occupy themselves or make a living, but he thinks that what any of them, including his most ardent admirers write, bears very little relation to what happens on stage while the music is playing. Though capable of expressing original and poetic insights himself in unguarded moments, he chooses—out of deep-seated principle, it would seem, or perhaps out of a canny intuition that so elusive an art cannot bear the burden of much theorising or solemnity—to talk about his work as seldom as possible and then only casually, playfully or in matter- of-fact technical terms. The numerous people who see grave sig- nificance and profound portents in his ballets get no encouragement from him. "When you have a garden full of pretty flowers, you don't demand of them, 'What do you mean? What is your signifi- cance?' You just enjoy them," he says. "So why not just enjoy ballet in the same way?" Of people who insist on seeing explicit meaning in ballet, he has said, in telling comparison, "People never seem to understand unless they can put their finger into things. Like touch- ing dough—when people see bread rising, they smell something and they say, 'Oh, is it going up?' And they poke their finger in it. 'Ah,' they say, 'now I see.' But of course the dough then goes down. They spoil everything by insisting on touching."

L

Despite his lack of solemnity, there is no mistaking his own or his company's dedication to ballet. "He doesn't do it by talking," a member of the company has said, "but he implies at every moment that there is a great art of classical dancing that all of us, including him, are serving." An unforgettable impression of this concentrated dedication was once made on a friend of Balanchine's—a pianist—when he went backstage at the New York City Centre during intermission one evening after a performance of Balanchine's early ballet *Apollo* to congratulate him and the dancers. It had been a triumphant performance, received by the audience with enthusiastic applause and repeated bravoes. The pianist had never gone backstage before, but on this occasion he had been so moved by the ballet that he felt impelled to offer his homage. When he got there the scene that met his eyes surprised him. He had naturally assumed that, on the heels of such success, he would find dancers and choreographer standing amid a throng of admirers and graciously acknowledging their praise. Instead, he discovered them hard at work. They were, it seemed, going over aspects of *Apollo* that Balanchine wished to improve. They were grouped near the lowered curtain and must have begun this impromptu post-mortem rehearsal the instant the last curtain call was over. The visitor stood in the wings watching as Balanchine worked first with Patricia Wilde, who had danced the role of the Muse Polyhymnia, and then Jacques d'Amboise, who had danced Apollo. He heard no harsh words spoken, no reproofs; when Balanchine finished making his point to Miss Wilde, the visitor saw her smile before she departed for her dressing-room and heard her thank Balanchine warmly for his help, as if she were a mere beginner, rather than a distinguished ballerina who had just received a public ovation. From her, Balanchine turned to d'Amboise, and the visitor could see them going over various sequences together—facing each other, like one man looking in a mirror, while both of them danced. Occasionally they would stop for a few words of comment. D'Amboise would nod vigorously. Balanchine would smile agreement at something d'Amboise said, and then they would spring into action again, face to face, about three feet apart. Time passed as they continued to work thus, and the backstage visitor watched them wonderingly. Dancers began to gather onstage for the next ballet, which was to be *Agon*. Bells could be heard ringing, announcing the imminent curtain. Stagehands hurried to their places. Totally preoccupied, Balanchine and d'Amboise ignored it all. When the pianist finally left, without having had a chance to congratulate anyone, they were still at it. They were gone from the stage, though, when the curtain went up on *Agon*. At the very last second, perhaps, the stage manager had taken each of them by an arm and led them off. The visitor, back in his seat, could not help wondering if they might not still be working away in the wings.

To visit the ballet company's studio while Balanchine is choreographing and to watch him get his "few ideas" and communicate them to a company of dancers is enjoyable and engrossing, and can be salubrious as well. Balanchine has a businessman friend who, whenever he feels oppressed by the tangle of his own affairs or the confusion of the day's news, likes to close up his office early and spend an hour or two watching Balanchine at work on a new ballet. He says it is the best therapy he knows. The peaceful, assured, workmanlike way Balanchine creates his dances has become legendary in the ballet world. Anecdotes concerning other famous figures of that world often revolve around some pyrotechnic display of temperament. The characteristic Balanchine story, on the other hand, has to do with some crisis or other in which Balanchine was to be found calmly and productively carrying on with his choreography, apparently unaffected by the chaos and hysteria around him. There are people who have worked closely with Balanchine for ten years or more and have yet to see him lose his temper or hear him raise his voice in anger.

When Balanchine is choreographing a new ballet, quite a number of spectators are usually present—seated on a bench that runs along the mirrored wall, leaning against the practice bars on the other walls, or standing around the piano, which is off to one side of the room. They observe Balanchine, they talk among themselves, they come and go. He pays no attention. His tolerance of visitors is exceptional among choreographers; most of them detest being watched and exclude from the room not only outsiders but any members of the company who are not required at the moment. Even so, by the nature of his art, a choreographer can never fully enjoy the pleasure of creating in solitude; eventually he cannot escape the dancers who are the medium in which he works. If he gets stuck and runs out of ideas, there they are before him, waiting—"with patient, drawn faces", as the choreographer Agnes de Mille has ruefully written—for him to find inspiration. As yet, none of the systems of notation which have been developed have gained such widespread acceptance as to permit the choreographer to do as a playwright or a composer does—that is, prepare his work at leisure on paper and hand the script or score to his performers for them to study before assembling for rehearsal. (So far, dance notation has been employed principally as a way of making a record of an occasional ballet after its creation.) Before coming to the first rehearsal, the choreographer may work out in his mind a number of steps and patterns for his ballet and jot them down on paper in some shorthand of his own, or he may write out in words a detailed libretto of the action, but, ultimately, to create a new ballet the choreographer must do what all the generations of ballet masters before him have done—get his dancers together in a large room and show them what he wants them to dance. The creation of a ballet has to be a public act. It is as if a composer had to assemble an orchestra (at a cost of hundreds of dollars an hour) and compose a symphony by standing in front of the musicians and making it up as he went along, first humming a snatch of music for the 'cellos to try, perhaps, and then turning to say, the woodwinds and humming a theme they might play at the same time. For all its sophistication, ballet is really a prehistoric kind of art. Lacking a widely accepted written language, it has been able to preserve its masterpieces only by devoted, laborious effort, passing them on from one generation to the next by direct communication, like folk legends. And, like legends, few ballets survive this process unchanged.

These conditions of the craft, which many choreographers find extremely trying, do not disturb Balanchine; he takes them for granted. In advance of the first rehearsal he makes no notes whatever. His way of creating a ballet is by extended improvisation under pressure. One of the fastest workers at this trade, he usually starts choreographing about three weeks before the date set for the première, though he has been known, in an emergency, to choreograph a ballet in less than a week. By the time he begins, the forthcoming ballet will have been announced in the press, the season's performances will have been scheduled, and the costumes and sets will have been ordered. Balanchine's advance preparation consists chiefly in studying the music he is to use until he has soaked it up completely. Sometimes, as part of this process, he makes his own piano reduction of the orchestral score. The son of a composer and the product of several years of advanced conservatory training as a young man, Balanchine is unquestionably the most musical of all choreographers, and he analyses an orchestral score the way a conductor does. At some point during his study of the music he has chosen for the ballet, he decides what dance quality is best suited to it—what palette of movement it calls for—settles on the size of the ensemble of dancers he will use and determines who his principal soloists will be. That is likely to be the sum of his preparations. All the rest must be done at rehearsal, with the dancers assembled and waiting and the large clock on the wall ticking away the costly minutes of rehearsal time and moving inexorably towards the production hour. When Tchaikovsky was asked, on one occasion, what conditions he required in order to be inspired to compose, he replied, "My Muse comes to me when I tell her to come." Asked the same question about his choreographing, Balanchine gives a paraphrase of this and says, "My Muse must come to me on 'union' time."

On the day rehearsals are to commence, Balanchine arrives at the studio shortly before the scheduled hour and changes into his working clothes—usually black pants, cut like sailor's pants, a T-shirt, and soft-soled dancing shoes. Even in that garb, he does not lose his air of elegance. He has aplomb, in every sense of the word. ("Aplomb", as defined by the French ballet master Despreaux in 1806, is a specific kind of dynamic balance fundamental to every position and movement in classic ballet.) Promptly on the hour, he comes to the front of the rehearsal room and, standing with the mirrored wall at his back, claps his hands lightly. The dancers, who have been warming up or standing about in the spectacularly impossible attitudes ballet dancers naturally fall into in moments of repose, gather before him. He greets them with ceremonious courtesy. A minute or two of banter may follow, and then, rubbing his hands briskly, he will remark, like a journeyman carpenter about to knock together a tool-shed, "All right. We begin."

Some choreographers, when beginning a new ballet, like to discuss their intentions at some length with the dancers, but Balanchine, who considers cerebration a deadly menace, prefers to engage in as little talk as possible. "You have to be vairy careful when you use your mind," he was once heard soberly cautioning a ballerina, "or you will get into trouble." In his cosmogony, dancers are like angels: they are celestial messengers who may communicate emotions but do not themselves experience the joys or griefs of which they bring tidings. The first thing he may do as he starts to work is arrange the dancers, in various poses, here and there about the room, in the pictorial composition they will form when the curtain rises. As they hold their places, he stands before them in silence, his hands clasped, head slightly bowed; he is listening to the first phrase of the music within him and summoning up in his mind's eye the dance phrase he will match to it—a phrase that may consist of five or six different movements by different soloists or groups at the same time. Standing there, he suggests a chess master planning a move. From the room next door, where other members of the company are rehearsing some other work, comes the sound of a piano thumping away, but it does not seem to penetrate Balanchine's concentration. As the dance ideas occur to him, his hands unclasp and his fingers come to life, as if they were dancing in the air. "All right," Balanchine says, stepping over to one of his soloists—the principal ballerina, perhaps—"you do like this." And he dances out for her the steps he has conceived, counting aloud each beat of the phrase as he does so. She immediately reproduces his movements while echoing his count. "And you," Balanchine says, turning next, perhaps, to the leading male dancer, "you do like *this*." In the same way, he produces sequences for the other soloists and the ensembles of the *corps de ballet*. When he has communicated in this way all the movements of the dance phrase, he will have the pianist play the few bars of music for it while the dancers put it together for his scrutiny. He may have them run through it several times more, and he may tinker with it or even discard it and try a fresh approach, but often it will be just the way he wants it from the start. With a brief nod, he murmurs, "Tha-at's right." The dancers store their steps away in their remarkable muscle memories, and Balanchine, in the same manner as before, takes up the next phrase.

So the work proceeds through the session. Every once in a while Balanchine will make a quick foray to the piano to check something in the score—peering at the notes through a pair of glasses that he keeps in his pants' pocket—or to show the pianist how a troublesome passage should go. Occasionally, some dance movement or sequence he has devised will make the dancers gasp with laughter or astonishment. Now and then, a dancer may say that he doubts whether he can master some particularly intricate or difficult passage. If Balanchine assures him that he'll be able to work it out with practice, he questions no more but says O.K., he'll try it. The dancer knows that later on, if the passage remains awkward for him, Balanchine will devise a variation to take its place—one probably no less intricate but in some way or other more congenial to that dancer's body conformation and dance style. Though Balanchine puts a continual challenge even to the most brilliant of the New York City Ballet's dancers, the choreography he ultimately provides is what each can dance best and most naturally. This is one of the things that Balanchine is noted for in the ballet world and that his dancers appreciate about him.

At the end of an hour of rehearsal there is a five-minute break, which Balanchine spends either at the piano with the score or chatting with some of the dancers. As soon as the five minutes are up, he claps his hands and everybody is ready to continue. Once more, all goes forward with a kind of simple, serious, unselfconscious concentration on the task at hand, as Balanchine serenely spins his web of dance, producing his delights and surprises as promised and on schedule. By the conclusion of the session, which usually lasts two hours, a measurable amount of progress will have been made—perhaps three minutes of ballet. The visitor who has sat in the studio while this was taking place often finds that a curious thing has happened to him. Whether or not he was familiar with the music before he arrived, he discovers that the steps and arrangements of movement that Balanchine has worked out already seem to him absolutely inevitable—as if the music itself had asserted a demand to be linked with just this pattern of dance and no other. Martha Graham, who is as eminent in the idiom of modern dance as Balanchine is in classical ballet, has said that she felt something of this sort when she visited Balanchine's studio one evening in 1959 and for the first time in her long career watched another choreographer at work.

As it happened, she and Balanchine were, in their separate studios, then engaged in a project that was to make dance history

in its way. Miss Graham was doing the choreography for the opening part of the ballet *Episode*, to the extremely difficult and atonal
music of Anton Webern, while Balanchine was handling the rest;
for once, those traditional foes, a classical ballet choreographer
and a modern dance choreographer, were working together in
amicable conjunction. The evening Miss Graham dropped in on
Balanchine, his studio, as usual, held an assortment of spectators,
among them the highly-regarded composer Leon Kirchner; Hershy
Kay, an arranger of orchestral works for ballet; and an old Russian-
émigré friend of Balanchine's who had dropped in to see what
Balanchine was up to. During the session, a brief mix-up occurred
when Balanchine inadvertently skipped a couple of bars in putting
two of his dance passages together. Upon discovering his lapse,
Balanchine coolly took it in his stride; there was no indication that
it bothered him to be discovered in such an error by an audience
containing a rival choreographer and a couple of musicians. First
he tried to see how it would go if he stretched out the preceding
dance phrase to incorporate the missing bars. "No, that doesn't
work," Balanchine said. "I'll have to make something new to put
in there." And he did, forthwith. Miss Graham—whose own
manner of choreographing is far more emotional and who, according to her friend Agnes de Mille, sometimes dismisses all the dancers
from the room when things are not going well and communes with
God and her soul—shook her head in wonder at this manifestation
of Balanchine's aplomb.

Throughout the rest of the session, she leaned forward intently,
following every move. At the end, after Balanchine had had the
dancers do a run-through of what he had choreographed so far,
she turned to the spectator beside her and said, "It's like watching
light pass through a prism. The music passes through him, and in
the same natural yet marvellous way that a prism refracts light, he
refracts music into dance."

During the weeks just before the season opens, when Balanchine
is not only choreographing new ballets but supervising the final
polishing of old ones, he works in the rehearsal studio every day
from noon to ten o'clock in the evening, with a little time off for
dinner. Because of the complexity of the company's daily rehearsal
schedule—its active repertoire during a given season consists of
some thirty or forty ballets, which have to be worked on in various

measure—Balanchine cannot count on having the full cast of any new ballet he is choreographing for more than a couple of hours at a time, so he is not able to work consecutively on a ballet from beginning to end. He has to make his ballets the way most directors make movies, working now on this section, now on that. As a further complication, he is often choreographing more than one new ballet at a time, so in alternate sessions during the day he may move back and forth between quite disparate works in progress— going, as he did in the memorable creative session of one recent season, from a complex, astringently witty, uncompromisingly *avant-garde* ballet like *Agon* to a sprightly, untroubled novelty like *Square Dance*, and from the romantic lyricism of the *Gounod Symphony* to the flashy brassiness of *Stars and Stripes*. The necessity of having to work in so disjointed a fashion provokes no complaint from him; he seems, if anything, to find the enforced variety refreshing to the spirit.

While Balanchine is working out his choreography and transmitting it to the dancers, he concerns himself little with nuances of performance. The last few days before the première, he usually concentrates on that aspect—on getting his ensemble to approach his idea of perfection. The style he has developed since coming to the United States is characterised by unusual precision and energy, and as he works on his dancers' performance techniques, he is constantly heard exhorting them to more vigour, to more clarity in their attack on every movement. "Audience must be made aware that leg is *your* leg and is going right *there*! Bam!" he will admonish them, slamming down his own leg to emphasise his words. The studio resounds, when he is engaged in this refining process, with "Bams!" and "Pows!" and similar exclamatory explosions, uttered in a voice that is charged with energy, though it does not go up many decibels in volume. If one were to hear these sounds and not see what was going on in the studio, one would hardly think that such a seemingly ethereal creation as a ballet was being prepared. Balanchine's intense vision of beauty as the end result of all this is always present, however, and no one is permitted to forget it. "Isn't it selfish of you," he chided one girl, "to expect three thousand people to sit and watch you lift your leg if you're not going to do it beautifully?" From then on, though she was far back in the ranks of the *corps de ballet*, she danced as if she were going to be alone onstage the night of the performance.

To make a point, Balanchine is capable of producing an apt illustration or a vivid, often surprising metaphor. "Don't forget," he said to a ballerina who he thought was getting too dreamy in her style, "that Carpentier was the most lyrical boxer who ever lived, but Dempsey knocked him flat in no time." She nodded her pretty head, apparently discerning a vital truth for herself in this odd bit of information, and immediately attacked her dancing with as much vigour as if she herself were training for a match with Dempsey. To bring home to another dancer, one of the company's leading ballerinas, the reason her performance of a particular passage was not altogether satisfying, even though she was dancing it absolutely correctly and in tempo, he told her a little story about Louis XIV, who one day, it is said, emerged from his palace with the intention of taking a ride somewhere and found that his carriage, instead of having long been drawn up awaiting his royal pleasure, was just arriving. It reached the palace door at the instant he came out. The King did not have to wait a second for it, or even slow down his stride, but he was nevertheless highly offended. As he swept into the carriage, he complained to the coachman, with majestic indignation, "You *almost* made us wait." The ballerina laughed at the story, and Balanchine said, "So you see, to be correct, to be perfectly on time is not enough. You must be *luxuriously* perfect if you want to satisfy."

On the whole, however, Balanchine's pedagogy, like his choreography, is essentially non-verbal. "You think, then," a dancer will ask him, "that it should go like this?" and she will perform the passage in question. "Yes," Balanchine will reply, "but maybe a bit more like this," and he will dance it himself the way it should be. In recent years he has been suffering somewhat from an arthritic condition, which manifests itself in a slight stiffness in his walk but, surprisingly, does not show up in his dancing or hinder him from dancing all day long at rehearsals. If this ailment ever got bad enough to prevent him from leaping about, or lifting a ballerina in the air when he wanted to show her partner how it is to be done, he would have to retire, he says, because he cannot imagine being a choreographer sitting down. When he performs a dance phrase for his company, he does not do the steps in full scale or finished form, but the effect is always astonishingly telling. He evokes an essence as easily as a master painter might with a hasty pencil sketch. Maria Tallchief says that when he was teaching her the role of the Swan Queen in his revised version of the second act of *Swan Lake*, she used to watch him do her part, and think, "I'll *never* look that beautiful." Similarly—though apropos of a very different kind of role—Jerome Robbins, who used to dance with the company as well as choreograph for it, and is at present its associate Artistic Director, recalls, "As a dancer, I got some of the best notices of my life for the role of Tyl in Balanchine's ballet *Tyl Eulenspiegel*, but I never came anywhere near the gusto and earthiness that he achieved when he was demonstrating it for me in rehearsal."

Eventually, in the course of preparing a new ballet, Balanchine will dance every step of all the parts—those of all the soloists and all the groupings of the *corps de ballet*. In a sense, when one witnesses a performance of the New York City Ballet, one is seeing a whole ensemble of Balanchine, in various sizes and shapes—and some critics consider this a fault or a limitation in the company. The matter is not so simple as this would suggest, however, for what a ballerina may pick up from watching Balanchine dance her part for her is a heightened awareness of her own special style and qualities, which his keen eye has perceived, and which he has rendered in clarified form for her. Still, there is no denying that all his dancers are acutely responsive in copying and appropriating the qualities he sketches out in dance for them. An instance of just how responsive they are occurred when he was choreographing *Bourrée Fantasque* a number of years ago. When he had the ensemble repeat for him a section that he had created the preceding week, he was perplexed to see that all the movements were being danced in a peculiarly cramped and agonised way. When he questioned the dancers they insisted that this was the way he had shown the steps to them. He could not figure it out until he recalled that the week before he had been suffering from bursitis; the company had apparently picked up all his aches and pains and magnified them into a bursitic *Bourrée Fantasque*.

Having done his best in the preparation of a work, Balanchine does not fret as the time for its première nears. "Somehow it will all work out all right," he says reassuringly when one of the usual emergencies arises shortly before curtain time, and, one way or another, it nearly always does. "Somehow" is one of Balanchine's favourite words. A recollection that Jerome Robbins sometimes summons up to help compose himself when he is getting jittery as opening night approaches is that of Balanchine a few hours before the première, in 1954, of his version of *The Nutcracker*—the costliest work the New York City Ballet had ever put on till then. At five o'clock that afternoon, with the curtain due to go up at eight-thirty, it was learned that the costumes were still not ready. Balanchine and Robbins hastened over to the workshop of Karinska, the noted costume maker, to see what could be done about this crisis. When they got there, Balanchine, discerning at a glance that everybody in the shop was working feverishly to get the job finished, spoke not a word of exhortation or reproof. He simply sat down among the seamstresses, took up an unfinished costume, threaded a needle, and began deftly stitching a ruffle. Robbins found himself following Balanchine's example. "After a while, I looked over at him," Robbins recalls. "Here it was only about three hours before curtain and there sat Balanchine, sewing away as if he didn't have a care in the world. I said to him, 'How can you be so calm?' He just smiled and went on sewing."

When the curtain rises on one of his new works, Balanchine usually observes what he has created from the rear of the centre aisle. Unnoticed by the audience, he slips into the auditorium after the lights have dimmed, and takes up a position just inside the door, where he stands among the ushers. As the curtain descends at the end of the ballet, he slips away backstage to his dancers, who, between curtain calls, are waiting to hear what he thinks of the way they danced. After everybody else has taken repeated bows— the conductor, the soloists, the *corps de ballet*—the audience may get a brief glimpse of Balanchine in the spotlight. Usually he emerges onstage in the grip of a couple of his dancers, like a culprit apprehended at the scene of his crime. His appearance always brings forth the most thunderous ovation of the evening, to which he responds with a quizzical smile, a shrug and a nod of acknowledgment. Then he quickly ducks back behind the curtain. People surmise that his diffident stage manner is a studied performance— like that of the nineteenth-century composer who, after the première of one of his operas, always had to be dragged bodily on to the stage, struggling valiantly to get away, while muttering to his captors, "Pull harder!" Those who know Balanchine some-what better disagree with this; the way he takes a curtain-call, they say, accords with the engagingly modest, unpretentious manner in which he invariably comports himself when they meet him off-stage. The few who know him very well, however, while agreeing that he does not put on an act and that his everyday behaviour is delightfully unpretentious, say that modesty is not the explanation but just the reverse—a kind of monumental self-assurance. He is so sure of himself and his work that he does not need to boast or to bathe his ego in applause. "He seems as soft as silk, but he's as tough as steel," says Lincoln Kirstein, the general director of the New York City Ballet, who for some thirty years has been Balanchine's most devoted patron and partisan. "He's the most secure man I've met in my life. He has authority to the nth degree." It is Balanchine's feeling that in seeing his new ballet the audience has seen exactly what he wishes to show of himself and that it is irrelevant, and also not very interesting, to follow the ballet with a display of his own person onstage. He feels about this rather as Joseph Conrad felt when he was asked by the *Bookman* for a photo-graph of himself that it could publish; Conrad replied, "My face has nothing to do with my writing."

FAMOUS PEOPLE
IN THE HISTORY OF BALLET

Clement Crisp

MARIUS PETIPA

Marius Petipa was born in 1819 in Marseilles into one of the several families of dancers who used to travel through Europe, dancing and staging ballets in various opera houses. By the time he was twenty-eight Marius had worked in France, Spain, Belgium and America; his father was a teacher and choreographer, and his brother Lucien was the most famous male dancer of the day. He then found work in Russia as a dancer at the Imperial Theatre, St. Petersburg, where he was to spend the next sixty-three years, destined to become the absolute master of the Russian ballet and chief architect of its greatness.

He danced in St. Petersburg for several years and was then given the opportunity to create a ballet; he was required to stage a spectacular five-act ballet called *Pharaoh's Daughter* in the incredibly short time of six weeks. It was a great success, and within eight years his ability to produce long ballets that pleased his audiences had won him the position of chief choreographer to the Imperial Theatres, responsible for ballet in both St. Petersburg (the capital and seat of the Czar's court) and in Moscow. In St. Petersburg the ballet was directly answerable to the Czar, and the performances were very much designed to please the court audience. Petipa had to produce at least one big ballet every year, containing four or five acts, and from 1869 until 1903 he managed to do just that, sometimes more.

Successes seemed to alternate with failures, but Petipa was a very astute creative artist and he tried to work out his ballets with the greatest skill so that they would attract his audience. At the same time he was deeply concerned with improving the standards of dancing, and in this he was successful, creating a school and generations of dancers who raised dancing to the highest peak it had ever known. The technical standards of the dancers were improved even more in the 1880s by the arrival of a series of brilliant Italian dancers whose extraordinary technical skill was a great inspiration to the Russians. The Russian style of dancing was a mixture of French, Italian and Danish teaching, and it produced the most gifted and most exciting dancers of the time.

It was during his later years that Petipa made his finest ballets (though a work like *La Bayadère*, which dates from 1877, is still performed and recognised as a work of genius). Towards the end of his career Petipa composed ballets to music by Tchaikovsky and Glazunov, and it is during these years that he produced masterpieces like *The Sleeping Beauty* and *Raymonda*, and—with his assistant Lev Ivanov—*Swan Lake*. Ivanov was responsible for the other Tchaikovsky ballet *The Nutcracker*, because Petipa had fallen ill and was unable to compose it.

In every one of Petipa's ballets that survives to-day we can see how great a genius he was; they are superbly worked out as entertainments, combining processions and national dances, solos and ensembles, *pas de deux* and dazzling variations. The stories of the ballets are sometimes foolish, but Petipa's genius added such excitement, and he devised such a wonderful flow of dances, that the ballets are still thrilling and important to-day. They are the treasure house of classic dance, which is the foundation of everything that is being done in ballet to-day.

MIKHAIL FOKINE

On the day that Mikhail Fokine graduated from the Imperial School into the Maryinsky Ballet in 1898 he was celebrating his eighteenth birthday. The Maryinsky Theatre, which boasted the finest and only really vital ballet company in the world at that time, produced only the huge evening-long ballet spectacles of Marius Petipa. They were splendid show-pieces, full of dances and processions and solos and *pas de deux*, but Fokine—who was a fine dancer—believed that there was a need for reform to create a newer and fresher kind of ballet. He thought that ballet should be true to real life, and that both design and music should be made to have a much more vital impact on the dramatic form of the ballets.

He started to make short ballets that expressed something of his ideals: that music, dancing and painting should be equal partners, that music should be of the finest quality (which it often wasn't at the Maryinsky), that there should be clear drama and historical truth where necessary. All this was a far cry from the complicated and improbable stories and the traditional processions and national dances that the Maryinsky audiences wanted and loved.

Fokine's chance to try out his ideas really came when Diaghilev invited him to make ballets for the first Paris season of Russian ballet. In 1909, and the next few years, Fokine produced a series of great works that guaranteed the success of Diaghilev's enterprise and also altered the whole history of choreography. *Les Sylphides, Le Carnaval, Petrouchka, Scheherazade, Prince Igor, Firebird, Le Spectre de la Rose*, were superb ballets that we still enjoy to-day, and they summed up all Fokine's ideals about the need for change in ballet. Here was the new form of movement, the vital and important stage design, the good music, the truthful mime and the dramatic sense that he sought. These ballets are now performed by so many companies—often with little feeling for their worth and with dancers who are far below the standard of the original interpreters—that their importance and greatness is sometimes obscured. But presented with loving care and a proper appreciation of their superb choreography—as, for instance, when the Kirov Ballet dance *Les Sylphides*—and the qualities of Fokine's creative genius are clear for every one to see.

Fokine raised the art of ballet from the doldrums into which it had fallen. His five years' work with Diaghilev has influenced every ballet-maker since, not least in insisting again on the importance of the male dancer and in giving a new seriousness to dramatic works. After he left Diaghilev, Fokine worked in Europe and America, but his later ballets never achieved the greatness and importance of his creations for Diaghilev. He died in New York in 1942.

ANNA PAVLOVA

Although Pavlova died in 1931, her name is still the most famous in the ballet of our century. The frail child who was born into a poor family in St. Petersburg in 1881 was taken as a treat to see the Imperial Russian Ballet at the Maryinsky Theatre in St. Petersburg when she was eight years old. Like so many little girls, this first view of a magic world of fairies and enchantment fired the youthful imagination; she *must* become a dancer, and two years later, despite her fragile physical appearance, she was accepted for the Imperial School of Ballet. While still at school her talents excited the interest of her teachers, and when she graduated into the company at the Maryinsky Theatre she was soon dancing solo roles.

Her lightness and delicacy, and that indefinable "something" that marks out the greatest dancers, earned her speedy promotion, and in 1905 she was given the title of ballerina, an official rank in the theatre and only awarded to the finest artists.

Two years later she made her first appearance outside Russia when she undertook a brief tour; every year thereafter she obtained leave of absence for a few months to dance abroad, and in 1909 she took part in the sensational first season of Russian Ballet organised by Serge Diaghilev for Paris. The attractions of touring to bring ballet to vast new audiences who had never seen a great ballerina before prompted Pavlova to resign from the Maryinsky Theatre in 1913, and from then until her death she toured the world with her own company.

Unlike the Diaghilev Ballet, which also toured extensively from 1909–1929, Pavlova did nothing to alter the actual nature of ballet. Diaghilev was an inspired impresario, bringing together artists, musicians, painters and choreographers to create a new theatrical form of ballet, producing constant novelties, influencing and changing public taste. Pavlova was a genius of the dance who performed throughout the world—she must have travelled half a million miles—dancing wherever there was a stage. She was seen by millions. To many she was their first contact with an art that had been previously reserved for the great cities and theatres. To all of them she was a messenger of joy and beauty and an inspiration to countless men and women who learned to love the dance and even became dancers because they had seen Pavlova. In Lima, Peru, a young boy saw her dance and knew that he had to make ballet his career: he was Frederick Ashton. Thanks to Pavlova, British ballet gained one of its greatest men.

To the millions all over the world who formed her audience, Pavlova *was* ballet; the magic of her artistry in important roles like Giselle, or in the brief *Dying Swan* solo that is for ever associated with her, made her the most popular and most influential ballerina of our century.

TAMARA KARSAVINA

Tamara Karsavina is a contemporary of Anna Pavlova: both graduated from the Imperial Ballet School into the ballet at the Maryinsky Theatre, but their careers took very different paths. Karsavina, born in 1885 into a family of dancers, had a very distinguished career at the Maryinsky Theatre, but in 1909 Serge Diaghilev invited her to join the group of dancers he was forming to take to Paris for that first dazzling season of Russian Ballet.

This event was to change Karsavina's career; she became the leading ballerina of the Diaghilev Ballet during its early seasons, and the choreographer Mikhail Fokine created for her many of the most important roles in modern ballet. Fokine's ballets were revolutionary because they turned their back on all the stiff old traditions of the long, complicated ballets like *Sleeping Beauty* that were danced at the Maryinsky. Instead Fokine made short ballets in which dancing, music and stage decoration were equal partners in creating a free and vivid stage action. Karsavina, with her partner Nijinsky, became the ballerina for whom Fokine devised several great roles that are still danced to-day. She was the first to dance the waltz in *Les Sylphides*, the Doll in *Petrouchka*, Columbine in *Le Carnaval*, the Girl in *Le Spectre de la Rose*, the *Firebird*, Chloe in *Daphnis and Chloe*, the Queen of Shemakhan in *Le Coq d'Or*, and Massine cast her as the Miller's Wife in *The Three-Cornered Hat* in 1919.

Karsavina was famous as a wonderful lyrical dancer and as a superb actress, besides being a fine exponent of the classical repertory of the Maryinsky Theatre, where she continued to dance until the Russian Revolution of 1917. Then, like so many other dancers, she fled Russia. She married an Englishman, and it is our good fortune that she should come to London, where she still lives.

This great lady has been an inspiration to many dancers, and when the Royal Ballet staged two of the ballets in which she had first appeared—*Le Spectre de la Rose* and *The Firebird*—it was Karsavina who coached Margot Fonteyn in the roles that she had been the first to dance. There is even a fascinating link with her career as a ballerina of the Maryinsky Theatre; when Sir Frederick Ashton came to create his own version of *La Fille Mal Gardée* he asked Karsavina to reproduce the mime scene when Lise dreams of marriage, which was also part of the ballet in St. Petersburg. This touching scene is now performed just as Karsavina used to dance it nearly sixty years ago. Not content with being one of the great dancers of our time, Madame Karsavina has also written one of the most vivid and enjoyable books about ballet: her memoirs of a marvellous career, *Theatre Street*.

VASLAV NIJINSKY

Nijinsky is a most tragic figure in the story of ballet; the loss to the future of ballet when this superb dancer and adventurous choreographer became insane at the height of his career is incalculable. He was born in Kiev in 1890 into a family of dancers; naturally he was entered for the Imperial Ballet School in St. Petersburg, and his extraordinary muscular ability soon excited comment. In her book of memoirs, *Theatre Street*, Tamara Karsavina tells how she was taken to see a class of boy pupils at work in the school; while they were practising jumps, "one boy in a leap rose far above the heads of the others and seemed to tarry in the air". When she commented on this extraordinary sight, the ballet master said: "It is Nijinsky. The little devil never comes down with the music."

People were soon to be aware that a unique male dancer had stepped on to the stage of the Maryinsky Theatre, but it was Diaghilev who really presented Nijinsky to the world. He was the principal male dancer of the first Diaghilev season in Paris in 1909, and soon Paris (and the whole Western world) was thrilling to the amazing gifts of this young man who, off-stage, seemed dull and unprepossessing, but who was transformed into a magical being of prodigious technical and dramatic power once he started to dance. Diaghilev realised that Nijinsky was an exotic being; all the roles that were created for him in the Diaghilev Ballet were strange, mysterious, out of the ordinary. Fokine devised a series of bizarre and beautiful roles for him: first the poet in *Les Sylphides*, then the Golden Slave in *Scheherazade*, then Harlequin, mischievous and heartless, in *Le Carnaval*. In 1911 Fokine made two of his greatest parts for Nijinsky: the Spirit of the Rose in *Le Spectre de la Rose*, in which eye-witnesses still speak of Nijinsky's sensational leap through the window at the end of the ballet when he seemed to hover in the air before disappearing into the night, and the tragic puppet Petrouchka. This ballet about performing dolls in a fair in old St. Petersburg was built around the tragedy of Pet-rushka, whose soul flickers weakly beneath the sawdust with which he is stuffed, and Nijinsky conveyed with uncanny skill the agony of the puppet in his love for the ballerina doll. Apart from being a dancer of genius, Nijinsky also showed evidence of being a choreographer with rare gifts. His first ballet, *L'Après-Midi d'un Faune*, showed a fascinating novelty in treating a Greek subject. In 1913 he created two ballets that excited great interest: *Jeux* was about tennis players and was the first modern ballet to show people wearing contemporary dress, and *The Rite of Spring* was an attempt to show the primitive rituals in old Russia that greeted the arrival of spring. It created a famous scandal; the first-night audience hooted and shouted and screamed and came to blows because both the choreography and the music by Stravinsky seemed too offensively modern to their staid and respectable ears.

Then Nijinsky broke with Diaghilev, who had been his guide and close associate for years. He started up a short-lived company of his own, led the Diaghilev Ballet on a disastrous trip to America, and on his return showed those first signs of the mental illness that soon ended his career. The last thirty years of his life (he died in 1950) were spent withdrawn from the world.

LÉONIDE MASSINE

Léonide Massine's great chance came in December 1913, and as with so many dancers and choreographers of that time, the chance came because of Diaghilev. He saw the young Léonide Massine at the Bolshoi Theatre in Moscow and was so impressed that he offered him the chance of creating the leading role of Joseph in a projected new ballet, *The Legend of Joseph*. Massine seized the opportunity, which was the start of his phenomenal career, for Diaghilev was a great educator of young talent, seeking to make them better and fuller artists by taking them to museums, playing them music, and introducing them to the major creative artists who surrounded him at all times.

The result of this education for Massine was that by the time he was nineteen he had made his first ballet, since Diaghilev was always on the look-out for new choreographers. This was in the middle of the First World War when the Diaghilev Ballet was at its lowest ebb; the impossibility of touring through war-torn Europe meant that the ballet had stopped functioning. But Massine took the opportunity to work hard; while in Spain he spent months learning Spanish dancing, and this enabled him to create one of his finest and most important ballets immediately the war was over and the Diaghilev Ballet could start functioning again. The ballet was *The Three-Cornered Hat*, a story of a miller and his wife, the best Spanish ballet that has ever been made, although it had a Russian choreographer working for a Russian ballet company! In the next few years Massine produced a series of ballets that are still performed and loved to-day: *The Good Humoured Ladies*, *The Fantastic Toyshop*, and many more.

When Diaghilev died, his ballet company could not survive its great creator, and his artists scattered all over the world. Massine, celebrated as both dancer and choreographer, became the most influential figure of ballet in the 1930s, and he created many important works for two Russian ballet companies that were formed to carry on the Diaghilev tradition, notably a series of six "symphonic" ballets that used symphonies by Berlioz, Tchaikovsky, Brahms, Beethoven, Schubert and Shostakovitch, as a basis for dancing. He also continued to make many short ballets—he special-ised in eccentric comedy works in which he often gave himself a fine character role—and after the war he revived several for the Royal Ballet at Covent Garden, and danced in London, for he was a tremendous stage performer. In recent years he has continued to make ballets, and also lectured and devoted himself to the study of writing down choreography—working for part of the time on the beautiful island that he owns in the Mediterranean.

GEORGE BALANCHINE

Balanchine is regarded by many ballet-goers as the most influential choreographer of our time; his tremendous output of ballets and the company he has created in America, the New York City Ballet, are evidence of his great importance. His career started in Russia; he was born in St. Petersburg in 1904, and he studied ballet there at the Imperial School. By the time he had graduated from the school the Russian Revolution had taken place and he joined the State ballet company at the Maryinsky Theatre. When he was nineteen he started making short ballets, though audiences found these too experimental for their taste, and in 1923 he left Russia with a group of five dancers on a short tour that eventually brought them to Paris.

There they were seen by Diaghilev, who invited them to join his ballet company which was now based in Monte Carlo. Balan-chine was soon staging ballets for the Diaghilev company, the most important and significant of these was *Apollo* in 1928. This ballet, to a Stravinsky score, was vitally important not only for Balanchine but also for the development of ballet in this century. For some years the works produced for the Diaghilev company had been very clever theatrical creations in which the actual dancing tended to be over-shadowed by brilliant designing and a desire to produce novelties for the audience. *Apollo* was a return to the essential element in ballet, the actual steps, and to the classical style of dancing that had been brought to its highest peak of perfection by Marius Petipa.

Apollo's theme was simple; Apollo, the patron god of the arts in Greek mythology, watches three of the nine muses—Calliope, muse of poetry, Polyhymnia, muse of drama and mime, and Terpsichore, muse of dancing—and teaches them their duties, choosing Terpsichore as the most perfect. At the end he guides all three to Mount Olympus, home of the gods. The true theme of the ballet was the importance and beauty of the classic dance, and this has been the theme of Balanchine's whole career. After Diaghilev's death in 1929, Balanchine worked for a few years in Europe, and then in 1934 he was invited to go to the U.S.A. to start a school of American ballet. From this school eventually developed the company that Balanchine now directs: the New York City Ballet, and through both the company and the school, Balanchine implanted the classic dance in America, where it has flourished.

The whole of Balanchine's artistic life has been devoted to the creation of ballets that insist on the importance of the classic dance. Very few of his works tell stories; the vast majority offer dancing—performed by artists in the simplest of costumes with little stage decoration—which needs no other aids to make it exciting and thrilling to watch. His first ballet in America, *Serenade*, was dedicated to showing how beautiful are the things that dancers do, it had no theme or dramatic incident to cloud the dancing, and to-day —some eighty ballets later—Balanchine's creations are still devoted to the same ideal. As long as the classic style of dancing continues, Balanchine's great classic ballets will always delight audiences.

BRITISH BALLET:
NINETTE DE VALOIS AND FREDERICK ASHTON

When we see how flourishing and splendid ballet is in Britain to-day it is hard to realise that British ballet is really less than forty years old. Of course, the British had ballet before that: there were periods in the past when dancing was immensely lively and popular in Britain, though it never flourished as it did in France and Italy and Russia. Ballet in Britain, as we know it to-day, owes everything to two women who worked with Diaghilev: Dame Marie Rambert and Dame Ninette de Valois, who each formed ballet companies. In the late 1920s Marie Rambert started a group that eventually became the famous ballet company that still bears her name. Ninette de Valois was determined to make a national ballet for Britain, and from her company—the Vic-Wells Ballet (later the Sadler's Wells Ballet)—grew our great Royal Ballet. Ballet companies need two essential things: a school and a choreographer, and Ninette de Valois started first with her school.

From the very first, in 1931, Ninette de Valois was determined that her company must be based in the classical traditions of the Russian Ballet: the ballets of Marius Petipa were to be a training ground for her dancers, and also, in a curious way, for her audiences who would learn to appreciate classical dancing from watching them. And so *The Sleeping Beauty*, *Swan Lake*, *Giselle*, *Coppelia* and *The Nutcracker* were the foundation stones upon which Ninette de Valois built her company. These ballets make tremendous demands upon the style and the classical technique of dancers, but if they can dance them well then everything else follows on naturally. They are also ballets that are so well constructed that it is possible to present them with the very limited numbers of dancers that Dame Ninette had at her disposal in the early days of the Vic-Wells Ballet. As her company grew larger, so the ballets could be expanded.

Dame Ninette is also a choreographer, and in her finest works, *Job*, *The Rake's Progress*, *Checkmate*, she showed a remarkable ability to create truly English ballets. But running a ballet company, directing its progress and planning its future meant that she needed

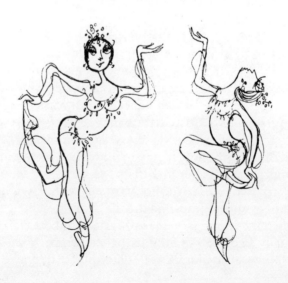

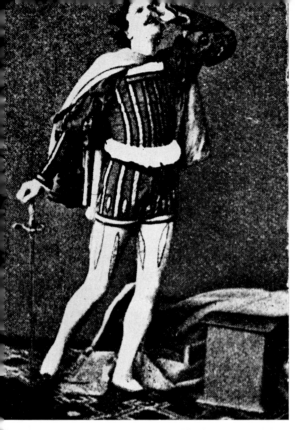

Marius Petipa in the role of Faust

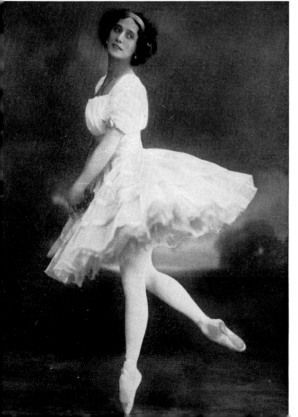

Anna Pavlova as the *Dying Swan*

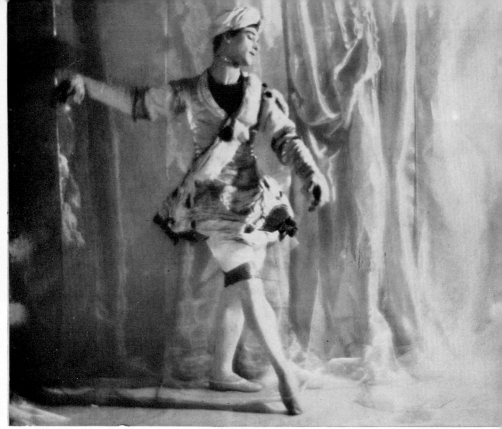

Vaslav Nijinsky

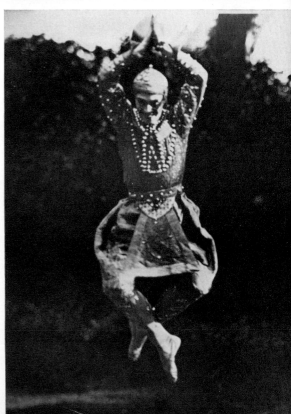

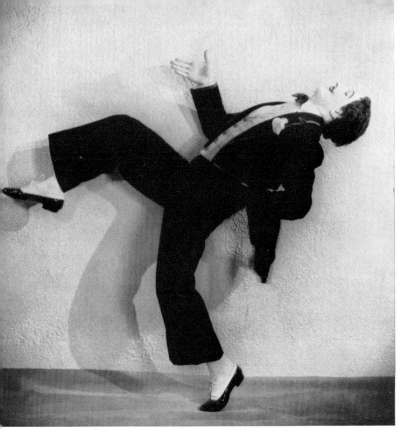

Leonard Massine in *La Boutique Fantasque*

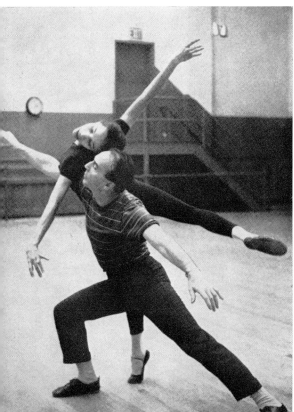

George Balanchine rehearsing Maria Tallchief for Gounod Symphony

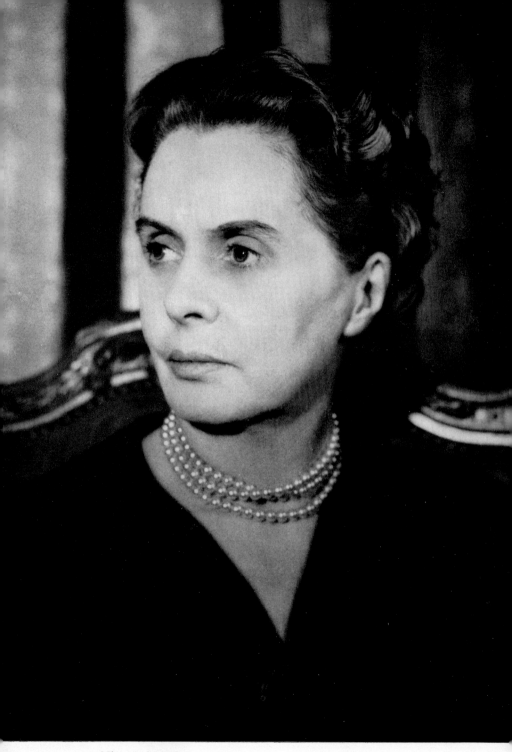

Ninette de Valois

another choreographer, and it was to Frederick Ashton that she turned.

Ashton had made his first ballet in 1926 with the Marie Rambert dancers, and he soon knew real success with works such as *Façade* and *Les Rendezvous*, both of which are still performed to-day. As the Vic-Wells Ballet developed, so did the opportunity for choreography, and Ashton started on that wonderful sequence of ballets that have helped to create the British school of ballet and the Royal Ballet's greatness. When the Royal Ballet moved to Covent Garden in 1946 and became even larger and stronger, Ashton created full-length ballets (of two and three acts) that were, in effect, the continuation of the classic tradition of the Maryinsky ballets which were the foundation of the company's strength. He wrote *Cinderella*, *Sylvia*, *Ondine*, *La Fille Mal Gardée* and *Les Deux Pigeons*, as well as continuing the collection of short ballets that had won such fame for him and for the company.

His ballets cover an enormous range; he can be tragic and funny, as well as producing wonderful ballets for pure dancing, like *Symphonic Variations*, that has no story. Ashton is a master-craftsman in the actual *making* of ballets, and his creations all insist upon the importance of classical dancing as the chief element. His works are a priceless heritage—as important as the Petipa inheritance—and they will delight audiences for many years to come.

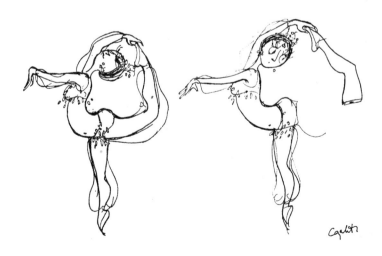

THE BLUE TRAIN

The Story of Anton Dolin

Joan Selby-Lowndes

1 The Family

A flight of startled birds wheeled up into the sky and circled over the tips of the trees clustered at the bottom of the garden. In the dusty shadows of the shrubbery below a thrush called shrill alarm. A violent rustling of leaves sent a nervous blackbird beak-first into the nearest holly bush, as a tree came suddenly to life, shaking its branches. High up a twig cracked and snapped.

"Bother," said a clear, young voice inside the tree, and the piece of dead wood went rattling down to earth.

"You'll have to climb up the other side," an older voice joined in. "Can you reach that bit?" Philip Kay, directing operations from the ground, watched his young brother Pat* through the tangled, black pattern of branches overhead.

For answer came a scuffle of feet and a spatter of broken bark on his upturned face.

Over at the house the tall, garden windows were swung open, and from the cool darkness of the drawing-room came a slender figure, graceful and slim-waisted in her long, summer dress. A wide, flower-decked hat shaded her face. Mrs. Kay moved swiftly on to the lawn.

"Philip! Pat!" She looked round the deserted garden, wondering at her sons' gift for disappearing.

"Philip! Pat! Where are you?" Her voice reached them faintly.

"We're here, Mother," an invisible Philip answered, and a few moments later she saw the tousled figure of her eldest son materialise from a laurel bush.

"Oh, Phil!" She came up to him. "What are you doing?" Her soft Irish voice was full of reproach. "Look at your clothes; those are your best school flannels."

Author's Note—Anton Dolin is the stage name of Pat Kay.

"I'm sorry, Mother, there didn't seem time to change." He gave a half-hearted scrape at the assorted smears of green and brown. She couldn't be annoyed with him for long though, not on the first day of the summer holidays.

"What a boy." Her quick laughter forgave him. "Hardly arrived home and you're up to mischief already. What have you done with Pat now?"

"He's up there." Philip pointed in the general direction of the sky.

"Here I am!" The upper branches of the tree shook violently and parted. The mischievous brown face of her second son Pat appeared among the leaves. "Watch me climb," he called down to her.

She waved gaily at him, but the colour had suddenly drained from her face.

"Phil, you shouldn't let him climb a tall tree like that, not by himself, he's such a little boy."

"That's the whole point," Philip explained carefully. "There's a nest up there and the branches wouldn't bear my weight."

"You and your birds' nests." She shook her head in despair.

"Pat won't fall," he consoled her. "He climbs like a monkey." He thrust his hands confidently into his pockets and together they watched the small figure wriggle his way up through the branches.

"I think I can reach it now," Pat announced, and the sight of him balanced on tiptoe on a swaying branch made his mother put her hand to her mouth as though to stop herself crying out.

Slowly, a bare, sunburned arm reached up to the nest, cradled in the fork of two slender branches above his head. Small, strong fingers groped over the edge to the soft lining where the eggs nestled.

"There's four," Pat's clear voice called down.

"Take one only," the instructions came back, "and mind you don't break it."

To Mrs. Kay, anxiously waiting below, it seemed hours before a small boy in a crumpled sailor suit climbed out of the laurel bush, and a pale, speckled egg lay in Philip's hand.

"Look, Mother, isn't it a beauty?"

But she was too relieved to have Pat safely on the ground again to be able to admire it.

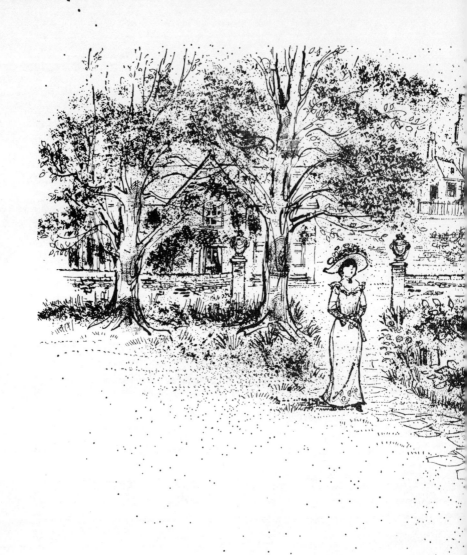

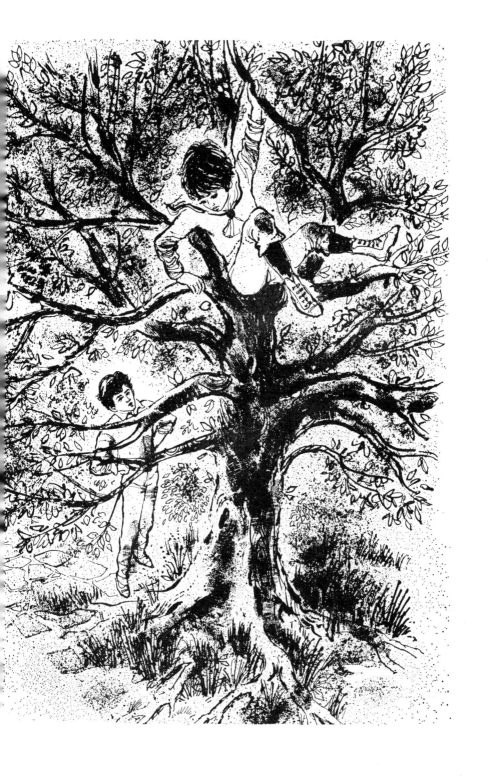

"Can I have it?" asked Pat.

"No, you can't. It's the only one I've got of this sort."

"I fetched it, so I ought to have it."

"You wouldn't have known where the nest was if I hadn't shown you."

"Yes, I would."

"No, you wouldn't."

Mrs. Kay decided that a change of subject was due.

"Pat, dear," she pulled her resisting small son towards her and tried to pick some of the bits of twig and leaves out of his hair. "Have you been for a swim to-day?"

"No, Mother." He wriggled impatiently. They weren't finished with the egg after all.

"Can't I have it because it's my birthday?"

"It isn't your birthday," said Philip.

"It will be—not to-morrow, but the next day. Won't it, Mother?"

"Yes, darling, it will—27th July." She made an attempt to straighten out the sailor suit. "Perhaps Philip will give you another egg for a present."

"I want that egg." Tears were threatening. Young Pat certainly knew what he wanted.

"I tell you what," said Philip. "We'll go bird-nesting on your birthday, and you can have all the eggs we find."

"Can we really?"

"Yes, it's a promise."

And, as Pat adored his elder brother, the bad moment passed and he was happy again. Besides, with this talk of birthdays a new idea had presented itself.

"Mother, you said when I was eight I could have a bicycle."

"Yes, darling, I did."

"I'm going to be eight the day after to-morrow."

"Yes, I know you are."

"Will I have a bicycle?"

"You must wait and see."

"If I have a bicycle on my birthday, can I take it to go bird-nesting?"

"You've got to learn to ride it first," said Philip.

"Is it difficult?"

"Father will teach you," Mrs. Kay gave up the crumpled suit as a bad job. "That reminds me, I wanted to know what you two boys were doing this afternoon. Father and I have to go out, and Anthony wants to go swimming."

"I'll take him." Pat, aged seven, considered he was quite grown-up enough to look after Anthony, aged four.

"No, darling, you know you mustn't go swimming alone." She was looking hopefully at Philip.

"I was going up to the schoolroom to rearrange my eggs," he said.

"Can I come and help?" Pat promptly inquired. He would give up even swimming if he could stay with his adored elder brother.

"Haven't you got something else you'd rather do?"

Pat hesitated, and then seemed to make up his mind.

"Yes, I have," he said rather loudly, and went trotting across the lawn.

"Pat! Come back!" His mother called out, but the independent small figure disappeared round the corner of the house. "Oh, Phil, dear, you might have told him that he could stay," she reproached him. "You know he loves being with you, and he's done nothing but count the days till you came home."

"He's such a nuisance in the schoolroom," said Philip. "He can never stay still for two minutes together."

"Couldn't you do your eggs later on?" she coaxed him. "I don't want to spoil your first day at home, but I'd feel much happier about going out if I knew that Pat and Anthony were with you."

"All right." Philip, who really loved his two baby brothers a great deal more than his birds' eggs, smiled at her and gave up his idea. "I'll take them on the beach," he promised.

It was a promise he was not to keep, however. Mr. and Mrs. Kay, on their way to Bognor, were happily unaware that poor Philip was running round the garden in search of two elusive small boys who had completely vanished.

"Pat! Anthony!" he called, but the garden, drowsing in the hot afternoon sunshine, lay mysteriously silent. "Little beasts must be hiding in the house." Philip gave up the garden search and went muttering indoors.

A bush near the front gate moved. A cautious head peeped out.

"He's gone." The rest of Pat climbed out, followed by Anthony, the youngest of the family.

"Come on." Pat caught hold of his brother's chubby wrist. "Run."

Out of the gate they went and down the lane; two small figures trotting along between the high, green hedges. Anthony's face soon turned red in the heat; he began to lag behind.

"Why do we have to run away from Phil?" he wanted to know.

"Because he doesn't want us with him." Pat looked round to make sure they were not being followed, and slowed down to a walk. "He wants to go and be with his eggs by himself, so we'll go on the beach on our own." And, as Anthony did anything Pat wanted, they went.

The beach at Felpham was a long golden stretch of sand cut by wooden breakwaters. There was the usual row of green bathing machines on big iron wheels. The large brown horse that pulled them into the sea rested in the shade at the back.

Dotted over the sands, little girls in floppy sunbonnets and white dresses played about with buckets and spades. Little boys in wide straw hats and sailor suits made sand-castles, while their nannies, very stiff and buttoned up, kept an eye on their charges, or mothers in long graceful dresses sat under shady parasols.

Pat and Anthony made their way down to the water's edge. They took off their sandals and went running through the curly, shallow waves shouting and kicking up the silvery spray. They fished for crabs, and looked for treasures among the shells in the wet sand.

"I say, Anthony, look at that." Pat's attention was suddenly caught by a noisy group of big boys playing about by a breakwater. They turned somersaults, and played leapfrog, and suddenly one was standing up on his hands.

Fascinated, Pat started to run towards them, but long before he got there the group had broken up and raced away.

"I'm going to see if I can do that." Pat put his hands on the sand, kicked his legs in the air—and fell over, sideways.

"It's not as easy as it looks," he informed Anthony who stood gravely watching him. Next time he fell over on the other side.

"What are you doing?"

Pat sat up. A dark-eyed little girl about his own age was standing quite close, looking at him as though he were a very strange animal.

"I want to stand on my hands." Pat tried again. This time he kicked too hard and fell over on his back.

"Let me try." Anthony, in faithful imitation, put his small behind in the air, but only managed to get one leg off the ground.

"What do you want to do that for?" the small girl asked.

"I want to see what it feels like," Pat told her. "Can you stand on your hands?"

"No." She shook her head.

"I climbed a tree to-day," said Pat. "Can you climb trees?"

"No. We don't have any trees at home."

"No trees?" Pat frowned. "How funny. Where do you live?"

"In London. It's all houses and streets."

"We live here." Anthony gave up his handstands and sat down.

"Why do you live in London?" Pat wanted to know.

"I don't know." She shrugged her shoulders. "My mother brought me there from our home in Hungary. It's a country far away from here. We travelled for days and nights in the train, and crossed the sea, and I was sick . . ."

"What's your name?" interrupted Anthony, who wasn't interested in travel talks.

"Maria. What's yours?"

"Anthony."

"I'm Pat. We're brothers. How old are you?"

"I'm ten," she twirled round on one foot.

"I'm going to be eight the day after to-morrow," Pat told her. "I'm going to have a bicycle for my birthday. Have you got a bicycle?"

"I'm not allowed to have one."

"Why not?"

"Because of my dancing. I'm going to be a dancer when I grow up." She turned round on the other foot. "In London I have lessons every day." She swung out a long straight leg and arched her foot.

"Dancing lessons?" Pat was interested. This sounded much more exciting than the reading and arithmetic lessons he did at school. "Do you like it?"

"I love it. I never want to do anything else." She danced about on her toes.

"What do you learn?"

"Ballet dancing, of course."

"What's that?"

"I can't explain." She shrugged her shoulders and her arms swept up into a graceful curve. "You must see it to understand."

"Dance something now," Pat demanded, and the small girl did a series of elementary ballet movements. Her full white dress flew out round her slim, golden-brown legs. She was very pretty and very graceful.

"I like that," Pat watched her carefully, "I can do it too."

"No, you can't."

"Why not?"

"Because you have to be taught properly how to hold your arms and legs."

"Well, I can jump in the air higher than you did."

"Come on, then, we shall see." They went running and dancing across the wet sand in a series of unrecognisable *grands jetés*.

"There, I told you I could jump higher than you." They stopped, out of breath.

"That's because you're a boy."

"I think I'd like to learn dancing." Pat looked at her. "Dance some more," but someone was calling.

"That's my mother." Maria turned and waved. "I must go." She went dancing away from him across the sands, her black hair flying out. Pat walked slowly and thoughtfully back to Anthony.

He was never to see little Maria from Hungary again, but the idea she had put into his head was never to leave him.

2 The Parcel

A big carrier's van came rumbling slowly along the lane, reluctantly pulled by a fat, brown horse.

"Whoa!" said the carrier.

The horse didn't need telling twice.

"Lazy lump of fat." As the carrier climbed down he sent a

malevolent look at his horse, who was already nodding in the shafts. "Not much chance you'll run away." He heaved a large crate on to his shoulders and went stumping along the path to the house.

"Parcel 'ere for the name of Kay." The carrier blew heavily through his overhanging moustache.

"Well, I never!" Rosie, the maid, stood on the doorstep gaping at the large crate on his shoulder.

"Is this the 'ouse?"

"That's right." Rosie's starched cap nodded vigorously.

"Where am I ter put it?"

"Oo! The mistress didn't say."

"Well, I ain't goin' to wait with this 'ere parcel on me back all afternoon while you make up your mind, see."

"It seems a bit large, but if it's a parcel I suppose it 'ad better go in the 'all, same as the letters."

The carrier dumped his offering at the foot of the stairs. Rosie fled into the kitchen to see if Cook thought she'd done the right thing, while up in the schoolroom in the far corner of the house, Philip, surrounded by trays of birds' eggs, remained happily deaf to the banging of doors, the scrunch of steps, and the distant sound of the carrier's horse moving reluctantly away.

In the hall, the large grandfather clock looked with disapproval at the intruding crate.

"Grrr!" it remarked, and, getting no reaction, struck five extra loudly.

Down on the beach, children, prams and nannies were on the move.

"Come on, Anthony, we'd better go home." Pat caught hold of his brother's hand.

The long sandy lane that led from the beach was sheltered and stifling. Anthony's short legs soon tired, and his feet dragged in the dust, getting slower and slower.

"Come on." Pat pulled him.

Anthony sat down in the middle of the lane.

"You can't stay there," said Pat indignantly.

"Yes, I can, Anthony's tired. Want Mummy."

"You can't have her, she's at Bognor." Pat tried to pull him up. "Come on, it isn't far now."

"You carry me," suggested Anthony, but Pat had a better idea.

"I say, aren't you hungry?" he suggested.

Anthony thought about this.

"It must be tea-time," Pat went on. "Cook said she might make chocolate cake to-day, and if we're late we shan't get any."

"Chocolate cake!" Anthony rapidly forgot he was tired. Hand-in-hand, they made good progress back to the house.

The hall was cool and dim after the bright sunshine outside. The light, filtering through a stained window, spilled untidy pools of red and green on the wooden crate standing at the foot of the staircase.

The patter of boys' sandals on the tiled floor stopped abruptly.

"Look at that!" Pat pointed.

"What is it?" Anthony hung back, afraid it might come to life and bite.

Pat tiptoed cautiously up to it. He looked at the labels pasted on the outside. There was no mistaking what the crate contained. The promise had come true. He fingered the rough wood and tingles of excitement shivered up and down his back.

"It's come."

"What has?" Anthony advanced cautiously.

"It's my bicycle. Mother promised I'd have one for my birthday and this is it." In rising excitement, Pat's fingers explored the gaps between the slats, trying to feel the shape of this exciting, hidden thing under the brown paper.

A sudden noise made him jump and whip his hands behind his back. The green baize door from the kitchen regions shuffled open. Rosie's face appeared.

"Oh! It's you, Master Pat and Master Anthony. I thought I heard the front door. You're late for tea. Now then, you leave that parcel alone. Don't you dare lay a finger on it."

Anthony looked at her doubtfully and put his finger in his mouth, but Pat's small, tense body didn't move. He didn't even look in her direction.

"You're not to touch it. Do you hear?"

Pat went on looking at the crate.

"Rude boy." She sniffed, and the green baize door sighed itself shut. In the silence that followed the muffled tap of Rosie's retreating feet, the tick of the grandfather clock repeated loudly, "Don't touch. Don't touch."

Pat and Anthony looked at each other.

"Where's Philip?" said Anthony.

"Philip! Of course. I wonder if he's seen it?" and the idea sent Pat suddenly chasing up the stairs.

"Philip!" His voice woke the echoes. "Philip? Where are you?" The sound of his feet pounding along the corridor broke up the sleeping stillness of the house.

"Philip!" called Anthony in shrill imitation.

"Philip, it's here, it's arrived." Pat burst into the schoolroom. "My bicycle, it's downstairs, in the hall. You must come and see."

No time for Philip to say, "Where have you been?" and "mind the eggs"; he was swept up in the general excitement and came racing down the stairs with them.

"But there's nothing to see," said Philip when he caught sight of the crate.

"Oh yes, there is." Pat began pulling at one of the slats.

"I don't think you ought to touch it," said Philip doubtfully, "anyway, not till Mother and Father come back."

"I only want to look at it." Pat had managed to wrench off a thin slat.

"You'll get into awful trouble."

"Never mind," Pat was recklessly tearing at the shrouding paper. "Do come and help." He pulled away a handful of straw packing and more paper. "Look!" The silvery curve of a handlebar stood revealed.

The sight of the treasure within reach was too much for Philip. He pulled out his penknife and got to work.

Wood cracked and split, nails creaked as the slats were prised off. Pat and Anthony ripped away the paper wrappings. Straw and wood-shavings spilled over the hall floor. No holding back now. They tore off the last cocoons of protecting paper, and there, in the wreckage of the crate, stood the gleaming new bicycle. It was shining black with a fine red line; silvery wheels and handlebars, and a shining leather saddle.

"It's a beauty," said Philip, and Pat wheeled it round the hall. The new rubber tyres made soft squeaking sounds on the tiles.

"What would happen if I got on?" He stroked the saddle thoughtfnlly.

"You'd fall off," said Philip.

"Wouldn't you hold it for me; just so that I could see what it's like?" he pleaded.

"Not in here."

Pat wheeled the gleaming bicycle out of the front door and down the step into the drive. Philip hoisted him into the saddle.

"It's just the right size for you."

"Do let's go down the drive, a little way."

"Hang on tight, then." Philip held him up and, with one hand on the handlebars and one on the back of the saddle, he pushed off.

The procession went wobbling down to the gate, Anthony trotting along in the rear.

"We'll try in the lane," suggested Philip. "It's less bumpy."

Up and down they went.

"Let go of the handlebars," said Pat as they turned to go up the lane a second time. "I want to steer myself." So Philip held on to the saddle and went jogging alongside, while Anthony sat in the grass on the bank and watched.

"I think it's lovely," Pat called out as the pedals spun round easily under his feet, and he watched the silver spokes of the front wheel flashing round. "I'd like to do this for ever."

"I daresay you would." Philip was getting out of breath and very hot. "But I'm going to stop for a minute."

"How does one stop?"

"Put the brakes on and steer for the side." Philip helped to ground the bicycle gently against the bank.

"Get off a minute while I rest," he said.

"Don't want to. Look, I can stay on by myself." Pat propped himself up with one foot on the bank.

"Well, don't fall off and scratch the paint." Philip flopped down on the grass beside Anthony.

Pat rocked the bicycle to and fro, wondering what it felt like to ride alone. He stretched a leg down as far as it would go.

"I can almost put my foot on the ground," he announced, but Philip, who was playing about with Anthony, didn't hear.

"I'll try a little way," Pat said to himself. "One, two, three— go." A strong push off the bank, and he was launched. His feet scrabbled on the pedals, the bicycle wobbled violently, but they were still moving; he hadn't fallen off. The wobble was almost under control. This was wonderful. He was getting his balance.

"Look, Phil! Anthony, look!" he shouted. "I'm riding it by myself."

He clutched at the handlebars tightly and, keeping his eyes on that wavering front wheel, steered a precarious course down the lane.

"Hi! Pat! Where are you going?" Philip's voice sounded a long way behind him. "Come back."

"I can ride! I can ride a bicycle all by myself," Pat shouted as he wobbled round the bend, and he rode it—straight into the arms of his returning parents.

3 First Appearance

"I still say that the boy should have had a damn' good thrashing." Mr. Kay, dressed for dinner, came in to see if his wife was ready. "You're too soft with him, Maude, that's the trouble."

"You have taken his bicycle away and sent him to bed early, don't you think that's punishment enough?" She was sitting at the dressing-table putting finishing touches to her hair.

"But the sheer impudence of it—breaking open the crate. Never saw such a mess as the hall was in, and then taking the thing out and riding it . . ." The enormity of the offence seemed to choke him.

"I think it was so clever of him to be able to ride it," said Mrs. Kay thoughtfully. "He must have an amazing sense of balance. I think he must inherit it from you," her gentle voice went on. "Do you remember the first time you put him on a horse? You remarked then that he had an extraordinary sense of balance."

Mr. Kay grunted, and came over to the mirror to see if his tie was straight. He wasn't ready yet to admit that secretly he, too, was rather proud of his naughty son.

Meanwhile, the subject of this conversation, shut away in the boys' bedroom at the end of the house, bounced about under the blankets and got his pyjamas twisted into a corkscrew round his wriggling body.

In the bed in the far corner of the room, Anthony, tired out with his day's adventures, was fast asleep. "Lucky thing," thought

Pat as he looked at the still lump under the bedclothes and heard his brother's quiet breathing. It made him feel more wideawake than ever.

Outside it was still light; a soft evening light that filtered through the closed curtains. Pat kicked the blanket back, waved his legs in the air and thought how horrid it was to have to be in bed.

He stared at the patterned wallpaper and saw again the scene downstairs; his father, stiff with angry disapproval, wheeling the bicycle; Philip and Anthony, very subdued, walking behind; and his mother keeping close to him and saying nothing. There had been worse to come when they arrived upon the wreckage of straw and paper in the hall. There was Rosie's horrified face repeating over and over again, "I told them to be sure and not touch it." His father's stern voice ordering him off to bed, and his own tears of rage.

"I shall take the bicycle away and lock it up," his father had said, "and if you don't behave yourself I shall give it to another little boy, and you will never see it again."

No more bicycle! Pat, however, was neither frightened nor subdued by threats. He thought his father was being unfair, and his Irish temper had come bubbling up inside him.

"No," he had yelled, "it's my bicycle," and he had gone running backwards on the tips of his toes, screaming at the top of his voice.

"Pat, be quiet." But his father's voice had had no effect, and Pat had yelled louder than ever.

"Pat!" He had felt his mother's arm go round him, and he had known by the look on her face that it was no use fighting. Fair or not, he had to accept his father's decision. So, the angry tears had dried on his cheeks and his mother had taken him upstairs to have supper in disgrace in the schoolroom while she bathed Anthony, and then bed.

"Anyway, I rode it," Pat defiantly kicked his legs up and pedalled an imaginary bicycle along the road. He didn't hear the door softly open.

"Pat! You bad boy! What are you up to now?" It was his mother's soft voice. "You should have been asleep long ago."

Her long evening dress rustled as she came into the room and the air was suddenly sweet with the warm fragrance of her perfume.

She leaned over Anthony's bed, smiling to see him happily asleep with a Teddy bear hugged in his arms.

"I can't go to sleep." Pat put himself the right way up. "What's the time?"

"It's about eight o'clock." She came and sat on his bed, the full skirts of her dress spreading their pale green folds of shining silk over the tumbled blankets. "What are we going to do with such a bad boy?" She pushed back the hair from his hot forehead.

"Mother!" Pat fingered the long coloured fringe of the shawl she wore. "Did Father really mean what he said about giving my bicycle away? I will really have it on my birthday, won't I?"

"You wait and see." She tried not to smile at the sight of his anxious face. "But remember, you've got to be good until then. No more playing truant either, running down to the beach."

She put the bedclothes straight and bent to kiss him good-night. Two very wideawake brown eyes watched her go.

"Good-night, darling," she called softly from the door.

"Mother."

"What is it?"

"Can I have dancing lessons?"

"Dancing lessons? Whatever for?"

"I met a little girl on the beach to-day who dances, and I want to be a dancer too when I grow up."

"We'll have to see. You just go to sleep now." Mrs. Kay went downstairs wondering at the curious ideas children get into their heads.

Bed was duller than ever after she had gone. Pat lay on his back and looked at the cracks in the ceiling over his head. He thought of the girl with dark hair who danced. He remembered the glorious feeling of running and jumping with her, flying through the air in great big leaps.

The sound of the gong reverberated through the house and from below came the sudden hum of voices. That would be Father and Mother and everybody going into the dining-room. He'd forgotten to ask who was coming to dinner to-night. He wondered what Father had said to Philip about the bicycle business. He wondered when Philip would be coming up to bed. Not for hours and hours if they were only just starting dinner. It was funny how one got sleepy all of a sudden . . . He didn't really want to go to sleep . . . he wanted to tell Philip about that girl on the beach. How pretty she looked when she stood on her toes and went twirling round and round . . . and round . . . and round . . .

The distant cascading notes of a piano wove their way insistently into the pattern of his dreams. The rise and fall of the melody turned into shapes, circles and curving lines, breaking and reforming. Now it shifted into a picture of a girl with flying dark hair on a shining bicycle; her feet whirling round and round, making the wheels spin faster and faster. He must catch her, he must run after her, but the music held him back. Faster, if only the music would hurry and let him catch up . . . with a jerk, Pat opened his eyes. The room was swimming in shadows, shadows that still moved. He frowned; he had been dreaming, yet he could still hear music. It was real. He sat up and the corners of the room came into focus, taking solid shape. What time was it? He looked across at Philip's bed. There was the familiar mound in it. It must be quite late.

"Phil." He called softly, but the tousled, dark head on the pillow didn't move.

Still the music went on. Pat was wide awake now, listening. It must be his mother. She often played in the evening to entertain her guests. Sometimes when they were alone, she played for him. He never tired of listening to the lovely sounds she drew out of the piano, sounds that sent tingles of excitement all over him and made him want to move, to jump, and wave his arms. Impossible to lie still now.

Pat got out of bed and tiptoed to the door. Softly, very softly, he turned the handle and pulled it open. The music suddenly poured through the gap.

Just across the corridor, directly in front of him, was the door that opened on to a flight of stairs curving down into the music-room below. Drawn irresistibly by those dancing notes, he crept down. Peeping through the banisters now, he could see the piano below, its top opened like a great bird's wing to let out those flying, golden notes.

His mother had her back to the stairs. He could see her slender fingers which seemed to dance over the white and black keys. Watching her, and absorbed in her music, Pat was quite unaware

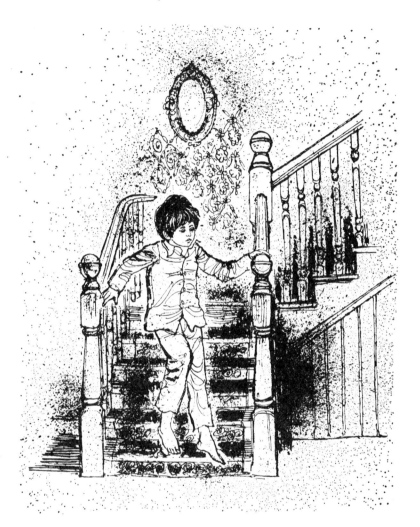

of the still circle of people sitting in arm-chairs grouped round the open windows at the far end of the room.

Noiselessly, he ran down the last few steps on to the wide expanse of polished floor. His bare feet made no sound as he danced, a small ghostly figure in white pyjamas. Like a puppet, pulled by invisible strings, he let the music shape the movements of his body.

There was a slow stir among the silent group of listeners. Someone had caught sight of that dancing white figure behind the piano. A second head turned, and a third. Glances were exchanged, and smiles.

At the piano, Mrs. Kay swiftly sensed that the quiet spell was broken. Her fingers faltered and stopped. Mr. Kay, whose head had been quietly nodding on to his chest, woke with a guilty start. He looked round and saw, to his horror, the small figure of his son, who had been sent to bed in disgrace hours ago, capering about in the middle of the music-room.

Mr. Kay was a man of action. Things happened swiftly. The apparition in white pyjamas was rapidly and forcefully removed. In the seclusion of the upper corridor, a sound spanking took place, and a subdued, small boy crept back into his bed.

So ended the first public appearance of Pat Kay, dancer.

4 Hove

"What is this idea of Pat's that he wants to dance?" Mr. Kay wanted to know. It was after lunch and they were sitting by the open french windows of the drawing-room.

"It seems that on the beach the other day he met a little girl who is going to be a dancer, and now he wants to do the same thing." Mrs. Kay, bending over her sewing, smiled as she listened to the distant shouts and laughter of her three sons romping in the sunlit garden. "He's quite serious about it."

"Nonsense," Mr. Kay rattled his newspaper indignantly. "Who ever heard of a boy wanting to dance?"

"I think it's just that he loves anything which makes him run about."

"Aren't games good enough for him, football and cricket?" Mr. Kay, sportsman, county cricketer, and master of hounds, dismissed dancing as a low form of amusement.

"You know he loves all games and sports," Mrs. Kay agreed, "but he's got this idea that he wants to dance too. After all, he does love music."

"Ridiculous." He went back to *The Times*.

Mrs. Kay said no more and, busy over her sewing, wondered again at the strange ideas of boys.

"Don't like this German business," her husband spoke suddenly from behind his paper.

"What about it?"

"They say here the Germans are building up a huge army and plan a fleet that will be bigger and stronger than the British Navy. Damn' cheek! Kaiser's getting very offensive these days. Bad sign."

"There's no danger of war, is there?"

"Can't tell." He shrugged his shoulders. "Don't like the look of things though."

"War!" she thought. "No, it would surely never come to that." Instinctively, she raised her head to watch those three sons of hers playing on the lawn like puppies, and in the security of that sunlit garden at Felpham in the summer of 1912, the possibility of war seemed very far away.

"Do look at them," she laughed. "Pat is doing a dance and the others are copying him."

"It's time that boy went off to boarding-school," said Mr. Kay fiercely over the top of his paper. "That'll knock the nonsense out of him. Dancing indeed!"

"I daresay it's just a passing fancy," said Mrs. Kay mildly. "He'll grow out of it. After all, he is only eight."

Pat didn't grow out of it. The desire to dance remained but, as there was nowhere to learn at Felpham, nothing could be done about it. So the desire remained unexpressed, half forgotten in the crowded days of childhood.

For two years life went on much as usual in the house at Felpham. Mrs. Kay saw Philip quickly growing up into a tall, broad-shouldered, serious member of the Senior School; while little Anthony was suddenly no longer a baby but a sturdy school-boy; and in between them her mischievous son Pat, already a vivid personality with a will of his own. He more than the others had inherited his mother's temperament. Impulsive, generous, quick to laughter or tears; the Irish strain ran strong in him, and perhaps for that reason he came closer to her, for she, better than anyone, understood his naughtiness, his fierce independence; the swift, strange moods that came on him, even as a small child, when he needed to be alone. She feared what the discipline of boarding-school would do to this proud, free spirit.

Happily, the time for that was not yet come, and Pat attended the local day school. He took solemn charge of Anthony each morning, pushing his unwilling small brother down the road, and keeping a fatherly eye on his activities until he brought him safely home again. The pair of them would count the days until the holidays should bring Philip home once more, and all three could romp their way through the glorious days of freedom.

So, school terms and holidays followed each other in the safe, ordered life of pre-war England. From time to time disquieting paragraphs appeared in the papers about the armed strength of Germany and her growing fleet; ugly rumours that were quickly dismissed and forgotten by most people.

"We shan't have war," they said; and Mrs. Kay, whose home, husband and three growing sons happily filled her life, agreed with them.

Then, early in 1914, something else came along to occupy her thoughts. Grandfather Healey became Family Problem Number One. Mrs. Kay's father was a widower and an old man.

"I do think he needs someone to look after him properly." Mrs. Kay, just returned from a visit to her father at Hove, was pouring out family tea. "He's not looking at all well."

"He's got that housekeeper person, hasn't he?" said Mr. Kay.

"Yes, but she finds him very difficult to manage nowadays. Pass the scones round, Phil, dear." She pointed to the big covered dish warming in front of the fire. "I feel that one of the family ought to be with him."

"Can't he come and live with us?" suggested Mr. Kay.

"I wish he could, but you know he'd never come here, there's no railway."

Pat decided that the conversation was getting interesting.

"Why does Grandfather have to have a railway?"

"He likes to see the trains go past." Mrs. Kay handed round the jam. "He used to enjoy shooting at the engine drivers. That's why he took this house at Hove. The railway goes along the bottom of the garden."

"Damn' fine shot, your father, Maude," said Mr. Kay suddenly. "Difficult target a moving train, especially with a revolver."

"I'd like to try that," said Pat. "Can I?"

"No, dear," his mother told him gently. "You see, Grandfather doesn't shoot at trains any more now. He nearly hit a driver once and the man complained so the railway people wrote and asked him not to do it again."

"In any case, he's been in bed for years," added Mr. Kay.

"What's the matter with him?" Philip asked.

"Nobody knew." Mrs. Kay passed the cakes. "He just decided to go to bed one day and he's been there ever since. It's a long time now—let me see. Pat was quite a baby. It must be nearly nine years."

"Do you mean he's been in bed for nine years without being ill?" Pat was horrified.

"Shall we say he is suffering from old age," his mother explained. "Now, who's going to finish up the toast?" She passed the dish round her hungry family. "His housekeeper complains nowadays that his room is getting so full of birds and cages that she spends all her time cleaning up after them, and he orders her about as though she were a regiment of soldiers . . ." She glanced up at the big gold-framed portrait of her father that hung on one side of the fireplace. It was difficult to imagine that the eccentric old man living alone in his house at Hove had once been the handsome, dashing young cavalry officer whose clear blue eyes looked steadily out from the painted canvas.

"That's Grandfather, isn't it?" Anthony pointed to the picture.

"Yes, darling, but he doesn't look like that any more. He's a very old man now. That was painted a long time ago just after he was married. The picture of my mother was done about the same time."

They all gazed up at the portrait of the young lovely Irish girl that hung on the other side of the fireplace.

"They met when Father's regiment was stationed over in Ireland," said Mrs. Kay, "and after they were married they lived just outside Dublin. That's where I was born and brought up."

"She's my grandmother, then," Anthony worked out the relationship.

"That's right. She never saw you though. She died many years before you were born."

"And Grandfather's lived by himself ever since, shooting at trains," Pat summed up the family story.

"That's about it," she smiled.

"Must do something about the old chap," Mr. Kay decided.

"Can't leave him there all alone if he's not being looked after properly."

Something was done about Grandfather Healey. As he wouldn't come to them, they must go to him. So, early in the spring of 1914, while Philip was away at school, the Kay family uprooted itself from Felpham and went to live at Hove.

They exchanged their quiet country house for the racket of trains running past the bottom of Grandfather Healey's long narrow strip of garden.

"No interesting birds' nests round here," said Philip gloomily when he came home for the Easter holidays. "Not with all these beastly trains about." Pat and Anthony were showing him round the garden.

"You don't notice them after a bit," said Pat, who was already getting used to his new life in a seaside town.

"What's your new school like?" Philip wanted to know.

"It's all right." Neither Pat nor Anthony could raise any enthusiasm for the process of being educated. One school was much like another.

"I want to go to a dancing school and have lessons," added Pat. "There are places here that teach it, but Father and Mother won't let me go."

"Dancing?" Philip stared at him. "What on earth do you want to learn that for?"

They were interrupted by the sound of a window opening, and a stentorian shout.

"That's Grandfather." Pat hastily straightened his suit and smoothed his hair.

"It's Saturday morning," added Anthony as he pulled up his socks.

"What about it?" asked a perplexed Philip.

"We have to go into his room on Saturday mornings." Pat did up a stray shoe-lace. "It's a parade."

"Shan't be long," Anthony called back as they ran indoors.

Their mother was waiting for them outside Grandfather's bedroom door.

"Are you nice and tidy?" She looked them over. "In you go then."

They opened the door.

There was a whir and a flutter of wings. As two rather awed small boys walked in, birds flew off in all directions. In the middle of the room Grandfather Healey sat up in a big bed looking very fierce. All round the walls and on the furniture were rows and rows of bird cages. Their doors stood wide open so that the inmates were free to fly in and out as they pleased.

Pat and Anthony, well trained by this time in their parade routine, lined up beside the bed, standing very stiffly.

"Shoulders back," barked Grandfather. "Heads up. Heels together." He looked them up and down, his blue eyes very stern under bushy, white eyebrows.

The birds, scattered over the room perching on cages, pictures and curtain rails, twittered and looked on.

"Very good. Parade dismiss."

Pat and Anthony relaxed. Grandfather groped among the clutter of things on the table beside him. The boys held out their hands and each received an orange, a shortbread biscuit and twopence.

"Thank you, Grandfather."

"Well! What are you waiting for now?" he barked at them.

"Will you make your birds fly for us?" asked Pat, who was not in the least afraid of the gentle old man who pretended to be so fierce.

"You like it, do you?"

"Yes. I'd like to have a bird of my own and teach it to do things like you do."

"You would, would you?" He looked hard at Pat. "How old are you?"

"I'm nearly ten."

"Well, perhaps I'll give you a bird one day."

"Thank you, Grandfather."

"Can I have one too?" asked Anthony.

"Not yet. You're too young. Wouldn't look after it properly. Now go over there and stand very still," Grandfather commanded.

The two boys tiptoed to the corner by the door. The old man crumbled some biscuit in his hand and whistled softly. His birds cocked their heads on one side, listening. Bright, round eyes watched the tempting handful of crumbs. He whistled again. There was a flutter, a little whir of feathers, and there was a chaffinch perched on one of Grandfather's big gnarled fingers. A bullfinch took courage and landed on his thumb. In a few minutes a whole lot of little birds were hopping about on his hand and arm, pecking crumbs. There was a gentle, faraway look on the old man's face as he watched them. He had forgotten all about his small grandsons. After a few minutes they tiptoed softly out of the room.

Their mother was waiting for them in the passage.

"What are you going to spend your money on this week?" she asked them as they showed her their treasures.

"Don't know." Pat jingled his two pennies.

"Toffee," said Anthony promptly. "Let's go down to the sweet shop now. Philip hasn't seen it yet. Can we go?"

"Yes, darling, if you like."

"I'll get Philip." Anthony went running into the garden, but Pat lingered.

"And what's my Pat going to do to-day?" Mrs. Kay put her arm round him.

"We're going to show Philip round." Pat thoughtfully nibbled the corner of his biscuit. "Mother?" He looked up suddenly. "There's a house down the road which says 'Dancing Lessons' on a board outside. Couldn't I go and learn dancing there next term?"

"You are a strange boy." She stroked his hair. "Still this idea of dancing. Wouldn't you rather be good at games?"

"Why can't I do both?" he asked. "I want to dance too."

"It's no good, darling, you know Father doesn't like the idea."

"Why won't he let me?" Pat looked at the ground, his eyes clouding with gathering tears. "I know if you asked him really hard he'd say yes. Please make him say yes."

"Supposing you try and forget all about this dancing idea," she suggested. "You just say to yourself that you're going to grow up into a big strong man who can run faster and play games better than anyone else."

"But I want to learn to dance as well." The angry tears were blinding him. "Other people dance so why can't I? It isn't fair," and Pat broke away from her and went running out of the house.

"It is extraordinary," Mrs. Kay was saying to her husband in the study a few minutes later. "He's got this idea in his head and he won't give it up."

The front door banged and through the window she watched

the three boys going down the road to the sweet shop. "I wonder if we shouldn't be wise and let him have dancing lessons, as his heart is so set on it. After all, it can't do him any harm."

"Waste of time and money," said Mr. Kay from his arm-chair.

"A few lessons wouldn't cost very much," she persisted. "He'll probably realise that it's not a bit what he thinks it is and it'll cure him of ever wanting to dance again."

And Mr. Kay, who was thoroughly sick of Pat and his dancing, finally agreed.

5 First Dancing Lessons

Outside a house in Hove, a painted signboard announced, "Miss Clarice James's Dancing Academy." Here, one Saturday afternoon, early in May, an excited small boy, accompanied by his mother, went up the steps to the front door.

"So this is Pat." Miss Clarice James welcomed her new pupil. She saw a lively, brown-eyed little boy, and her professional eyes noticed his well-proportioned body and strong, straight legs. "I'm very pleased to have another boy in my class."

The class was already milling about in the big front room that served as a studio. There were girls of assorted sizes and shapes in coloured party frocks and ribbons; a thin sprinkling of boys, scrubbed clean and put into best clothes.

Mrs. Kay joined the row of mothers and discarded outdoor clothes on chairs against the wall. Pat put on his new dancing shoes. The traditional black slipper with cross-over elastic.

The class began.

Miss Clarice James was young. It was not long ago since she had been a pupil herself, studying under Grace and Lily Cone. She wanted her children to enjoy their dancing as much as she had, and enjoy it they did, to a series of lively tunes from the piano.

Beginners were gently initiated into the mysteries of the five positions of the feet in classical ballet. They did their first *pliés* and *battements* at the bar, then to more exciting free dancing. They were elves and fairies; they were butterflies and birds, and the whole class ended up in a romping polka.

"It was lovely." Pat hopped and skipped all the way home. "I do love dancing," and he went off to find Anthony to teach him the polka.

There was no question of curing him of the idea. Dancing was served up at every meal for days. Saturday afternoons were marked up as special red-letter days.

"Extraordinary!" said Mr. Kay, and resigned himself to the idea of having a son who enjoyed dancing.

It didn't take Pat long to discover that Miss James held ballet classes on Wednesdays for more advanced pupils.

"It's such a long time to wait till Saturday," he pleaded with his mother. "Couldn't I go on Wednesdays as well?"

Mrs. Kay went to see Miss James.

"I think it would be an excellent idea," she said. "I've already noticed that your Pat is very promising. He has a good ear for rhythm and a remarkably developed sense of balance. I should be very pleased to have him in my Wednesday class. He will soon catch up with the work."

On Wednesdays Pat met the more serious ballet pupils. To the beginners' *pliés* and *battements* were added *ronds de jambe*, elementary *adagio* and *allegro*.

"What funny-looking shoes." He watched some of the older girls changing into blocks for the last part of the class.

"It's for point work," they told him.

"What's that?"

"Dancing on your toes." One of them demonstrated.

"Is that difficult?" Pat was very intrigued.

"Yes. You have to practise ever so hard."

"Do it again." Pat watched carefully. "It's not all that difficult," he said at last. "I think I can do that."

"You can't, not in a soft shoe. You have to have special blocks."

"I'm going to try, anyway." Pat went up on his toes and stayed there.

"Look at that!" The girls clustered round.

"Have you done it before?"

"No." Pat was moving about, getting used to the feel of his toes.

Miss James came over to see this phenomenon.

"You must have real dancer's feet, Pat," she told him. "Very strong. It's most unusual."

"Can I get a pair of block shoes too and do the exercises with the others?" he wanted to know.

"No," she laughed, "it's only girls who dance on their points."

Which, however, did not deter Pat from practising on his own to amuse himself.

The summer days lengthened into June. Hot, golden days that made the gathering rumours of war seem more unreal than ever. Pat and Anthony made new friends at school, and on the beach, where groups of sun-browned children spent long happy hours swimming and playing.

Grandfather remembered his promise and Pat became the proud owner of a song-bird in a cage. It could also do one trick—a backward somersault.

"We'll teach it others," the old man had said. "I'll show you." But he never did.

There were suddenly no more Saturday morning parades. Then for a few days the house was hushed and quiet with blinds drawn down, and everyone in black speaking in whispers, while little birds twittered and hopped about, looking in vain for the gentle, gnarled old hands that gave them crumbs.

To Pat and Anthony, Grandfather's death had an unreal quality. He just wasn't there any more. It was difficult to associate the old man sitting up in bed feeding his birds, with the flower-covered mound of earth in the cemetery up on the hill.

"I don't think he minded dying," their mother told them. "He was such an old man, and very, very tired."

Grandfather and his birds quickly faded into the half dream world of remembered things, like the house at Felpham and the little girl on the beach who danced. Disconnected pictures, some vivid, some blurred, strung haphazardly together, making up the tumbled pattern of childhood's memories.

Meanwhile the future beckoned, and the immediate future for Pat was Miss James's dancing display.

"I'm giving a show at the end of term," she told Mrs. Kay. "I would so like Pat to take part in it for I look on him as one of my most promising pupils. Do you think you could let him come for extra practice and rehearsals?"

"I expect that will be all right," said Mrs. Kay. "I will have to see what his father says."

"I do hope he will agree."

Mr. Kay had now to resign himself to the idea that not only did his son enjoy dancing, but that he had definite talent for it.

He even accompanied Mrs. Kay and Anthony to the Hove Town Hall to see Pat dance.

"Can't think what people see in this dancin' business." He looked at Miss James's little ballet pupils in white and pink tutus, hopping rather nervously about the stage.

"There's Pat," said Anthony loudly.

"Sh!" his mother warned.

"Young devil doesn't even look nervous," remarked Mr. Kay. "Looks as though he's enjoin' himself up there, eh, Maude. What do you think?"

But Pat's mother watched her son dance and kept her thoughts to herself.

Before the dancing academy closed for the summer holidays, Mrs. Kay had a long talk with Miss James, who agreed that it would be well worth while to give Pat a more serious training. She suggested her own teachers, Grace and Lily Cone.

"They have a school in London," Miss James explained. "But they come to Brighton twice a week to hold ballet classes. I shall certainly be very sorry to lose Pat, but I realise I can't give him the training he needs in my little classes. There is no doubt about it that he has a great natural gift for dancing."

So it was quietly arranged that next term Pat should start with the Misses Cone.

The autumn, however, was still far away. Now the summer holidays were upon them. The end of July brought Pat's tenth birthday and Philip home from school, a strong, grown-up young man of fifteen.

Mrs. Kay was busy packing trunks for they had planned a family holiday on a farm in Berkshire.

"It'll do us good to get away for a bit," Mrs. Kay had decided, "and like this we shall escape the August holiday crowds."

"Probably won't be any crowds this year," remarked Mr. Kay. "Judging by the way things are going." He rattled the paper. "News getting worse every day."

"But Germany keeps saying she wants peace," said Philip.

"She means she wants to be left in peace to overrun Europe," he snorted.

"If you men would stop thinking about Europe for a minute and tell me if there's anything else you want me to pack." Mrs. Kay interrupted them. "I wonder if two big trunks will be enough?"

The next day they left for Berkshire.

In the sunlit peace of the remote farm the menacing war-clouds receded. Far away in Germany soldiers might be massing on the frontiers, and in London tired, anxious statesmen might be working long hours into the night in a last effort to avert disaster, while servicemen all over the country were hurriedly recalled from leave; but here, in the peaceful heart of Berkshire, the heavy crops ripened to gold in the sun, the air was fragrant with the last of the new hay gathered on to the ricks, and cattle moved lazily through rich green fields.

Here it was easy to push back the haunting spectre of war. School, lessons, everything was forgotten but the glory of the moment, as the boys explored their new territory. There were trees to climb, haystacks to slide down, streams to play in, big cart horses to ride, calves and baby pigs to watch, dogs, kittens and chickens, and all the exciting freedom of a farm.

Philip and Pat planned a long bird-nesting, tree-climbing expedition. Anthony, the proud owner of a pop-gun, had other ideas.

"I'm going to find a rabbit and shoot it," he announced, ramming the cork firmly in the end of the barrel. "Then we shall have rabbit pie for supper."

He tucked his gun under his arm as he had seen the farmer do, and went stalking off, all proud and independent.

"Let's take our gun out with us," said Pat. He and Philip shared a handsome air-gun.

"Good idea." Philip went and fetched it.

"I've found something to shoot at," Pat called out to him. He was leaning on the fence that railed off the orchard. "I'm going to see if I can hit that fallen log over there, beyond the pear tree."

"Where?" Philip followed the pointing finger. "That's not a log," he said suddenly. "It's a pig lying down."

"I'll make her get up in a hurry," Pat squinted along the barrel. "I won't shoot her dead, will I?"

"No. Not at this range."

Pat fired.

"Missed," said Philip.

Pat fired again. Nothing happened.

"What a rotten shot you are." Philip took the gun over. Three more slugs went whining on their way. Still no reaction from the target.

"Who's a rotten shot now?" Pat laughed at him.

"It's funny. I could have sworn I'd hit her."

They climbed through the rails and came nearer to investigate. There was a sudden grunt from their target. Two leathery ears and an inquiring snout appeared. With a vast effort the large, fat pig heaved herself on to her trotters and stood looking at them.

"We can't miss her at this range." Philip raised the gun and aimed for the middle of the pig.

"This'll make her run," Pat chuckled.

It didn't. Philip fired and the pig went on looking at them. The awful conclusion was forced upon them.

"She doesn't feel a thing. Her skin's too thick."

As the boys came up the pig walked unhurriedly away.

"Look!" Pat stooped down. Scattered over the grass they found their bullets, squashed flat. "They've all bounced off her."

"She must be armour-plated like a rhinoceros." Philip loosed a parting shot after the retreating back.

"Hi, there!" A voice was calling them.

"Who's that?" Pat spun round quickly.

"Perhaps they don't like us shooting at their pig." Philip hastily lowered the gun.

It was their father.

"Come here," he called.

They found a little knot of people gathered at the farmhouse door. A red-faced lad on a bicycle seemed to be the centre of attention.

"What is it?" Philip and Pat looked round the circle of serious faces.

"War," said Mr. Kay quietly. "Germany has invaded Belgium, and at midnight we declared war on her." His solemn words struck a cold chill to the heart.

"Yes. I saw it as I were comin' through the village." The red-faced lad spoke up. "They were puttin' up the placards." He had already learned the piece by heart. " 'A state of War exists and mobilisation has been ordered.' That's what it says."

"Mobilisation." The thud of endless marching boots. Armies on the move. Sounds that made the heart beat faster with mingled fear and excitement. "War." The little group of people stood wondering deep in their hearts how this war would touch their lives. It was Philip who voiced the unspoken thought.

"What happens now?" he asked. "What do we do about it?"

There seemed no answer to this. They looked at each other, and the slow-voiced farmer at last spoke his mind.

"The way I see it," he said. "War is a job for the professional soldier." He shifted his weight from one foot to the other. "I don't see how it touches us here. War or not, people must have food; cows have to be milked, the harvest got in, and the stock cared for. That's our job and I reckon we go on doing it." Which piece of countryman's good sense made everyone feel much better.

"He's quite right," added the farmer's wife, looking at her own sons. "There's nothing any of us here can do, except go on with our work." She looked at Mrs. Kay. "Thank God your lads are not old enough to be needed. So don't let it spoil your boys' holiday."

It didn't; for Pat and Anthony, still too young to be touched by the shadow of war, drew Philip back into the charmed circle of their own vivid, childhood's world, and August 1914, the last carefree holiday of the whole family together, was to remain for them all a golden, sunlit memory they would treasure all their lives.

6 Charity Show

"Ready at the bar, everyone. In the first position for your *pliés*." The long line of pupils rose and fell to the measure of the music.

"Keep your heels on the ground as you go down. Body straight." Miss Cone came slowly along the line. "Pat, press your knees farther out . . . Good! Now rest everybody. Ready for *pliés* in second position."

No playing about in Miss Cone's class. No more frilly dresses and romping polkas. This was serious ballet with girls in business-like black practice tunics and boys in plain shirts and shorts.

"How is Pat getting on?" Mrs. Kay asked Miss Cone after the first few lessons.

"He is a very promising pupil," Miss Cone assured her. "He has quite a natural talent, and if only he will work hard he should do very well."

"Doesn't he work hard?"

"Not all the time, I'm afraid," Miss Cone smiled. "You see, he wants to dance, now, at once, and sometimes he gets bored with the dull exercises he has to learn. Those are the bad days when I can't make him work at all."

"I am sorry." Mrs. Kay was surprised and disappointed. "I'll talk to him about it."

"I think it would be better to leave him." Miss Cone was wise in the ways of artistic children. "If he really has got it in him to dance he will do it. It is natural that he should get bored sometimes with the routine work. Do you know what he did the other day to play a joke on me? He got the others to dress him up as a girl and bring him in as a new pupil. There he was in a little tunic, dancing on his points. I had to be cross with him at the time for he was disorganising all the class, but how we laughed afterwards, my sister and I."

"The young devil." But Mrs. Kay couldn't help laughing too. "Isn't that just like his mischief."

"He was very sorry afterwards," Miss Cone went on, "and worked twice as hard to make up for it. I know he really wants to learn, and if he has the patience to go through with his training he should make a very fine dancer."

At home, Mr. Kay was more concerned with the war news than his son's progress at dancing class. In the study whose walls were hung with sporting prints, and trophies, treasured relics of his active, sportsman's life, Mr. Kay, submerged in a deep leather arm-chair, studied newspapers and maps, and grew restive because he was too old to take part in the war.

Philip was too young, or so they all thought, until he suddenly announced his intention of joining up.

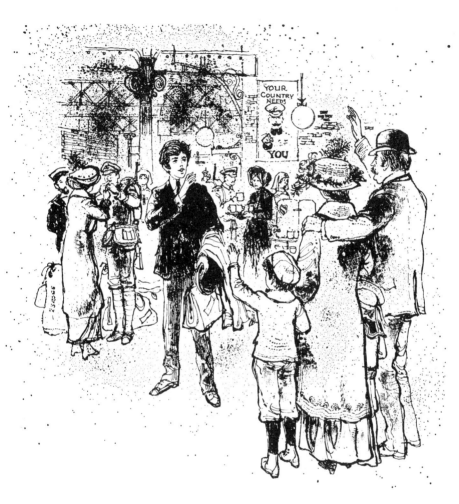

"Everyone says the fighting will be over in six months," he told them. "I don't want to miss it."

Shortly afterwards his call-up papers arrived with orders to join a Training Unit, and Pat and Anthony were saying good-bye to a grown-up soldier brother.

"I'll be back before long." Philip's courage was high as he left them. "We'll soon finish off those Germans."

"Wish I was going with him," his father sighed as he watched him go.

"I'm glad you can't. It's enough to lose one of you." Mrs. Kay hugged her two younger sons close to her and thanked God that at least the war couldn't take these from her. How proud she felt of her eldest son, and how afraid for him too.

All over the country young men like Philip were disappearing from the civilian scene, to be turned into drab, khaki figures with packs on their backs and rifles in their hands.

But while the great machinery of Mobilisation slowly gathered speed and strength, everyday life at home went on, much as usual. There were still houses to be run, meals to be seen to, the shopping to do, children to go to school.

Pat came home from dancing class one Saturday, bubbling with excitement.

"Miss Cone is to give a display and she wants me to dance in it. It's going to be in a real theatre."

"That's a great honour to have been chosen, darling. Especially your first term."

"She told me what she wants me to do." Pat was full of enthusiasm. "It's to be a surprise and a secret, but you must know about it because you'll have to help."

It turned out that the display was really a Charity Show Miss Cone was getting up; for even dancing pupils could do their bit for the war. Pat, encouraged by his mother, worked hard for it, going to extra practices and rehearsals. She herself worked hard making his costumes and selling tickets to all her friends.

It was to be at the Hippodrome at Brighton.

"I hope you're coming to see him dance." Mrs. Kay produced tickets for her husband and Anthony. "I shan't be able to sit with you as I have to be at the back to help Pat change."

The theatre was well filled on the great night. Down in the stalls, Anthony, very proud to be out alone with his father, sat up especially straight and talked loudly about Pat.

Behind the shrouding velvet curtain, backstage was the usual excited confusion, inseparable from a children's charity show. The two Miss Cones hurried to and fro, trying to be everywhere at once, and succeeding.

"Don't wriggle, Pat, or I'll get this lipstick smeared." Mrs. Kay was trying to colour up his mouth. "There you are, I've done the outline, now smooth it in yourself."

"It's all right like that." Pat took a quick look in the glass. He saw a pale face with large brown eyes, very bright in the lights, and a vivid mouth. He was already dressed in his first costume, a navy-blue and white sailor suit. "Do you think it's time to go down?" He danced about practising a few steps of his sailor's hornpipe.

"Come here and let me tidy your hair." Mrs. Kay grabbed him and held him still with one hand while she combed his dark hair smooth with the other.

Miss Grace Cone looked in.

"Ready, Pat?"

"Yes, Miss Cone." He ran forward for inspection.

"Is he all right?" Mrs. Kay asked.

"Yes, he looks very nice," she replied. "You'll have plenty of time to come up here and change before your second number." She looked at Pat's costume hanging up on the stand, smiled, and wished him good luck.

"They're starting." Anthony wriggled excitedly in his seat as the house lights faded and the footlights blazed into action.

The heavy curtain swung off the floor, and to the music of "The Nutcracker" Suite, on to the stage came a long line of Miss Cone's *corps de ballet*.

"Aren't they sweet." The friendly audience welcomed them in. Never mind if some of them were rather wobbly on their points, and others didn't quite keep time, they looked so young and pretty it didn't matter.

"When's Pat coming on?" Anthony whispered loudly as the *corps de ballet* floated unevenly into the wings.

"Sh!" said Mr. Kay, and they watched two older girls do their *pas de deux*.

The music changed and a row of little girls in white blouses, pleated navy-blue skirts and cheeky sailor caps ran on to the stage.

"There's Pat!" Anthony clutched his father's arm.

Out in front of the row of girls ran a saucy sailor boy, and the rhythm of the hornpipe set everyone's feet tapping.

"Good tune that." This was something Mr. Kay could appreciate. "Plenty of life about it."

The rest of the audience liked it too and the dancers went off to a good round of applause.

The show went on, and in the interval Mr. Kay bought Anthony a lemonade.

They both laughed over the antics of two comedy dancers. Somebody sang, a little boy recited a poem, and a group of girls in bare feet and white tunics danced a Greek legend.

"Want to see Pat again." Anthony was growing impatient.

"He'll be on soon, I expect."

"Perhaps this is him." Anthony sat up as the tune changed for the next number. "Oh no!" He sank back. "It's another girl."

To the strains of Mendelssohn's "Spring Song", a golden-haired little girl came floating in from the wings. Her small oval face was very serious as, poised on her toes, she danced. The fluffy pink ballet dress stood out in a cloud round her legs.

"Isn't she sweet," said a lady behind Anthony.

"Very graceful indeed," said another. Mr. Kay and Anthony, however, were not particularly interested in a little girl dancing.

"Do you think Pat will be on next?" Anthony whispered as the "Spring Song" came to an end. The little girl sank down in a low, graceful curtsy before the applause she had won.

"Well done," people clapped. "Very nice." The clapping faltered. There was a gasp as the little girl rose up again. Her pink ballet frock had fallen to the ground. The golden wig had suddenly vanished, and there was the cropped dark head and thin body of a boy.

"It's Pat!" Anthony suddenly shouted. "Look. It's Pat!"

The audience loved it. Applause and laughter echoed round the theatre as Pat, clothed only in a pair of pink knickers, picked up his dress, waved his wig at them, with a mischievous grin, and went running off into the wings where his mother waited for him.

"A very good show, Pat." Miss Cone came into the dressing-room after the performance was all over. "Our secret was a great success."

There was a knock on the door and a man came in. Miss Cone introduced Mr. Boardman, the manager of the theatre.

"I just looked in to congratulate your boy, Mrs. Kay," he said. "Very good little number he gave to-night. The public loved it. Good idea that, dressing him up as a girl."

"I got the idea from Pat himself." Miss Cone smiled at Pat as she retold the story of the practical joke he had played on her.

"I must say it's the first time I've seen a boy dance on his toes," said Mr. Boardman. "And it comes natural to you?"

"Yes."

"He's always been keen on dancing ever since he was a small boy," added Mrs. Kay.

"Does he want to do it professionally?"

"I don't know." She looked at Pat doubtfully.

"He should do," said Mr. Boardman. "Your boy has talent, Mrs. Kay. Believe me, I've seen enough youngsters on the stage in my time to recognise the real thing when I see it."

"We've never really taken Pat's dancing very seriously," Mrs. Kay explained. "We only let him go to classes because he was so keen on it, but if he really has talent for this sort of thing . . ."

"There's no question about it," Mr. Boardman was emphatic. "Your boy has a natural gift for the stage. I would strongly advise you to have him trained and let him make it his career."

"I quite agree with you," added Miss Cone.

"Yes, but how does one go about it?" Mrs. Kay looked from one to the other, sensing that a cross-roads had been reached in Pat's life and that a far-reaching decision would have to be made.

"He needs proper training."

"If I could have him at our school in London," Miss Cone suggested, "he could have full-time training and the chance of work in West End theatres."

"Miss Cone's right," Mr. Boardman nodded his agreement. "I'd say London is the place for him."

Mrs. Kay, faced with this sudden inrush of new ideas, looked to her son for help.

"What do you think about it, Pat?" But even before she asked, she knew what the answer would be. It was shining in his eyes.

"London," he said.

7 London

It was a clear summer dawn, and two large, snub-nosed motor vans were chugging purposefully along the road to London. At the back of one, perched among the piled-up furniture, Pat watched the ribbon of road slipping away under the solid rubber tyres. Beside him, in a large open packing-case, was his bird-cage. High above the clatter and fuss of the engine poured the clear notes of a bird's song.

"He's singing for me," said Pat to himself. "He's singing because he's happy we're going to London," and his own heart seemed to rise with happiness to the bird's song. "You'll bring me luck," he said aloud, and at the sound of his voice the bird stopped singing, hopped on to his swinging perch, turned a backward somersault and cocked his head on one side to see if his master was looking.

"Go on then," said Pat, "do another." The bird swung over again and again; round and round he went, and as Pat watched he seemed to see his grandfather again, teaching him to do the trick. That made him think of the house at Hove, deserted now, all the rooms empty and unfriendly. He wondered who would go and live there; if anyone would feed the birds in the garden. Then he thought ahead to the new house in London and tried to imagine what it would be like. He wished Anthony was with him, they would have had a wonderful time together in the van, climbing over the furniture and waving to the people as they passed. Poor Anthony was at boarding-school this term. Pat remembered the day he had gone off, looking rather self-conscious in his new uniform and school cap, and very determined not to cry.

It was funny how quickly things happened. It seemed such a little while ago since last summer when they were all together on the farm, sliding down haystacks and shooting at the pig. Anthony never did get a rabbit after all. Now everything was suddenly different with Philip away in the army and Anthony gone to school, while dancing had become the most important thing in Pat's life.

He thought of his first appearance at the Hippodrome in the pink ballet dress and the golden wig. He remembered too, as he had come on to the stage, the sudden glare of the footlights had dazzled him so that he had forgotten his steps. He could still hear Miss Cone's urgent whisper from the wings.

"That's right, Pat, dear, now do a *pas de chat*, turn round on your toes, now *glissade* and *ensemble*. Repeat, dear, that's a good child."

Luckily the audience hadn't seemed to notice anything.

He'd got used to the footlights now, for the little girl with golden hair had since made several successful appearances at charity shows, as well as the small boy Pat Kay, who danced, and even sang or recited poems that his mother taught him.

"I shall recite you a poem," he shouted at his bird through the vibrating roar of the engines. The bird stopped turning somersaults and listened politely, with his head cocked on one side.

"Did you like it?" Pat inquired. "I like reciting poems, but I'd rather dance." He stretched his legs out on the top of the packing case and looked at his bird through his knees.

"I want to dance." He wriggled his toes about. "I want to dance like those people Miss Cone tells us about." He frowned, trying to remember. "Pavlova. That's right, and Karsavina. They're very famous. And who was the wonderful man who could jump higher than anyone else . . . what was his name . . . Ni . . . Nijinsky. Yes, I'm going to dance as well as he did. Mother and Father keep telling me that if I go on the stage I ought to be an actor," he confided to his bird. "But I'd much rather dance to lovely music." His bird bobbed about on its perch in agreement, and went spinning round in another series of back somersaults.

Pat yawned suddenly and wondered what time they would arrive, and whether Father and Mother would get there first. They were going by train. He had been allowed, as a great treat, to travel with the furniture. It had meant getting up at half past four, a horrible, cold, middle-of-the-night feeling, dragging oneself, half asleep, out of a warm bed to stand shivering in the chill, grey morning air, pulling on one's clothes and feeling slightly sick. A welcome, scalding hot cup of tea, and by five o'clock they had been on the move. The big vans had gone rumbling through the deserted streets, past the quiet, sleeping houses. A last glimpse of the sea, a misty blue-grey line beyond the roofs and chimneys, and they were clear of the town, and away in the open country. The sun had come up, turning the sky to blue and gold, with all the promise of a glorious summer day, and the long ribbon of road stretched ahead of them.

He wondered what the time was now. It seemed they had been travelling for hours and hours. They had stopped three times on the road already, to put water into the engines and tea into the men. Pat felt sleepy, but it was too bumpy to do anything about it for every time he laid his head on something it got jolted off again, so he sang songs to his bird or watched the road, and the throbbing engine shook him into a dazed, half-awake state.

One more stop before the spreading tentacles of the London suburbs reached out to them, and soon the open fields and gardens were crowded out, as the miles of grimy brick closed in. How did anyone find their way about this tangle of streets, Pat wondered. They all looked alike, a squalid, dingy muddle of cobbles and tram-lines, factory walls, sooty houses, and rows of huddled shops.

Then, quite suddenly, they had come out of the clanking traffic and the crowds that swarmed through the sprawling, brick wilder-ness of south London; they were on an open bridge, with the wide, brown Thames shining below.

A few more twists and turns and the vans came to a stop.

"Well, sonny, here we are." One of the men came round to lift him down. "Safe and sound at your new home."

Pat stood on the pavement and looked up at 49 Bishops Mansions, Fulham.

The front door was open and the men from the first van were already carrying in the furniture.

"Aren't you going in to look at your new home?" one of them asked. Pat shook his head. The house suddenly didn't interest him. He wanted to be away, on his own. He turned and wandered along to the end of the road, where he found the park that fringed the bank of the Thames. In the far corner was a railing. Here he sat, a small, solitary figure, looking down at the wide, shining river sliding past.

"I'm in London," he said softly to himself. "We've come to live in London, and all because of me."

He looked along to the strings of barges moored out in the stream. He saw the distant huddle of wharves, and beyond them the crowded, smoky skyline that held the pulsing heart of the Capital. London was to be his home. A new life was beginning, like a new chapter waiting to be written. What did the future hold for him?

He looked up. Overhead, slow, white clouds drifted over the smoky grey pall of the city. He watched them, his mind crowded with dreams and half-formed ambitions; but through them all beat the steady determination to make his own way in life, to do something that mattered, to be someone who counted in this great city.

London seemed to fling out a challenge. He accepted it.

8 The First Job

"Dear Anthony . . ." Pat, kneeling on a chair, sprawled over the table, pen in hand. "It's been very dull since you went back to school . . ."

He stared at the rest of the blank page in front of him thinking over the summer holiday. It had been fun having Anthony home, showing him the new house and exploring their own bit of London. They had enjoyed being together, but they had both missed the old free life with the garden and the sea. It wasn't really much fun being in London in August when the hot, sunny days made one long to go running down to the beach for a swim.

Though neither of them had said much about it, they had missed Philip badly. It was their first long summer holiday without him.

"Philip thinks he'll be coming home on leave soon," he wrote. "I hope it'll be in the Christmas holidays, then you'll see him too . . ."

How lovely it would be for the three of them to be together.

Pat felt very alone now that Anthony had gone back to his boarding-school.

". . . I hope you have a good term . . ." He chewed the end of his pen thoughtfully and a blob of ink fell on to the page. "I go to dancing classes every day at Miss Cone's. I love it. I have a governess now, called Miss Etwell. She has red hair and very long eyelashes. I thought she stuck them on but I looked through the keyhole and she doesn't . . ."

He looked over his shoulder as the door opened, and there was Miss Etwell coming into the schoolroom. She was slim and pale, in a white blouse, a long black skirt, with a broad, shiny black belt pulled very tightly round her waist. She frowned as she saw the sprawling figure of her pupil.

"Pat, what are you doing?"

"I'm writing a letter." He looked at her out of the corner of his eyes, wondering if she could see what he'd put.

"Sit down on the chair properly," she told him.

"I write better like this."

"Nonsense," she insisted. "Sit down."

"She's just come in . . ." Pat's spidery writing went on, as he reluctantly got into the required position. The letter was hurriedly finished.

"Have you learned your poem yet?" Miss Etwell settled herself in the big arm-chair and picked up the paper. "Your mother wants to go over it with you this evening."

Miss Cone's Charity Shows were still with them.

"I know most of it." Pat sighed, picked the book out of the untidy pile on the table, twisted himself into a new knot on the chair, and began to study.

The silence in the schoolroom was broken only by the crackle and fall of the coals in the fire and the rustle of Miss Etwell's paper. Pat fidgeted uneasily, muttering his poem to himself, Miss Etwell read through the war news. No signs of peace yet in this daily record of battle and death. How wrong they had been at the beginning when they had all said the Germans would be finished off in six months. It was already October 1915. The war had been going on for over a year.

Miss Etwell sighed, and turned over the page in search of something that made more cheerful reading. A little paragraph caught her eye.

"Oh!" she exclaimed. "There's something here that might interest you, Pat. Boys and girls are wanted to take part in a play."

"Let's see?" Pat came and looked over her shoulder. " 'Auditions will be held for a forthcoming production by Mr. Seymour Hicks,' " he read out. "Who's that?"

"Haven't you heard of Mr. Hicks? He's a very famous actor."

"I wonder what sort of a play it is." Pat's interest was aroused.

"The auditions are on the 28th." Miss Etwell looked at the advertisement again. "That's the day after to-morrow. At the Prince's Theatre."

"I don't see why I shouldn't try for that. I'll show this to Mother and see what she thinks." Pat went running off to find her.

Outside the Prince's Theatre a lugubrious commissionaire with a white moustache was standing on guard.

"Brought your little boy for the audition, lady?" He gazed mournfully at Mrs. Kay. "Not in 'ere. Round the back." He jerked a thumb. "Stage door."

"Audition, lady?" The stage door keeper glared at them disapprovingly. "Through that door there."

Pat and his mother found themselves on a stage, bare of scenery and swarming with people.

"Do you think they've all come for the audition?" Pat gazed at this alarming, churning crowd of girls and boys.

A harassed-looking stage manager trying to make his way through was besieged.

"What time does it begin?" One mother pulled at his sleeve.

"Where can I change my little girl's dress?" Another closed in, plucking at his coat.

"Where is the pianist?" A third waved a sheaf of music under his nose. "I want him to go over my little boy's song."

"Will we have to wait long?"

"I don't know." The stage manager looked desperate and fled. Mrs. Kay drew Pat aside.

"We'll just stand here and wait until they tell us where to go."

"Is Mr. Hicks here?" Pat wanted to know.

"He's over there." A nearby mother overheard them. She pointed.

Pat, standing on tiptoe, caught sight of two men surrounded by a swirling tide of mothers.

"That one on the left is Mr. Hicks," he was told. "The dark man with him is Mr. Wolheim, his manager."

"What play is it?" asked Mrs. Kay.

"It's a revival of *Bluebell in Fairyland*. It's several years now since Mr. Hicks has done it. Lovely play for the kiddies. He wrote it himself you know."

Someone clapped their hands.

"Clear the stage, please."

Parents and children were herded into the side. Mr. Hicks and Mr. Wolheim made their way down to the stalls.

The audition began.

One by one the children were called out to do their piece. Some recited, some sang, others danced. Pat's mother had made him prepare two or three of the recitations he had done at charity shows.

"Which shall I do?" he whispered urgently as the boys were called out and it began to look like his turn soon.

She didn't answer for she was watching a mournful-looking boy on the stage plodding his way through a mournful poem.

"That will do, sonny." Mr. Hicks interrupted him after two verses. "You can go." He turned to Mr. Wolheim beside him, and Mrs. Kay overheard him say: "No good, too sentimental."

"Next, please."

The stage manager looked over the line of boys.

"Your turn," he signed to Pat.

Mrs. Kay bent and whispered quickly:

"Recite Dan Cupid."

Mr. Hicks looked up as Pat walked on to the stage.

"What's your name, sonny?"

"Pat, sir. Pat Kay."

"How old are you?"

"Twelve, sir."

"Done any stage work before?"

"Yes, sir." He hoped he wouldn't be asked for details.

"What are you going to do now?"

"Recite a poem."

"All right. Go ahead." Mr. Hicks smothered a yawn.

"Dan Cupid," Pat announced. The poem was short. It was comic. There was a pause.

"All right, sonny," Mr. Hicks told him. "Go and stand over there, will you, and wait."

Mr. Wolheim, who was taking notes, leaned over and said something.

"Well, at least he speaks the King's English," replied Mr. Hicks loudly.

Pat's hopes rose as he crossed to the other side of the stage to join the lucky ones who had also been told to wait. He caught his mother's eye and winked at her.

The audition went on, it seemed, for hours. Gradually the crowd thinned out as the unsuccessful were packed into coats and outdoor shoes and taken away.

"Is that the lot?" Mr. Hicks called out at last.

"Yes, sir." The stage manager bobbed into sight.

"Bring these others on." He waved towards the survivors. There were about forty of them in all. They were fetched on stage again, lined up and looked over. Two or three more were sent home. Finally the chosen bunch were paraded into the stalls. The long line of them queued up in the centre gangway.

They moved slowly along to Mr. Wolheim who was taking names and addresses.

It was the turn of the small boy in front of Pat.

"The part of the Fish Boy," they heard Mr. Wolheim say. "What salary do you want?"

Pat nudged his mother urgently.

"What do we say?"

"I don't know." They looked at each other doubtfully, wondering what on earth one should be paid for a job on the stage. Then Mrs. Kay heard the "Fish Boy's" father ask for £2.

"We'll ask for the same," she whispered.

"Pat Kay, 49 Bishops Mansions," Mr. Wolheim wrote it down. "For the part of Peter, the Black Cat, £2. There will be twelve performances a week," he told them. "We'll send you on the contract. First rehearsal Monday, ten o'clock."

Pat and his mother were walking on air as they left the theatre. A contract for a West End theatre. How important it sounded. £2 a week when one was only twelve years old.

"I'm rich," said Pat.

He spent the journey home planning all the things he would buy for the family with his new fortune.

The first rehearsal saw a collection of thirty children and a sprinkling of adults assembled on the stage before Mr. Hicks. Mothers were banished into dark corners out of sight. Someone handed out scripts. Mr. Hicks explained what the play was about, and Pat discovered that Peter the Black Cat was quite a leading part, most of it with Bluebell herself.

"Who is playing Bluebell?" he whispered to a big boy standing near him.

"Miss Terriss, of course, she always plays it."

"Who's she?"

The boy stared down at him, wondering where this ignorant new arrival had sprung from.

"Mr. Hicks's wife, of course. She's over there talking to the stage manager."

Pat had a quick glimpse of a beautiful, expressive face.

"We will walk through Act I with books this morning," Mr. Hicks was saying. "The rest of you Fairyland people who aren't in Act I go now with Mr. Farren to learn your dances."

The stage was rapidly cleared. Only a few of them remained. Miss Terriss, self-possessed and charming, came over to where Pat stood by himself, feeling rather lost.

"I hear you are to be my cat, Peter," she smiled at him.

"Yes." Pat looked up at her and thought how lovely she was.

"Is this your first show?"

"Yes, it is really." He felt one didn't mention charity shows when one was in a real professional West End theatre.

She looked across to where her husband was talking to some of the men from the cast.

"Come over here in a corner," she whispered. "I'll explain what you have to do before they start."

The rehearsal trailed through the long hours of the morning.

"All right. Break for lunch. Back at 2.30 this afternoon. We'll go through the same act." Mr. Hicks dismissed them.

"Isn't Miss Terriss a wonderful person?" said Pat enthusiastically as he joined his mother.

"I was asking Mr. Wolheim what happened about your school lessons." Mrs. Kay, at that moment, was more concerned with Pat's education. "We can't have you missing your school work every day like this. He tells me they engage a governess to teach all you children here, on the spot, so that you can fit in school with the rehearsals."

Pat, however, thinking about the beautiful Miss Terriss, wasn't listening, and Mrs. Kay went on talking to herself.

"I wonder if Miss Etwell would be interested to apply for the post."

Miss Etwell was. She applied; Mrs. Kay recommended her highly to Mr. Wolheim, and she got the job. What a job too!

In a makeshift schoolroom set up over the L.C.C. Swimming Baths opposite the theatre, she faced, each day, her unruly class of thirty rowdy, high-spirited boys and girls.

The rehearsals dragged out their tedious length. Through

tears and temperaments, curses and praise, boredom and delight, Bluebell and her fairy world were slowly and painfully brought to life.

There were the days when things went well and Mr. Hicks was charming.

There were the other days.

"No! You little fool." Mr. Hicks raged at Pat. "Think what you're doing. My God, the boy's got no brains." And Pat, paralysed with fright, hadn't.

"Go through that bit again, and remember in this second act you're no longer just an animal, you've become human."

How complicated it was, to be a cat and a human at the same time.

"Not so fast," Mr. Hicks screamed from the stalls. "Watch your timing. Now, go back and take it again."

Pat, near to tears, took it again.

"All right, go on."

"Don't worry, Peter, dear, you're all right." Miss Terriss whispered to him. "It's coming on well." Pat adored her.

At the end of the rehearsal Mr. Hicks called him over.

"Yes, sir." Pat ran across the stage wondering what fresh horrors lay in store.

"Here, sonny, catch!" A coin flicked across the footlights, a silver half-crown landed in Pat's hand.

"Go and buy yourself a box of chocolates." Mr. Hicks, without waiting for Pat's startled and incoherent thanks, turned away to talk to someone else.

Pat looked up from the half-crown and saw Miss Terriss smiling at him.

"Do you think it's all right to take it?" he asked anxiously.

"Of course, take it, Peter." She always called him by his part name. "Take anything you can get."

"But I worked so badly to-day. I mean, Mr. Hicks was so annoyed with me."

"That's his way of showing you that it's all forgotten." She came and put her arm round him. "You mustn't let it worry you so much when he gets cross. You see, he gets impatient because we've done Bluebell so many times before he knows exactly how he wants each bit played, and you can't always manage it first time,

or even second time. After all, you're very young and you just
haven't had the experience, but he forgets that. I know it seems
very hard, but you take my advice." She leaned closer to him. "Try
not to mind about the shouting, but take notice of all these things
he tells you. You can learn such a lot from him."

Her gentle words poured healing into Pat's sore heart, giving
him back his confidence in himself.

He smiled up at her, finding no words to express the swelling
gratitude for her understanding and encouragement.

His day, however, was not finished. Mr. Farren had still to have
the last word.

"Rehearsal Act II, same time to-morrow." The stage manager
came on. "Will those of you who dance in Act I stay behind, please.
Mr. Farren wants to run through the dances now."

The children involved looked at each other and sighed. Dance
rehearsals provoked nearly as many storms as the others.

"Peter, on stage, please," Mr. Farren called Pat out. "We'll go
through your minuet. Can you remember the steps from last
time?"

"I think so." Pat had done it only once.

The music started.

"No." Mr. Farren stopped him. "Two paces to the right, bow,
and then turn to the left."

Pat tried again and didn't seem able to get the hang of it.

"No," Mr. Farren came on stage. "Follow me now. Do it like
this. One, two—bow, and turn to the left." He demonstrated.

Pat, tired and flustered from the storm of his other rehearsal
with Mr. Hicks, took two paces, bowed and turned to the right.

Mr. Farren's blood pressure rose.

"Left, I said, not right," he shouted.

A bored pianist in the wings thumped out the bars again. Pat,
panic stricken, forgot his bow.

That finished it.

"Leave it alone." Mr. Farren strode off the stage in a fury.
"You may make an actor, my lad," he shouted for all the world to
hear. "But my God, you'll never be a dancer."

Pat felt he had now heard everything.

"Here's your costume, duckie." The wardrobe mistress brought the black cat's skin into the dressing-room and hung it on the stand. "I want to see you in it before you go on."

"Yes," said Pat.

"Now where's the Fish Boy? I want you during the interval." She made her way through the crowded room and was promptly waylaid by excited boys.

"Lor' luv a duck!" She covered her ears. "You're worse than the girls."

The door opened and Mr. McKay, one of the men in the cast, looked in.

"Is Peter the Cat in here?"

"Yes." Pat, half undressed, twisted round on his chair.

"I've been told to come and make you up." Mr. McKay did not appear to relish the idea.

"Do I finish getting changed first?"

"No. Always make up before you put on your costume." Mr. McKay was young, tall and elegant and obviously had no time for little boys.

Pat presented his face and Mr. McKay ungraciously covered it with an assortment of colours.

"Can't think why they don't teach you little beggars to make yourselves up before you start on this profession." He squinted down a greasepaint stick at Pat's eyebrows, and went on grumbling as he worked.

"Well, there you are. That'll have to do." He gave a final dab of powder. "It's a straight make-up. I suppose that's what they want."

"Thank you very much."

Pat turned and looked at himself in the glass. At least, he supposed it was himself, for an entirely strange object was staring back at him. He saw a startling pink face, two black eyes, a red and rather shapeless mouth and two George Robey eyebrows.

Mr. McKay had gone.

"I say," Pat asked his neighbour, the Fish Boy, "am I meant to look like this, do you think?"

The Fish Boy gazed at him without flinching.

"I expect it'll be all right in the lights," he said.

Pat got into his costume. The cat's skin was all in one piece, buttoning up the front. He had big padded paws at the end of his arms and legs, and a moulded cat's head which left just a hole under the jaw, where his face appeared.

The call-boy rapped on the door.

"Overture and beginners, please," he called in his sing-song voice. They went trooping down the stairs to the stage.

Miss Terriss, a radiant-looking Bluebell, was standing in the wings, as calm and untroubled as always.

"How's my Peter feeling?" she smiled at Pat, and whatever she thought of Mr. McKay's efforts on his face, she tactfully gave no sign.

"I'm all right, thank you, Miss Terriss." He thought how young and lovely she looked. She didn't seem to have any make-up on at all.

"Not nervous?" she asked him.

"No." He shook his head. It had never occurred to him to be nervous. Looking at her face more carefully, he could see now how she had put on her make-up. He noticed the careful eyeshadow, and the rouge of her cheeks that blended into the deepened colour of her skin. Pat resolved to make up his own face next time.

"Is your mother out in front to-night?"

"Yes, and my father too."

Mr. Hicks came upon them. He was tense with nerves.

"Ah! There you are, Ellaline," his presence charged the atmosphere with electricity. "You won't forget that new business in the second scene? You! Peter . . ." He jabbed a finger at Pat, "don't hurry that minuet . . ." He broke off as he noticed Pat's face. "Good God, what a make-up. Get someone to show you how to do it next time . . . Oh, Eric!" He caught sight of Mr. Wolheim and went charging off before Pat could explain about his face; not that Mr. Hicks would have listened anyway.

"Why is he so nervous?" Pat wanted to know. "I mean, he's been on the stage before so he ought to be used to it."

Miss Terriss laughed.

"Lucky boy," she told him. "You don't know yet about first-night nerves."

"But you're not nervous."

"That's very sweet of you to say so. You see," she confided in him, "I am really, inside of me, but I try not to let it show. It's enough to have one in the family with nerves!"

The stage manager came by.

"Ready, Miss Terriss?"

"Yes." Her hand rested a moment on Pat's arm. "Good luck, Peter."

To Pat, all this first-night business had a strangely unreal quality, like a game of make-believe at a party. In spite of rehearsals, or perhaps because of them, he still had only the most confused idea of what the whole play was all about. His own part, he thought of merely as a string of things to be said and actions to be done, exactly as Mr. Hicks had taught him, without in the least understanding why.

Meanwhile, the curtain went up. The play had begun.

"Ready for your cue, Peter?" Someone whispered to him in the darkness of the wings.

"Yes, I'm ready." He crouched down on all fours, close to the window, timing his entrance. This was it—now!

The Black Cat jumped through the window and on to the bed, just as he had learned to do at rehearsals.

"Don't hurry it." He could almost hear Mr. Hicks's voice beside him. "Stay on the bed a moment. Give the audience a chance to see you before you jump down and cross to Bluebell." Automatically Pat carried out his instructions. He crouched on the bed, looking round, but, as he paused there, he suddenly realised it wasn't his imagination. He could really hear Mr. Hicks's voice. An angry, hissing whisper was coming from the wings, and it was directed at him. What was he doing wrong this time? He jumped hastily off the bed, and in the panic of the moment got up on his hind legs and walked across to Bluebell on two feet instead of four paws.

The vicious whispering was plainly audible now.

"Get down on all fours, you little fool." The full force of Mr. Hicks's rage hit him. "Don't show your face to the audience. What do you think you are doing?"

Poor Peter. The magic and excitement had fled, and a terrified small boy dropped on to his hands and knees. His mouth opened and a sad, pitiful "Miaow" came from his choked-up throat. Thank goodness he had managed to get that sound out in the right place.

This was Bluebell's cue to turn round and see her cat—a cat who was vowing to himself at that moment that nothing would induce him ever to go on the stage again. Then he saw Bluebell's face. She gave him a special look and a smile. He came and rubbed his head against her, stroking her dress with one paw. The audience loved it, and the Cat decided that the stage wasn't so bad after all.

The rest of Bluebell's first night went without a hitch.

After the show was all over his mother and father came round to the dressing-room.

"It was wonderful, darling," his mother hugged him.

"Very good, my boy." Mr. Kay, tall, slim and sporting, looked quite out of place among the clutter of the boys' dressing-room.

"Did you see when I went wrong at the beginning?" Pat, still worked up, found relief in talking. "Mr. Hicks shouted at me from the wings, it was awful."

"I didn't notice anything," his mother reassured him.

"You must have done. I walked across the stage instead of going on all fours."

"Oh that!" she said easily. "Nobody would notice, or if they did they wouldn't remember."

"The whole thing looked all right to me," said his father. "Very good play. Fine actor, Mr. Hicks."

"What a charming Bluebell Miss Terriss is," said Mrs. Kay. "I thought it was altogether a beautiful production."

The first night was over. The revived *Bluebell* was welcomed back into theatreland. Box office business was good. Mr. Hicks was charming and everyone breathed more easily.

Bluebell settled down to her task of taking two audiences a day into the charmed world of fairyland that waited behind the big velvet curtains.

For the children in the cast, the run of *Bluebell* was one long frolic, starting in the morning when the whole rowdy, romping crowd of them collected in the classroom over the swimming baths, with one idea only in mind; to have as much fun and as little school as possible.

By lunch-time Miss Etwell may have been worn out, but not her lively charges. Fortified with sandwiches, buns and milk, they swarmed happily into the theatre to get ready for the matinée, and invaded the dressing-rooms with noise, laughter and practical jokes, most of which were attributed to Pat.

At intervals an outraged stage manager read the riot act and threatened to have them put out of the show.

"But I didn't mean to drop it on the stage." Pat, full of virtuous indignation, stood before the stage manager. "It was a mistake."

The subject of dispute was a stink bomb that had made hideous the whole of the first act.

"Oh! And where did you mean to drop it, may I inquire?"

"In the girls' dressing-room."

"You did, did you?" And the stage manager, suddenly seeing again the faces of the cast as they had acted their way through a stench of sulphurous decay, had to turn away quickly to hide a laugh.

The stink bomb incident was followed by the ink episode.

"No, I didn't put ink on the other children's clothes," Pat defended himself hotly against the wardrobe mistress's accusations. This was quite true, he hadn't, but he got blamed for it anyway. How unjust!

Slightly less unjust was the rage of one of the actors, Fred Buckstone, who came storming into the boys' dressing-room, his eyes red and streaming.

"Which of you has been messing about with my moustache? You . . ." he caught sight of Pat. "I suppose it's . . . Ah! . . . Ah! . . . Ahtishoo!" A mighty sneeze shook him from top to toe. There was a riotous giggle from the boys.

"You—just wait till I get hold of you . . ." Another sneeze shook him.

Pat didn't wait. He fled to hide in the wings, where a delighted bunch of children gathered to watch poor Fred Buckstone struggle through his part fighting the itching, tickling, sneezing powder that Pat had thoughtfully sprinkled in his moustache.

So it went on. *Bluebell* ran for three happy months at the Prince's Theatre, and all too soon came the sad day in March when they gave the last performance and were saying good-bye.

"See you next year," they all said to each other, for surely there would be another *Bluebell* next Christmas time.

"What are you going to do after this?" one of them asked Pat. "I don't know." He shrugged his shoulders. "Ordinary lessons again, I suppose." How dull and flat it would be he thought. Lessons by himself again with Miss Etwell.

It didn't work out like that, however, for at home his father was to ask the same question.

"What are we going to do with Pat now this is over?"

"Nothing, dear," Mrs. Kay was surprised. "I mean, he'll go on with his dancing and school lessons as before, won't he?"

Mr. Kay, however, had been doing some serious thinking.

"It's all very well, this acting business, but the boy has got to have a proper education," he announced.

"He gets a proper education from Miss Etwell," said Mrs. Kay mildly. "I'm sure she's very good with him."

"A boy of his age needs a man to teach him and proper school discipline." Mr. Kay spoke very firmly. "He's been running wild these last months and hasn't learned a thing. I tell you, Maude, the boy should go to a boarding-school like his brothers."

They had had discussions like this before, but Mrs. Kay realised that this time her husband really meant business. He was deeply concerned with Pat's lack of what he called proper education.

"What about his dancing lessons if he goes away to school?"

"Look here, Maude, you're not going to spoil the boy's chances for the future because of this idea that he likes dancing." Mr. Kay spoke with great decision. "After all, he's only twelve, we don't know if he's going to do any good on the stage when he grows up. We've got to give him a decent education to fit him to earn his own living."

Mrs. Kay had, unwillingly, to admit that his reasoning was perfectly right. Pat should have a proper schooling. Why, then, did all her instincts cry out against making this drastic change in his life?

"We've sent Philip to a good school, and Anthony too. We'll do the same for Pat," said Mr. Kay, and she knew her cause was lost.

"Will you send him to the same school as Anthony?" she asked him.

"No," he replied. "Anthony has settled down very nicely on his own. We don't want Pat to arrive and lead him into mischief. We'll find somewhere else." He was determined to have his own way, and he got it.

So it came about that, at the beginning of the summer term, a cross and miserable Pat was put into a uniform and dispatched to a boarding-school.

10 "*A Proper Education*"

"I hate it here, when can I leave?" Pat wrote with unfailing regularity to his parents, and his mother wrote back with equal regularity, but without conviction.

"You must be patient. I'm sure you'll like it when you've got used to it."

A half-term report informed them that Pat's progress in education was practically nil, whereas his performance at games and sports was remarkable.

"Looks as though he'll turn into a fine sportsman." Mr. Kay read this part of the report with high approval. "Much better life for a boy, proper healthy outdoor activities."

"I thought you sent him away to be well educated," suggested Mrs. Kay with gentle malice. "His school work doesn't seem to be advancing much."

Mr. Kay's reply was inarticulate.

"We had the school sports on Saturday," Pat wrote later on in the term. "I won two races and got the silver cup for high jump, second prize for long jump, and first prize for gym. I like gym. I'm learning to walk on my hands, and I can do somersaults in the air off the springboard."

Mr. Kay, who was reading the letter, looked up.

"Damn' fine show, Maude, winnin' all those prizes." He was very proud of his son's achievements.

He was less pleased, however, with the rest of the letter.

"Only eighteen more days to the end of term," it went on. "Can I have dancing lessons during the holidays? I do miss them here."

T.W.B.   Q

"Dancing lessons!" his father snorted. "What is this nonsense? I thought he'd forget all about that business. Can't understand the boy at all."

Poor Mr. Kay, puzzled and hurt that his son who showed all the promise of being a fine athlete and sportsman should still cling to this absurd idea that he wanted to dance.

"If he was no good at anything else, Maude, I'd understand it." He shook his head. "But for a boy who gets prizes . . ." He appealed to her, and Mrs. Kay, who loved and knew them both so well, realised that he never would understand the wild Irish spirit that Pat had inherited from her. He never would be in sympathy with this strange urge to dance.

"I can't explain it," she said. "I think it is just one of the things about Pat that we must accept without understanding."

"Thank goodness we don't get this trouble from Anthony." Mr. Kay tossed the letter aside.

Mrs. Kay smiled, said nothing, and quietly went off to see whether Miss Cone could give Pat dancing lessons during August.

The end of July brought Pat home; a thinner, taller, quieter Pat. A couple of days later, Anthony, released from his establishment, arrived back; a very self-possessed schoolboy now, of a year's standing.

Pat's quietness wore off rapidly, and the house echoed to rowdy, schoolboy noises. Pat set out his sports prizes on the mantelpiece and turned the bedroom into a gymnasium, where he and Anthony tried out doubtful and highly dangerous experiments in acrobatics. In these, Pat found a slight consolation for his lost dancing.

"Do be careful, Pat, dear." Their mother looked in, in the middle of one of these sessions. "Anthony! Mind your feet on the wash-stand. Don't break the basin!"

"Mother, you must watch this. It's a new one." Pat climbed on to a chair at the foot of the bed, grasped the bedrail and carefully did a handstand.

"That's very clever." She was genuinely amazed at his skill and control. "What else can you do?" She sat down and watched him, wondering again at his unerring sense of balance.

"I say, Mother." He came wriggling up beside her. "If I get a bad school report, do you think Father will let me leave?"

"We'll have to see," she pushed back his dark hair. "Do you think it will be bad?"

"Oh yes!" he replied cheerfully. "I didn't learn a thing, and I was always being punished for playing about in class. I say, is there any chance of having dancing lessons in the holidays?"

"I went to see Miss Cone, and she told me she was very sorry she couldn't have you because the school is closed during August."

"Shall we go away to the seaside this year?" Anthony wriggled up on the other side.

"No, dear, I'm afraid not. It's too difficult with the war; besides, we can't really afford it. You see, everything is getting so expensive nowadays, we have to be careful about spending when prices are going up all the time."

"I'll earn lots of money and make you rich, Mother," Pat promised her. "Do you think I'll get a part in *Bluebell* again at Christmas? Oh!" The brightness had suddenly gone from his eyes. "I'd forgotten school. Please, Mother, you won't keep me there, not while *Bluebell* is on? I couldn't bear it. I think I should run away, I really would. If you knew how I hated it you wouldn't make me go back."

"I think I know, darling," she held him close to her, and she knew also by the look on his face when he spoke of school that something would have to be done. She must get him away somehow. "Let's forget all about it for now, shall we?" she chased away the nightmare for him. "I really came in to tell you something nice."

"What is it?"

"A visit to the theatre. Miss Cone said that I was to be sure and take you to the ballet to see Astafieva. She is dancing at the Coliseum with the Swinburne Ballet."

"Oh!" Pat's eyes lighted again. "Who's Asta . . . whatever you said?"

"Astafieva." She smiled. "Well, I must confess I didn't know, but Miss Cone tells me she is a very fine Russian dancer. Apparently she has a school of her own here, in London, and it's not often she actually appears herself on the stage. Miss Cone says you really mustn't miss it. Would you like to go?"

There was no need to ask. Theatre and ballet were magic words that spelled music, beauty and movement, and sent his blood racing.

All the old urge to dance, that school life had forced into the background, came flooding up again in full force.

"Let's go soon."

They did.

A few nights later an excited boy sat beside his mother in the Coliseum waiting for the curtain to go up. To Pat this was like coming back into the world again after long exile. His whole being responded to the sights and sounds around him; the gilt, the plush, the lights, the shuffling crowds filling the house, the buzz of voices, the orchestra tuning up. School life faded into a dim, grey background, and he felt alive all over.

"Serafina Astafieva." Her name made a bit more sense now that he saw it on the printed programme in front of him. "Did you say she was Russian?"

"Yes, darling. Miss Cone was telling me that she was trained at the Imperial Ballet School in St. Petersburg."

"And she's got a ballet school of her own here?"

"Yes, she has a studio somewhere in Chelsea. Apparently she is a wonderful teacher as well as being a very fine dancer herself. Miss Cone says she was dancing with Diaghilev's Ballets Russes before she came to London."

"Who's Diaghilev?" Pat asked, but there was no time to know the answer—then. The lights dimmed and the buzz of talk faded into silence.

The curtain rose.

To Pat's young and uncritical eyes, ballet was a world of enchantment that lifted him out of himself like the soaring flight of a bird.

To-night, as the ballet began, he had a dreamlike impression of floating white dancers, grouped like some quivering flower, to be suddenly blown by a gust of music that scattered the white petals and laid bare the living heart: a single, delicate figure, poised on her toes. No need to ask who this was. With Astafieva, a living force had come on to the stage. No dreamlike impression here. Pat sat up, sharply aware of her. She commanded and held his whole attention. Here was a personality as well as a dancer. There was fire in her movements. The sparkle of a *pirouette*, the flash of a *grand jeté*, the scintillating brilliance of a string of *fouettés*, seemed to light up the stage. She clothed the music with shimmering movement, and beside her the others paled to insignificance, at least, to the young boy who sat, still and tense, in the darkness, the colour drained from his face, and his eyes, large and brilliant, fixed on that one dancing figure.

He was seeing for the first time the beauty and strength of pure classical dancing. It was a revelation. The perfect control that creates the flawless curve of an *arabesque*, the clean-cut precision of an *entrechat*. The style and polish that only come from years of training, glittered through every movement.

It was over. The clatter of applause broke up the enchantment, letting in reality. Pat was filled with an unbearable excitement. As surely as if someone had spoken it aloud, he knew now where his own road lay. He turned to his mother.

"I want to learn to dance like that," he told her. "I will, must learn to dance at Astafieva's school."

If Mrs. Kay hoped that this new idea was a passing fancy, she was wrong. The impression Astafieva had made had gone too deep ever to be forgotten.

"It's no good, dear," Mrs. Kay came into her husband's study a week or two later. "I've done everything I can to persuade him to give up this idea, and it's impossible. Since he has seen Astafieva he is absolutely convinced that he wants to leave school and study under her. He pesters me all day about it."

"I gave him a good talking to in here." Mr. Kay leaned against the mantelpiece and put his hands in his pockets. "He's a wilful young devil."

"I really think it would do him a lot of harm to force him to go on at boarding-school." Mrs. Kay sat sidesaddle on the arm of a chair. "You know yourself, dear, how it is when you are training a spirited young horse, you can bend him so far to your will, but there comes a moment when you have to let him have his head. I believe Pat really would do something desperate if we sent him back to that school."

"Too damned independent for his age." Mr. Kay stared at the carpet as though hoping to find a solution there.

"He has shown us that this wanting to dance isn't just a passing fancy," Mrs. Kay persisted. "After all, it's nearly three years now since he started, and he's keener than ever, and everyone who has taught him says he is unusually promising."

"M'm," Mr. Kay admitted. "The boy certainly knows what he wants and sticks to it. I'll say that for him."

There was a long silence. Slowly, he looked round his study. He was seeing the photos on the walls, cricket groups, pictures of his favourite horses, himself as M.F.H. with a pack of hounds; the case of silver cups he had won at school for sporting events, hunting horns, foxes' masks; treasures that evoked for him the scent and sound of summer days, of cricket matches and tennis, or winter, and long hard days riding to hounds. These were the good things of life, the things he had enjoyed himself and wanted his sons to enjoy in their turn. But his simple ideas for them weren't working out. First the war had come and taken Philip away into the army. Now Pat was in revolt against boarding-school, and all because of this hare-brained idea that he wanted to learn to dance.

Mr. Kay shook his head wearily, remembering Pat's tears and entreaties, and his passionate rages when he was refused, and Maude sided with the boy, seemed to understand him. Well, he had forced his will on them both and sent Pat to school. He'd been so sure the boy would settle down and like it, but he hadn't. Perhaps he needed longer to get used to the idea of school. Perhaps he never would get used to it. Mr. Kay sighed heavily. It was all very difficult.

"In my day, all boys went away to school," he said slowly, "and that was an end of it."

"I think our Pat is different from other boys," said Mrs. Kay softly. "He has got this artistic streak in him. I think we should be wise to let him follow his own instincts over this."

"He's got your Irish blood in him, you mean," Mr. Kay looked at her. "You understand him, Maude, and I don't." He straightened his shoulders, and looked away, out of the window.

It was not easy for him to admit he was wrong, that school was a failure. He was a sportsman, though, who knew how to take a defeat, however bitter the disappointment might be. He looked again at his wife.

"There is one thing I insist on," he said. "No more governesses. If he leaves school he must go to a proper tutor."

She stood up close to him.

"I don't think you will ever regret this," she said softly as she kissed him.

The battle was won.

11 *Astafieva*

A boy in a brown velvet coat, brown velvet knickerbockers and thick black stockings, walked with his mother along the King's Road, Chelsea.

"This must be it." Mrs. Kay stopped outside a gracious old house set back a little from the road, behind a white stone archway. "Miss Cone said it was over 'the Pheasantry.' "

"Oh, I see!" Pat pointed to the row of tall windows with curved, iron balconies on the first floor. He wondered what lay in store for him up there, and his heart beat fast as they climbed the stairs.

At the top they became aware of a confused murmur of voices.

"But darling, I tell you I put them down in that room . . ." reached them loud and clear in broken English. "I cannot go without them . . ." The door swung open abruptly. A surprising apparition in trailing scarves, long strings of pearls, and loose clothes untidily bunched up round her stood before them.

"Madame Astafieva?" Mrs. Kay inquired.

"Yes. That is me. You want to see me?" She looked round like a cornered bird seeking escape.

"Yes," said Mrs. Kay. Could this really be the same immaculate white figure they had seen on the stage of the Coliseum? "My son Pat is very keen to come to your classes."

"My classes?" Astafieva's mind was still darting about among her lost gloves. "This is your son?" She looked him up and down, knickerbockers, black stockings and all. "He wants to be my pupil?"

"Yes, please," said Pat.

" 'Ave you found them, darling?" she called to an invisible maid. To Astafieva, everybody was "darling".

"Not yet, Madame." A harassed-sounding voice replied.

"Come in 'ere," she told Pat. "Let me look at you. I 'ave not much time now. You 'ave danced before? Yes? What can you do? 'Ow long 'ave you been dancing?" Rattling off questions, she led the way into the long, light studio. "What makes you think you can dance? Don't you know that to be a dancer it takes much work, long training for many years . . ." She kept on walking round him, and Pat wondered if she expected him to provide any answers.

"We saw you dancing at the Coliseum three weeks ago," Mrs. Kay managed to put in. "Ever since then, Pat has given me no peace till I brought him to you."

"I have learned dancing at Miss Cone's school for two years," added Pat. "I'm thirteen."

"Ah!" Astafieva hitched a drooping scarf over her shoulder. By contrast to her trailing clothes, her movements had grace and precision.

"Shall I dance for you now?" he suggested.

"Dance?" she suddenly remembered. "No. I 'ave no time. I am late. I 'ave to go and be photographed." She precipitated herself suddenly out of the studio.

"What about Pat?" Mrs. Kay pursued the darting bird into the passage. "May he join your class?"

Astafieva collected her scattered thoughts.

"I will see 'im dance to-morrow," she twirled round. "Let 'im come to my class in the morning. Eleven o'clock." Her hands fluttered in a helpless gesture. "What is the time now? Three o'clock? I shall be late! Yes, Madame, to-morrow I shall see what 'e can do . . ." And she was gone, scarves and perfume trailing in her wake.

Pat slept badly that night. Dancing feet chased through his dreams; a mocking, smiling face half-hidden in swathing scarves lured him on. He reached out his arms and went leaping after it. He knew he must catch it, that he could never rest until he held that elusive dancing shadow.

He woke sweating, the dream still vivid in his mind. It was not the first time he had chased this shadow in his sleep. Even waking he felt always that he was reaching out for something that was still just beyond his grasp. What was this unknown power that lured him on? Was it the veiled vision of his own future? Or the haunting spirit of his own ambition? He could give it no name, and it gave him no peace.

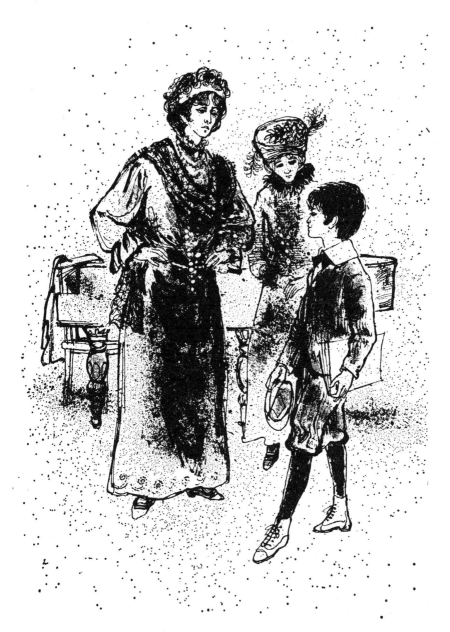

There were voices and laughter in the big studio next morning
as the class assembled. The girls were in plain tunics, some with
their hair tied back in the severe, classical style with bandeaux,

others with short, bobbed heads. They stared curiously at the boy who had appeared among them. Boys were in the minority.

There was silence as Madame Astafieva arrived to start the class. If anything, she looked even more haphazardly dressed than the day before. Her beautiful head was swathed in a silk bandeau, the lovely lines of her body hidden in a shapeless tunic and short black skirt. The whole outfit seemed to be held together with knotted scarves and safety-pins. White stockings covered her legs, and on her feet she had tiny pink ballet slippers. In her hand she carried the traditional symbol of the ballet mistress—a long jewelled stick.

"At the bar, everyone." She rapped the floor sharply.

Pat took his place in the long line of pupils.

The class began.

Madame worked them hard. She demanded intense concentration. Nothing escaped her sharp eye. As she passed along the line of pupils her long stick would flash out to hit any legs that were not working properly.

Demi-pliés, pliés battements, ronds de jambe, they went through all the routine of work at the bar. In the far corner by the piano, Mrs. Kay sat and watched. She soon realised that here was a teacher of rare quality. Astafieva not only taught, she inspired. She was putting into her pupils her own fiery spirit. She poured out her energy to give these boys and girls her own unquenchable love of the dance.

Adagio and *Allegro* in the centre. The pupils were called out in twos and threes. It came to Pat's turn.

Mrs. Kay, watching Astafieva, would have given much to know what she was thinking as she saw him dance before her. She made no comment.

When the class was over, Pat joined his mother. Together they came over to Astafieva.

"What do you think of him?" Mrs. Kay asked. "Will he make a dancer?"

Astafieva's dark eyes were thoughtful as she looked at the eager, upturned face of the boy standing before her. Was she seeing into the future? Seeing a small figure dancing through the years ahead, and growing all the time in stature, greater, and even greater?

"I don't know," she said slowly. "We shall see later. He will have to work very hard."

With that Mrs. Kay had to be content, but Pat was completely happy for he had got his desire. He became a regular pupil at the studio, and his legs became regular targets for that flashing, jewelled stick. He adored his temperamental teacher who called him Patté and sent him home covered with bruises. Through her own radiating energy she was giving him his first living contact with the inspiring tradition of the great Russian Ballet Schools. This was the teacher he wanted. For her he was prepared to work till he dropped.

At home now there was peace. Dancing was accepted as an inevitable part of Pat's life. His education was taken over by a tutor. In September Anthony went back to school.

From the war, Philip, who was now an officer, wrote scrappy letters mostly talking about his next leave, and wondering gloomily when the interminable fighting was going to end. Two years they had had of it now. Mr. Kay, watching his income slowly drowning in a sea of rising prices, wondered too, how much longer it would go on. No question now of giving his boys the leisured, sporting life he had known. His great worry nowadays was whether he would be able to hold out financially until they were old enough to earn their own living.

For Mrs. Kay the days became one big problem to keep the home going, to make the housekeeping money go round, to keep the maids and to provide meals for her family.

In November a letter arrived for Pat one breakfast time.

"It's from Mr. Wolheim," he waved it about excitedly. "They're going to do *Bluebell* again this Christmas and he wants me to go along for the audition. It's at the Palace Theatre."

"How lovely, darling," said Mrs. Kay. "When is it?"

"Twenty-fifth November—that's to-morrow, ten o'clock."

"To-morrow," she repeated thoughtfully. "I don't think I can come with you. I have to get the rations, and that means queuing most of the morning."

"I shall be all right alone," said Pat airily. "I wonder if all the others will be there too."

They were, or at least most of them. There was an excited and noisy reunion of last year's *Bluebell* gang.

"What time is this audition going to start?" they began asking when the gossip flagged. "We've been here an hour already."

"Let's find out what is happening." Someone went to investigate and came back saying, "We've just got to wait here."

The gossip and reminiscences started up again. As Pat talked and joked with the others, he became aware of a man making his way over to him.

"May I talk to you a minute?" The man beckoned him aside. Pat followed him suspiciously, a little apart from the others.

"I wondered if you would be interested in a job. I think I could offer you a good part." The man looked him up and down. "Yes, you're just about the right size."

Pat frowned at him, finding all this most odd.

"Thank you very much but I don't want a job," he said. "I expect I shall be playing in *Bluebell*. I played in it last year, and they wrote and asked me to come here to-day."

"Yes, quite," said the man slowly. He paused a moment, as though he were going to say something more but changed his mind. "Well." He raised his hat. "In that case, I'm sorry."

Funny man, thought Pat, as he joined the others, and then he wished he'd asked what the job was.

They hung about for another hour before Mr. Wolheim appeared.

"I'm very sorry, boys and girls, but there won't be an audition to-day, after all," he told them. "Will you come back again next week? Yes, to-day week, here, at the same time."

What an anti-climax. All the excitement and waiting, just to be told that. Disappointed, the groups began to break up.

"You'd think they might have made up their minds before bringing us all here," Pat grumbled as they went down to the stage door.

"Excuse me," said a voice at his side, and there was the mysterious man again. "I would like to give you my card." He pushed it into Pat's hand. "Just in case you change your mind about my suggestion. Think it over."

"Who is that?" another boy asked as they came out into the street.

Pat looked at the name on the card.

"Kreimer," he read out. "Theatrical Agent and Impresario."

"Never heard of him," said the boy.

"Nor have I." Pat put the card in his pocket. "I say, why do you think they've sent us away for a week?" They walked along together.

"I heard a rumour that it's not at all certain whether they will put on *Bluebell* this year after all."

"Oh!" Pat stopped short. That was different. His fingers felt the square card in his pocket. That explained a lot of things. If there was no *Bluebell* . . .

He turned and ran back through the stage door.

"Yes, young man," said Mr. Wolheim as Pat came hurrying across the stage to him. "What is it?"

"Is it true that *Bluebell* may not be put on this year after all?"

Mr. Wolheim raised his eyebrows, wondering at the speed at which rumours travel.

"Who told you that?"

"One of the boys."

"I'm afraid I can't answer your question. We shall know more about it next week."

"I've been offered another job." Pat trotted out his half-truth with a convincing air. "What shall I do about it?"

"Take it and be thankful," said Mr. Wolheim, who was a busy man.

"I think you did quite right," said Mrs. Kay when Pat told her about it. "I should go and see Mr. Kreimer as soon as possible and find out what he has to offer you."

There was a smile on Mr. Kreimer's face as Pat was shown into his office the next morning.

"So you have thought it over."

"I just came in to ask you what the job was," said Pat.

"It is *Peter Pan*," Mr. Kreimer told him. "They are looking for a boy to play the part of John. How old are you?"

"Thirteen and a half," Pat told him.

Mr. Kreimer asked him some more questions about himself and scribbled something on a pad.

"Can you be at the New Theatre at 5.30 to-day?"

"Yes, I think so." Pat rapidly decided that tutors and dancing classes should be slung overboard for the occasion.

"Good. You will go for an audition there with the producer, Mr. Boucicault. He will want to hear you recite. Have you something ready?"

"I will have," said Pat.

Events were crowding in thick and fast. He rushed home to tell his mother the exciting news, and spend the afternoon feverishly rehearsing his poems, and watching the clock, with that screwed-up feeling of adventure, until quite suddenly he was caught up in it and found himself standing on the stage of the New Theatre facing a dim group of people in the stalls, who seemed altogether hostile. They interrupted his poem, one man flung questions at him, another pushed a script of *Peter Pan* into his hand and told him to read parts of it. Could he sing? they wanted to know. Could he dance? Pat felt that he was being dragged through a large machine that was slowly tearing him into little pieces.

Miserable and frightened, he obeyed the summons to come down into the stalls. He wondered why they didn't throw him out at once.

"I think he'll do," he heard one man say to another. "Inexperienced, but possible."

One of the dim faces loomed closer to him.

"We can offer you the part of John."

Pat opened his mouth in such surprise that no words came out.

"At a salary of £4 10s. a week," the voice added.

Pat shut his mouth and swallowed. His brain unfroze and began to calculate. Four pounds ten shillings was more than twice his salary in *Bluebell*. But what about *Bluebell*? In spite of what Mr. Wolheim had said, could he just walk out on *Bluebell*?

"Thank you very much, sir," he fetched out at last. "May I talk it over with my mother first?"

"Yes, but we must have your answer to-morrow. Before twelve o'clock."

Thirteen-year-old Pat was feeling extremely grown-up as he left the theatre. The terror of the ordeal he had been through gave way to the rising elation of success. He'd been offered a contract.

There were two parts to choose from now. "John" in *Peter Pan*; or the "Black Cat" in *Bluebell*. *Peter Pan* or *Bluebell*. "John" or the "Black Cat".

The two chased each other round in his head all the way home. He felt he was faced with the most important decision in his life.

"What do you think, Mother?" he asked her gravely.

"I think it's wonderful, darling."

"Yes, but which shall I take?"

They discussed it all the evening.

"I think the best thing is if I ring up Mr. Wolheim for you first thing in the morning," suggested Mrs. Kay. "Then we can find out just what is happening about Bluebell."

"I will ring him up." Pat, still feeling grown-up, insisted on conducting his own business.

"Is that Mr. Wolheim?" He perched on a chair in front of the wall telephone next morning.

"Yes, Mr. Wolheim speaking," came the muffled voice over the wire.

"This is Pat Kay here. Can you tell me if you really are putting on *Bluebell* this year?"

"No, I can't," the muffled voice sounded annoyed. "As I told you when you asked before. There's nothing definite."

"Would you have me as the Black Cat again if it was put on?" Pat insisted.

"I expect so."

"Well, how much would you pay then?"

A muffled snort came over the wire.

"Four pounds," said Mr. Wolheim. Pat made a face over his shoulder at his mother, holding up four fingers.

"Five." He bargained.

"You little devil," the voice rattled back. "Come and see me to-morrow then, and we'll fix it up."

Mr. Wolheim rang off. Pat thoughtfully hung up his own earpiece.

"It's not certain about *Bluebell* and it's not certain they'll pay me more than £4." He looked at his mother.

"What a real businessman you're becoming." She tried not to show how amused she was at his important, serious air. "Conducting your own affairs over the telephone."

"I think I'll take the *Peter Pan* offer." Pat made the great decision.

"I think you're very wise," she told him, and before twelve o'clock they were both in Mr. Boucicault's office. The contract was signed.

"*Peter Pan*. First rehearsal. Thursday, ten o'clock." The call was sent out. The company assembled on the stage of the New Theatre. For many of the actors *Peter Pan* was an annual reunion.

"Hallo, old man, how are you?" Veteran Pirates and Indians greeted each other. It was all a big family party.

Pat, standing alone, felt homesick for his friends in *Bluebell*.

"Is this your first time in *Peter*?"

He looked round and saw a flaxen-haired girl, smaller than himself, standing beside him.

"Yes."

"It's mine too. I'm Michael Darling."

"Oh! Are you? I'm your brother John." They introduced themselves. "I say," Pat went on. "Do you know the play well?"

"My mother brought me to see it last year, but I don't remember much about it except the flying."

"I wonder how they do it." Pat gazed up at the flies over his head as if hoping for an immediate solution to the mystery.

A young man joined them, introduced himself as the Crocodile.

"Were you in it last year?" they asked him.

"Yes. Unity Moore was Peter."

"Who's Peter Pan this year?" Pat wanted to know.

"Fay Compton. Look! She's standing over there, talking to Mr. Boucicault." They turned to see the already famous young actress with glorious auburn hair that framed the most attractive, heart-shaped face.

"It's awfully hard being Peter," said the Crocodile, "because Pauline Chase was so wonderful in the part that critics have decided no one can ever be quite as good again. You see, she played it eight years running."

"Goodness! It's an awfully old play, isn't it?"

"It's been played every year since 1904."

"That's thirteen years!" Michael was very impressed.

"Who's the other one?" Pat asked. "The one next to Fay Compton?"

"She's Stella Patrick Campbell," the Crocodile knew all the

answers. "She is the daughter of the famous Mrs. Patrick Campbell."

"What is she playing?"

"Mrs. Darling."

"Oh!" said Michael and John together. "She's going to be our mother." What a young and charming-looking mother too.

"And do you see that man talking to Fay Compton now?" the Crocodile whispered urgently.

They looked, and saw a frail-looking, little man who had just joined the group. He was chiefly remarkable for a drooping, untidy moustache, and a high, domed forehead with deep-set, sunken eyes that gave him a melancholy, brooding air. He looked rather out of place, they thought, between the two beautiful actresses.

"Is he in it too?" asked Michael.

"That," said the Crocodile, in an awed whisper, "is the author of the play, Sir James Barrie."

"Oh!" Pat and Michael looked again at the small, unassuming figure of the great man. He was smiling now at something Fay Compton was saying. What a change had come over him with that smile. His whole face seemed to light up. He looked quite boyish.

"I never thought he looked like that," said Michael. And Pat, who had never thought of him at all, said nothing.

"I say, what do those do?" Michael was looking at a group of girls talking and laughing together on the side of the stage. "I don't remember seeing a lot of girls in it last year."

"They're the lost boys." The Crocodile laughed at the sight of their surprised faces. He broke off to wave as one of the "Lost Boys" had caught sight of him looking in their direction.

"Were they all in it last year?" asked Pat.

"No, but most of them are Conti children so I know them."

"What's that?"

"Haven't you ever heard of the Italia Conti Stage School?" He was surprised. "Miss Conti trains children for the stage. We nearly all come from her."

"What sort of things do you learn there?" Pat was interested, but there was no time for an answer.

"Stand by everybody," the stage manager called out.

They saw the short, energetic figure of the producer come into the centre of the stage.

Mr. Boucicault took over the company and work began.

At the beginning, Pat, already tempered in the fire of a Seymour Hicks production, felt that he had been through the worst and was ready to face anything in the way of rehearsal temperament. Mr. Boucicault, however, lost no time in changing his mind for him.

As rehearsals followed, day after day, the atmosphere became steadily stormier. Where Mr. Hicks barked his displeasure, Mr. Boucicault roared, and the New Theatre and everyone in it trembled with the sound. Where did such a little man pack such a volume of rage, most of which, it seemed, was directed on the unfortunate Pat?

"Don't worry, my boy." One of the Pirates consoled him after a long and trying ship scene. "He always picks on Johns. Never did like 'em."

"That's all this morning, thank you." The stage manager dismissed them. "This afternoon, 2.30. Return Nursery Scene. Will Wendy, John and Michael stay behind now for flying practice."

Pat wondered unhappily what new horrors were in store.

"Cheer up." His sister Wendy came over to him, smiling. "Flying is lovely. Mr. Kirby takes us and he's ever so nice."

"Not Mr. Boucicault?" Things were looking a little brighter.

"No," she laughed. "He won't be there."

"Who's Mr. Kirby?"

"He's the person who invented flying especially for *Peter Pan*."

The stage hands were putting up the Nursery Scene. In the wings, the Kirby men were disentangling ropes and wires and calling up to invisible comrades in the flies over their heads. The three children stood about waiting, until a quiet-voiced man came up to them.

"Will you come over here to get your harness?" Mr. Kirby led them to the back of the stage. Here stood the big wooden crates with "Kirby Flying Apparatus" stamped in bold, black letters across their sides.

They were initiated into the mystery of their harness, a curious collection of straps that buckled round and over their bodies, tying them up like a parcel.

"None of this is seen, of course, under your pyjamas," Mr. Kirby finished tightening the straps. "There is a special slit in the jacket for the wire."

"I think this is rather frightening," whispered little Michael as she and Pat were led into the middle of the Nursery, and the wires were clipped on the saddle-shaped pads on their backs.

"Does it ever break?" Pat walked about cautiously, looking up at the long shining thread to which he was attached that disappeared into an unknown darkness above.

"It'll lift half a ton, so you don't need to worry," Mr. Kirby smiled as he led Pat over to a place by the bed. "Now stand here. We'll give you a straight lift first. Hold on to my hands. Don't try and jump. Let the wire do the work. All right, Tom," he called. "Take him up."

Pat, clutching Mr. Kirby's hands, felt himself slowly lifted off the ground. His feet were now level with the middle of Mr. Kirby's waistcoat. He felt like a sack of potatoes dangling there. Looking across, he saw Michael dangling a few yards away. They smiled at each other.

"Good." Mr. Kirby had him lowered again. "Now try by yourself."

Up and down they both went, growing more confident with each lift. The flying men heaved on the ropes, and the two of them were hoisted up higher and faster.

"It's fun," Michael squealed and wriggled about on the end of the wire.

"I like flying," Pat flapped his arms wildly.

Wendy arrived, her harness modestly hidden under a long nightdress. A third wire came down and she joined the dangling figures in the air.

"Now for some real flights," said Mr. Kirby. "I want you to remember children that while your wires are on you must only move where I tell you, otherwise you will get them crossed." He walked about drawing chalk marks on the floor. "John, come over here." He led Pat into a corner and stood him on a large "J". "This time, instead of going straight up and down you will fly across the Nursery."

"How do I make myself go there?" asked Pat.

"You don't," Mr. Kirby told him. "We see to that for you." They did. Pat was lifted into the air. High over the bed he swung in a graceful curve to land gently by Nana's kennel. He looked back and there were Michael and Wendy floating across the width of the room.

"That was lovely," Pat called out. "Can I do it again?"

"Wait till Michael and Wendy are back in their places."

Small figures went swinging through the air under Mr. Kirby's careful eye. All over the Nursery they flew, and all too soon the practice was over and they were clamouring for the next one.

"I can't tell you yet." Mr. Kirby, who had been giving *Peter Pan* children the thrill of their first flights for thirteen years, smiled sympathetically as he took the wires off. "It depends on Mr. Boucicault. To-morrow I'm rehearsing Peter by herself, and then you will all do it together."

For Pat, flying remained the nicest part of rehearsals. Even Mr. Boucicault's shouting couldn't spoil the thrill of soaring through the air. Besides, one felt so superior sailing about over Mr. Boucicault's head.

The rest of the rehearsals, however, had become a daily misery. Pat came to dread each new day.

"You must just stick it out, darling," his mother tried to give him courage. "It'll be better when the play is on and everyone has settled down."

"I don't think it ever will go on," said Pat gloomily. "Not with me in it; when he shouts at me I just forget everything and that makes him more angry and he shouts louder. If I don't understand what he wants straight away he just catches hold of me and drags me round the stage."

"It's not much longer now till the opening night." She wished she could give him comfort. "Think how proud you will be playing a big part in Barrie's famous play. It'll all seem worth while then."

So, Pat, grateful to her, but unconvinced, counted the days until the opening on Christmas Eve.

13 Peter Pan

Christmas Eve 1917; a theatre full of excited children with their parents, and the curtain going up on the firelit Nursery. There was the big cuddly Nana busy on bed-time preparations.

Outside the Nursery door waited a nervous Michael in little white blouse and shorts, a nervous John in a black Eton suit, and an equally nervous Wendy; all of them uncomfortably aware of the flying harness buckled tightly under their clothes.

Nana came to the door to fetch Michael.

"Good luck," they whispered as he climbed astride the white woolly back, and Michael was carried into the lights, shouting:

"No, Nana, no! I tell you I won't go to bed."

John and Wendy watched him through the fake picture on the wall. As they waited for their cue, Pat thought suddenly of that other first night in *Bluebell*, and Mr. Hicks hissing at him from the wings.

"If I make a mistake out there and Mr. Boucicault shouts at me, I shall dry up," he whispered panic-stricken, "I know I will."

"John, dear! What an idea! Of course he won't shout at you." Wendy squeezed his hand. "You won't make any mistakes. Come on, it's us."

John and Wendy moved into the lighted Nursery.

Down in the stalls, Mr. and Mrs. Kay and Anthony had the thrill of seeing their Pat take the stage in his first straight acting part.

"No, Nana. No, I won't be bathed, I tell you, I won't be bathed." To roars of delight from the sympathetic young in the audience, he was chased round the arm-chair by a growling Nana, and pursued into the bathroom in his turn, to do a quick change into pyjamas and slippers.

Nerves had gone now, excitement only remained. The hardest part he found was having to go to bed on the stage and lie very still for hours and hours, or so it seemed. Only later in the run of the play would he and Michael think of taking bags of toffees to bed with them to pass the time. On this first night, however, one was on one's best behaviour. John lay quite motionless while Mother tucked them up one after the other. His bed was on its own by the fire. He lay under the covers with his back to the audience, hoping that his make-up wasn't getting smudged on the pillow. The Nursery was dimly lit now by the nightlights over each bed.

In the wings a man waited with a mirror in his hands to send the michievous Tinker Bell dancing into the room, while his mate stood behind the curtained window with a rope of bells, and Fay Compton crouched on a mattress ready for her take-off.

The audience were very still now, watching that hushed Nursery. From where Pat lay he could just see the window. He saw the curtains shake violently and heard the jangle of bells as Tinker Bell flashed into the room. One after the other the night-lights flickered and went out. Only the glow of the fire remained, spreading a mysterious red light in the room.

Soft music wove a mysterious spell, mounting in excitement till the air tingled with it. On a swift climax the windows burst open, and out of the night sky, high over the rooftops, Peter Pan flew into the Nursery, a brown, elf-like figure in the glow of the fire. Another flight to the bathroom door, then high across the room to land on the mantelpiece. Back again to the corner. Cue for the sleeping children to toss and turn, and send Peter flying to hide behind the curtains to have the wire taken off.

After this, a long, dull wait for John lying without moving while Wendy woke and she and Peter went through their business of sewing on the shadow, exchanging thimbles and releasing Tinker Bell who had got shut in a drawer.

There was a big laugh when Peter pushed John out of bed and he rolled on the floor. Not so funny for John who landed awkward-ly with his head on the fender and his legs twisted and had to stay like that, bundled up in bedclothes "sleeping", until he was officially awakened by Wendy.

"I shall get cramp and I shan't be able to move," he thought. Cautiously he straightened a leg, hoping that no one would notice.

It seemed hours before Wendy came and shook him.

"Wake up, John. Get up. There's a boy here who is to teach us to fly."

Another laugh for John as he sat up, rubbed his eyes, found himself on the floor and remarked:

"Oh! I see I am up already."

After that, quick action. The alarm of Nana barking and the children scattering to hide so that Kirby men could quickly clip on their flying wires. Tremendous laughs from the children in the audience as Wendy, John and Michael tried to fly off their beds and landed flat on their backs on the floor. The thrilling moment when

Peter put the secret of flying on them, and the roars of delight as they went up, John's arms and legs threshing wildly about, Michael doing a vigorous breast stroke through the air, and Wendy hovering gracefully over her bed, while out of sight in the wings three men heaved on the ends of their ropes.

Swiftly followed the decision to emigrate to the "Never Never Land" where Wendy could exercise her maternal instincts on Peter's collection of "Lost Boys". John and Michael, lured by the promise of Pirates and Indians, ran to stand on their chalk marks ready for the take-off. Tinker Bell swung the windows wide, and away they went, the brown figure of Peter, the white Wendy, John in pyjamas and top hat, and lastly little Michael.

"Keep well down," someone whispered at them as they landed on the mattress below the window-sill. They crouched waiting while Mrs. Darling rushed into the Nursery too late to bring her children back, and the curtain came down on the first act to the ringing sound of applause.

"Well done, nice flights." The Kirby men came hurrying round to release them from their wires.

"I do think Pat is good," Mrs. Kay was clapping as loudly as she could, "he looks so natural."

"Got a good voice for it," said his father. "I must say that flying business is very effective."

"I think flying is the best part," Anthony fidgeted about excitedly. "I do want to know how it's done. I wish Pat would tell me."

All round them children were wanting to know the same thing. Many of them, probably, were secretly resolved to try on their own, just as soon as they got home to their own nurseries; for the unsophisticated young of 1917 firmly believed in magic and the world of fairies where everything was possible.

"It's hard to believe that it really is Pat." Anthony swung his legs, kicking the seat in front. He felt so proud of his brother that he wanted to tell everybody.

"Don't talk so loudly, dear," his mother stopped the kicking.

"What comes next?" Anthony rummaged for the programme under a big box of chocolates already half empty. "Will they fly again?"

He was soon to find out, for the curtain rose and they were carried away into Peter Pan's Never Never Land; to the Frozen River; to the Mermaid's Lagoon; to the exciting Home under the Trees where the Lost Boys lived, guarded by the friendly Indians.

Breathlessly they followed the terrible adventures with Pirates; battle, treachery, and the Capture of the Lost Boys.

Even Anthony was pale with excitement as the curtain rose on a real sinister Pirate Ship, and the evil Captain Hook walked the deck in his own green light, flashing his curved steel finger as he gloated over his chained captives.

John's big moment came in this scene when Captain Hook said he had room for a Cabin Boy. It was tempting.

"I'd rather like to be a Pirate," John confessed every small boy's dream. "I thought of calling myself Red-handed Jack." A confession that brought a roar of derision from the real Pirates, and the dream was rudely shattered when John discovered that being a Pirate meant swearing "Down with the King".

"Well, I won't." John, a courageous and loyal subject, shook his chained fists at Captain Hook's face and defiantly started a rousing chorus of "Rule Britannia"; a brave and hopeless gesture, for it was swiftly drowned by the yells of the infuriated Pirates, and the enraged Captain Hook condemned the lot of them to the terrible death of walking the plank.

This was altogether too much for some of the audience who were removed, screaming with fright. The brave who remained, however, saw Peter's dramatic arrival and the rescue, ending in a glorious battle as the boys swarmed down from the rigging, sword in hand, to surprise and attack the Pirates.

"This is one of the best bits in the play," thought Pat as he chased a large Pirate across the deck at the point of his wooden sword and sent him screaming overboard.

The battle was over. The villains were defeated and the audience relaxed to the Return Nursery Scene where Mr. Darling was now to be found living in Nana's kennel, while Mrs. Darling played the piano and mourned for her lost children.

A last flight for Wendy and John who carried Michael on his back. They came sailing in through the window for a glorious reunion. The Lost Boys moved into the Darlings' home. There was a last glimpse of Peter and Wendy in the House in the Tree Tops among the fairies and birds, and it was all over.

Curtain-calls and applause.

"Well done, Pat," Mrs. Kay's voice was lost in the storm of clapping, but she felt she had to say it.

Anthony was tremendously proud as he saw Pat line up on the stage with the principals to take his bow. He thought it was fearfully grand to have a brother who was a real actor. He'd be able to swank about it like anything to the other boys at school next term.

"Is Pat famous?" he asked his mother suddenly.

"Not yet, dear," she told him. "But he will be."

They had a celebration family supper after the show. A first night was, after all, an important occasion, Mr. Kay decided. He felt really rather proud of his actor son.

"I told you so," Mrs. Kay smiled at Pat as she drank to his success.

"What?"

"I told you it would all seem worth while once the show was on."

She was right. The dark and dreadful days of the rehearsals were well and truly over.

Already by the second day the atmosphere backstage had become relaxed and friendly. Nobody shouted at John and life began to be worth living again.

"I think I'm going to enjoy *Peter Pan* after all," Pat was saying to himself as he was in his dressing-room changing for the Underground Scene on the second day.

There was a knock on the door. Wendy looked in.

"There's a tea-party in Mrs. Darling's dressing-room. Everyone's invited."

The big room that Stella Patrick Campbell shared with Doris McIntyre, the first twin, was already crowded. Pirates, Indians and Lost Boys were perched on chairs and hampers. Wolves and the Crocodile sprawled on the floor.

"Come along!" Mrs. Darling welcomed her "children" into the family. "I'm so glad you're here."

"Help yourselves," Doris waved a hand in the direction of a

table covered with plates of cakes and sweets. "I'll just get you some tea."

They found a space on the floor with the Wolves. There was a knock at the door and a sudden silence. It was Mr. Boucicault.

"So this is where all the company get to after the Lagoon Scene," he said severely, looking round the crowded room.

They all waited rather guiltily for a storm to break.

It didn't, Mr. Boucicault was suddenly laughing.

"I thought I'd frighten you all," he told them. "Well, Stella, I think this is a splendid idea of yours. Very nice of you to invite me."

A chair of honour was found and he joined the party. As he stayed talking and joking with them, the atmosphere rapidly warmed up again, and all too soon the call boy was hammering on the door.

"Underground beginners, please."

"Who'd have thought it?" Pat remarked as he and Michael went down to the stage. "The old dragon is quite human. He was actually nice to me."

"I hope it lasts," rejoined Michael.

It did. Now that *Peter Pan* was well launched, Mr. Boucicault was a changed man. It was as though all the pent-up fire in him had burned itself out. He was calm and friendly. An atmosphere of peace pervaded the backstage world.

The tea-party was the first of many. In fact, Mrs. Darling's dressing-room became a happy gathering place for most of the company. *Peter Pan* was a thoroughly happy family. All too soon, it seemed to Pat, the six weeks' run had come to an end and he was hanging up John's Eton suit and flying harness for the last time.

"What happens next?" was the question that hung heavily in the air.

"Isn't it horrid that there's no theatre to go to to-day?" He trailed disconsolately round the house next morning. "I wish they'd let *Peter Pan* run longer. *Bluebell* will be going on for another month at least. They don't finish till March."

"Do you wish you'd done *Bluebell* this year after all?" his mother asked.

"No." Pat was quite decided. "I love *Peter Pan*, and I love being

John. It's a much better part. Why does Peter always have to be a girl?" he was pursuing an idea of his own.

"I suppose it would be too difficult to find a boy each year who was good enough."

"Fay Compton was wonderful. I love her voice. It's just my idea of the way Peter would talk, but I still think it should be a real boy. I wish I could play Peter." He began doing the shadow dance. "I say, Mother, I am out of practice," he stopped again.

"It's hardly surprising as you've had to miss so many classes."

"That's the only thing I'm pleased about the show being over for. I am free to go to Astafieva's again. Oh, Mother, I do want to be a dancer!"

14 "What Happens Next?"

The question "What happens next?" loomed very largely in Mrs. Kay's mind during the days that followed. She had hoped that *Peter Pan* would lead to another engagement, but nothing so far had materialised. She wanted to encourage Pat with his acting. Dancing was all very well, she thought, but she couldn't see much future in it for him.

The world of 1918 seemed to present very little opportunity for a ballet dancer, especially a man. After all, Pat had got talent for acting. She felt he needed a proper training for the stage, but where? and how? What was the best thing to do for him? What did happen next? Mrs. Kay, puzzling over the problem, realised that the time had come to get professional advice and help for Pat's future. She talked it over with her husband.

"Who do we know in the theatre? I feel we should go to someone who could advise us what is the best thing to do to have him trained."

"You're right, Maude. Want an opinion from a really first-class man in the profession," he agreed with her. "Someone like Beerbohm-Tree."

"Yes, except that he's dead," said Mrs. Kay. "He died last year. All the big actor-managers seem to be disappearing," she realised with a shock. "Kendal died last year. Forbes-Robertson has been retired two or three years. There's Sir Charles Wyndham, he's a very old man now. I should think he must have retired too. Henry Ainley, he's away in the war. There doesn't seem to be anyone taking their places."

"Who's that man at the St. James's Theatre?" said Mr. Kay suddenly. "Your cousin was talking about him the other night at dinner."

"Which cousin?" She searched vaguely among their more recent guests.

"You know . . . what's her name? Lady Pontifex."

"Oh!" The light broke in. "I remember. She was talking about Sir George Alexander."

"Alexander, that's the man. He must be getting on in years. Why, I remember seeing him at the St. James's when I was a young man. Very fine actor."

"He's very active still," said Mrs. Kay, "I remember Mary was telling us what wonderful work he is doing for the war, organising charity matinées to raise money for the Red Cross. She's on a lot of those committees herself. I think she knows him quite well. I wonder if she would help us?"

She did. She gave them an introduction that opened for them the well-guarded doors of the St. James's Theatre.

Through that stage door they passed into one of the last strongholds of the great actor-manager tradition.

For nearly twenty-eight years Sir George Alexander had reigned over this theatre.

Mrs. Kay and Pat were ushered into the presence of the great man in his dressing-room. More like a drawing-room, Pat thought, sitting up rather straight and on his best behaviour, on the edge of a chair, while his mother and the great man exchanged polite preliminaries.

As Pat looked round he could not help comparing this with his own bare dressing-room at the New Theatre. What a contrast! Here were heavy brocade curtains, a soft carpet, and arm-chairs. A silk screen went across one corner, hiding, perhaps, the make-up table. A bright coal fire in the grate sent flickering, golden lights over the dark, polished furniture. Everywhere he saw books, photographs, pictures, old programmes, souvenirs; treasures gathered during the quarter of a century that this dressing-room had been Sir George Alexander's home.

Pat gazed with awe at the famous and distinguished-looking man who had reigned over the St. James's Theatre for so long. How little could he guess that the reign was so soon to come to an end; that this courteous and handsome actor was fighting a silent, losing battle against incurable diabetes. Before the year was out, this dressing-room would stand, forlornly empty, and Sir George would never see the brilliant destiny of the boy who now sat before him.

These things still lay mercifully hidden behind the veil of the future, as Sir George spoke to Pat asking him questions about himself and his work in *Peter Pan* and *Bluebell*. He was a charming and kindly person.

Pat, obeying his mother's instructions, did not mention dancing. They spoke of various ways of starting a stage career.

"In my young days, of course, a boy joined a company and started with walking-on parts," Sir George told him. "It was up to him to pick up what knowledge he could and make good. That was learning the hard way." A smile lit the tired lines round his eyes. "Nowadays, it is much easier for you youngsters. There are schools which train young people." He looked at Mrs. Kay. "The best advice I can give you is to send your boy to Italia Conti. You couldn't do better than to let him go to her school."

Words that suddenly fitted on to all that Pat had already heard about this school in *Peter Pan*. He knew that this was the right answer for him.

"I'd like to go," he told his mother afterwards. "I've heard a lot about her."

"I've always heard that it is an excellent school. We'll have to find out what the fees are. I hope we shall be able to afford it." Mrs. Kay was thinking rather anxiously of the tutor's bill and Astafieva's fees. "One thing," she went on, thinking aloud rather than talking to Pat, "as they give an all-round training, I daresay you'll be able to carry on with your ballet there, and give up Astafieva."

Pat looked at her in horror.

"Give up Astafieva?" he repeated. "No! No!" he said violently. "I won't ever give up Astafieva. Never. I won't learn dancing anywhere else, and if it means giving her up then I'd rather not go

to the Conti School. Promise me you'll never make me give up
Astafieva."

"All right, darling, of course I won't. Not if you feel like that
about it." Realising what a mistake she had made, she tried to
quieten this passionate outburst and reassure him.

"I don't mind learning to act," Pat went on, "but I don't ever
want to stop dancing."

"Nor you shall."

With this assurance Pat relaxed, while his mother wondered
again at this relentless urge to dance that drove him so insistently.

"When can we go and see Italia Conti?" he asked.

"I'll write her to-day," Mrs. Kay promised.

15 The Conti School

"I've accepted a new pupil for next term," Italia Conti came into
the office where her younger sister Evelyn sat at a littered desk
trying to keep the confused and swiftly moving affairs of this lively
school in some sort of order.

"What rhymes with apple?" Third sister, Bianca, came to life
behind a pile of books tumbled over a table in a corner of the
crowded room.

"Grapple," suggested Italia, crossing to the mirror to rearrange
her hair. "What's it for?"

"The Red Cross show we're doing next month. I want three
of my babies in the beginners' Elocution Class to act a poem."

Italia stopped arranging her hair.

"But I told you I want them to do a Romeo and Juliet scene,"
she said over her shoulder.

"Dapple . . ." Bianca's fingers drummed the metre of her poem
out on the table. "I decided that it is too advanced for them to
learn."

"Nonsense, Bianca." Italia's voice went several shades deeper.
"Of course they can learn it. A child can learn anything by heart.
Besides, tiny children look so sweet playing Shakespeare, it's a good
advertisement for the school."

"You can train them yourself in that case," Bianca was obstinate.

"I'm not going to waste all the time of my class teaching toddlers to recite long passages of Shakespeare that they're much too young to understand."

The atmosphere was piling up for a storm.

"What's the new pupil's name?" Evelyn now had found a pen and the right book.

"What did you say? Oh yes! The new pupil." Italia left the battle pending. "It's a boy. Kay—Pat Kay. I've got his address somewhere." Her beautiful and helpless hands rummaged in her handbag. "Ah yes!" She produced Mrs. Kay's card. On the back she had written, "Elocution and Acting."

"He'll be coming to several of your classes, Bianca."

"To learn Shakespeare, I suppose," she flashed back.

"Of course he's to learn Shakespeare," Italia screamed at her, "and the earlier they start the better."

"You've got to teach a child things it can understand," Bianca opened up in full volume. "It's actors we want, not parrots."

The walls of the office rang to the shrill sounds of battle, while Evelyn went on placidly entering up Pat's name and particulars in the book. The noisy clash of personalities was a frequent and familiar event. Evelyn took no notice.

"How old is this boy?" She made herself heard through the vocal tumult.

"Thirteen and a half," Italia tossed back at her.

"What's he done before?" asked Bianca suddenly.

"Played John in *Peter Pan*." Italia stopped abruptly. "That reminds me, Bianca. I wonder if one of those boys of ours would do for John or Michael next year?"

"Do you mean one of the Livesey brothers?"

"Yes."

"I thought you were keeping them for *Where the Rainbow Ends?*"

The battle was ended as quickly as it had begun by a sudden switch of mood. They discussed amicably the respective merits of young Roger and Barry Livesey.

Evelyn carefully blotted the new name she had added to the fast-growing list of pupils and put the book away. That was in March.

For several weeks the name of Pat Kay was forgotten in the day-to-day activities of the busy school.

The Conti sisters, brilliant and temperamental, owed the rising success of their school to Bianca's magnificent teaching and to Italia's unerring instinct for recognising raw talent, developing it and seeing that it got its chance on the stage.

It was less than seven years since the first band of Conti children had gathered in the hired studios in Great Ormond Street, but already, in 1918, the hallmark "Conti" on a young actor or actress stood for quality in the theatre world.

This was the school, then, to which Pat Kay came as a new boy in the summer term.

"Evelyn . . ." The ill-used office door crashed open. "Get me the Kays on the telephone." Italia filled and dominated the room. "I must speak to Mrs. Kay at once."

"Shut the door!" Evelyn spread her arms over a threatened snowstorm of papers.

"Where's Bianca?" With a regal gesture Italia closed the door.

"She hasn't come up from her class yet." Evelyn relaxed off her papers and glanced at the clock. "She ought to be back any time now."

"She must hear him." Italia paced up and down the office. "It was beautiful, most moving."

"What was?"

" 'Mother o' Mine.' That boy Pat Kay has just been reciting it in my class. Excellent," her expressive hands underlined her words. "Such feeling."

"Are you going to tell his mother about it, then?" inquired the practical Evelyn.

Italia stopped walking to and fro and leaned over the top of the desk.

"That boy has talent." A sensitive forefinger probed in Evelyn's direction. "I want him under contract—to us. Get Mrs. Kay on the phone for me—darling."

"I'm trying to do the accounts," Evelyn grumbled.

"It won't take you a minute just to do the telephone for me." Her voice was soft and persuasive.

Evelyn never could resist Italia's charm. She pushed aside the long column of money she had been trying to add up and searched for the number.

Bianca came in and the office echoed to the name of Pat Kay.

"We can do a lot for that boy, I feel it." Italia's wide gesture sketched a brilliant future.

Evelyn dropped her hand over the mouthpiece of the telephone. "Mrs. Kay is on the line."

Italia went into action. All the charm of her deep expressive voice went over the wire . . .

"Mrs. Kay is going to think it over." Italia smiled as she hung up the receiver again. "She wants to talk it over with Pat. There is some difficulty apparently because of his dancing. The boy goes to dancing class with Astafieva and doesn't want to give it up." She looked round at her sisters, her shrewd, business mind working fast. "I don't think it need make any difference to us."

"No," said Evelyn, "as long as the contract makes it clear that all his stage work is handled by us he can go on with his dancing lessons."

"There'll be plenty of work for a boy of that type," put in Bianca.

"His mother is coming to see me to discuss it," Italia remembered.

She saw Mrs. Kay the next afternoon and the result was a contract. Pat Kay, with the exception of his dancing classes, became the exclusive property of the Italia Conti School.

Pat himself was delighted, as were his parents. His career seemed to be taking shape. His days became a busy round of school with his tutor, dancing with Astafieva, and stage classes at Conti's.

His mother, watching him absorbed and happy in all the unfolding promise of his young life, sent up a prayer of thankfulness that the war had not touched him.

The war—that horrible monster—was dragging its hideous length through its fourth year of destruction and death. The daily casualty lists darkened long columns of the newspapers, and Mrs. Kay, like thousands of other mothers, did her best to hide her constant, gnawing fears for her eldest son. Philip was far away these days in Egypt, serving with General Allenby's Forces. Better there than in the trenches of Northern France, she told herself, as she prayed for his safety, finding it hard to believe sometimes that this dreadful war would ever end. She wondered what the future held for this eldest son of hers who had given four long years of his young life to his country. She tried to find forgetfulness in busy, crowded days, and was glad that Pat claimed so much of her attention.

He was taking his acting very seriously and needed her help and encouragement to unravel the endless passages of Shakespeare and the long poems he had to study and learn by heart.

"Why do I have to learn all this stuff, Mother?" He sat in the old schoolroom plodding through a heavy piece of *Hamlet*. "I don't see what use it is going to be."

"I suppose Miss Conti knows what is best for you and that it is all good training," she suggested.

"Miss Conti is a wonderful teacher," said Pat enthusiastically, "so is Mrs. Murray, that's Bianca, her sister. She's the one who takes me for Elocution. It's a wonderful school."

"Yes, I'm very glad you're there, darling, I hope they'll do great things for you."

Now that Pat's acting career was in Italia Conti's skilled hands, things soon began to happen. He had been in the school scarcely three months when Miss Conti was ringing up.

"Would you be prepared to take Pat on tour?" she asked, and Mrs. Kay, who had never thought about it, heard the charming and persuasive voice in her ear, "I can offer Pat a very good job . . ."

Pat, who was listening over his mother's shoulder, jumped about with excitement.

". . . They want a boy to play the part of David in the musical comedy *Betty*. I can tell you, Mrs. Kay, it's one of the best parts for a boy that has ever been written in a musical comedy. I think Pat would be just right for it."

Pat nudged his mother, making frantic signs to say yes.

". . . They're sending a first-class company out," the voice went on smoothly. "Very good names in it."

"How long is the tour?" Mrs. Kay managed to ask.

"It'll be about twelve weeks, starting at Scarborough. I haven't the list here but I know they plan to do a fortnight in Ireland, going to Belfast and Dublin . . ."

Dublin! Mrs. Kay's childhood home. She hadn't been back there for years. Dublin! Her eyes were bright with excitement as she looked at Pat.

"Go on, say yes," he urged her in a whisper.

"When does it start?" she asked.

"They are beginning rehearsing at Daly's Theatre next week and plan to be on tour by the beginning of September . . ."

Italia, at the other end of the phone, smiled as she heard Pat's urgent prompting in the background, and Mrs. Kay's rather startled consent.

"Well, that's fixed." Italia dropped the receiver back on its hook. "Evelyn, dear, can you get someone to send a letter off to Mrs. Kay with the details of the rehearsals for *Betty*, and the contract? I want it to go at once before she changes her mind."

Mrs. Kay hung up her receiver more slowly, wondering what she had done. She had just agreed to go off with Pat for twelve weeks. But what about the house? Her husband? Domestic problems crowded in, and then another thought.

"Bother!" she said. "After all that, I never asked what salary you'd be getting."

They looked at each other and laughed.

"How like us!"

"Never mind." Pat caught his mother round the waist and waltzed her in a mad circle, "We're going on tour, and we're going to Ireland, and it's all terribly exciting."

16 *"Betty"*

Bulky theatrical hampers were packed; scenery loaded on to lorries and dispatched in advance; musical instruments crated and labelled, and one Sunday in September 1918 the Touring Company of *Betty* started out on its travels, heading north in a grimy, crowded train. No reserved carriages to be had in these war-time days, so the company scattered to find their own places as best they could.

Neither Pat nor his mother knew anything about touring, and no one had thought to tell them.

They arrived in Scarborough station, dazed, dirty and tired.

"I thought there would be someone from the theatre to tell us what to do." Mrs. Kay stood like an island in the stream of people flowing towards the ticket barrier.

"Hallo! Lost your luggage?" A couple of men from the company, loaded with suitcases, parcels and mackintoshes, came staggering by.

"No. We were wondering where to go," Mrs. Kay replied.

"I should go and get settled in your digs first," one of them told her. "We shan't be wanted at the theatre till to-morrow morning." He broke off, seeing the blank look on Mrs. Kay's face. "Aren't you fixed up with digs?"

"No."

"You'll have a job to find 'em, especially on a Sunday," said the old trooper cheerfully, and they went on their way.

Mrs. Kay and Pat made their way to a hotel.

"This is all right," said Pat as they were shown into their rooms. "I wonder why the others don't do this."

They discovered the answer soon enough when the bill was presented at the end of the week.

"One thing is quite clear," Mrs. Kay declared. "We can't go on living in hotels. Not on the £5 a week you're earning."

They lost no time in getting addresses from people in the company and wrote round to book cheap rooms in advance like everyone else.

As they travelled week by week over England, Pat and his mother had their first experience of theatrical digs. They moved through a succession of dingy houses in back streets, sleeping in airless little bedrooms whose brass bedsteads invariably had knobbly mattresses. There was the inevitable marble mantelpiece with dreadful ornaments in coloured glass, a chipped wash-basin and jug on a marble-topped wash-stand, and a dim, flickering gas-light. They received indifferent food served on thick, coarse plates.

"Can't 'elp it, dearie, it's the war," the landladies never failed to tell them. "Things are very difficult 'ere."

"I don't mind it," said Pat, and he didn't. It was all new still and a great adventure. Besides, there was always the hope that next week's digs would be better.

He enjoyed his part in *Betty*, there was the rewarding satisfaction of being in a first-class musical comedy that played everywhere to good houses.

"Manchester this week." Mrs. Kay gaily packed their suitcases on a Sunday morning. "Then to Ireland. No uncomfortable digs in Dublin," she laughed. "We shall be home."

All the way in the train to Manchester, Pat made his mother tell him again of her childhood over there; of the big house near the River Liffey and the millstream where she used to play when she was a little girl, or where she would just lie and watch the big mill-wheel turn, sending the sparkling water racing through it.

"I always loved watching anything that moved," she told Pat. "I still do. I can remember when I was quite small how I would lie for hours on my back on the grass under the trees and watch the pattern of moving leaves, or the clouds drifting overhead. I always managed to turn them into shapes of people or animals, and I used to make up stories about them. My favourite ones were all about circus riders, horses and dancers."

Pat remembered how he used to watch the moving shadows in the nursery when he was a small boy, and how they came to life for him and danced.

"I used to get dreadfully teased." There was a far-away look in her eyes as she relived some of these childhood moments. "I was always dreaming and I was never any good at school lessons or games. My sister was just the opposite. She was good at everything. How tall and graceful she was, just like Father with her black hair and blue eyes. She could dance beautifully. We often gave balls at our house and she was the one all the young men wanted for a partner. I never could dance, but I loved watching it. I think I was born to be a looker-on and just enjoy other people."

"Shall we go and visit your old home?"

"Sure we shall," she told him with a twinkle in her eyes and an Irish lilt to her voice that Pat loved to copy. "And many other homes besides. There's all the cousins who'll be wanting to see you."

"Grandfather wasn't really Irish, was he?" asked Pat.

"No, the Healeys were an old Lincolnshire family. Father's regiment was stationed in Ireland for a long time though. I think that when he fell in love with Mother, he fell in love with Ireland too, and so they made their home over there until she died."

"I like being Irish," said Pat. "I always feel I'm more Irish than English."

"I think you are," his mother smiled at him. "You have the dark Irish eyes, and the wayward Irish heart in you."

"And an Irish voice when I've been to Dublin." He laughed.

Meanwhile Manchester waited; a damp, depressing Manchester. on a drizzling October evening.

Pat and his mother went through the half-blacked out streets on their way to the theatre.

"Wait a minute," Pat suddenly held her arm. A poster had caught his eye. "Look!" He pointed to a name. "Do you see? 'Boucicault.' Do you think it's the same man who produced *Peter Pan*?"

They went over to read it. The poster advertised a play at another theatre in Manchester. "Dion Boucicault" stood out in bold letters.

"Yes, it must be the same," said Mrs. Kay. "What a curious coincidence. His play is here all this week too."

The coincidence gave Pat an idea.

"I could go and see him," he said thoughtfully. "What do you think? If he's producing *Peter Pan* this year I might get the part of John again. They'll be starting rehearsals next month." He looked at his mother. "Supposing I went round to see him to-night?"

"I think it would be better to write first, darling," Mrs. Kay reined back his impatience.

Between them they composed a letter, and a couple of days later Pat was invited round to see Mr. Boucicault.

"He was ever so nice to me," he came hurrying back to pass on the good news. "He says that as soon as I'm back in London after the tour I'm to go and see him at the New Theatre and he'll give me my contract."

"Darling, that's wonderful!" She was as delighted as he was. "It's all fixed then, I am pleased."

She caught sight of the paper Pat was carrying. "Is that the evening paper you've got there?"

"Oh yes! I bought one on the way back, but I was too excited about *Peter Pan* to read it." He handed it over.

The first headline that caught her eye as she opened it was, "Disaster in the Irish Channel."

A ship had been torpedoed and sunk by a German submarine.

When they reached the theatre everyone was talking about it.

"What a terrible thing."

"They won't send us to Ireland now."

"But we're due to sail in three days. We can't let the people down over there, not at such short notice."

"Perhaps the shipping company will cancel the sailing so we can't go."

"I hope they don't. I can't afford to be out of work for two weeks."

The discussions went on all over the dressing-rooms and back stage. Finally a harassed management decided that the company would sail for Ireland on Sunday as arranged, but that those who preferred not to go would be given leave and could rejoin the tour in two weeks' time at Leeds.

This decision started up the discussions all over again. In the end, only two or three decided not to go.

"What shall we do, Mother?" Pat asked.

"I don't think we should go," she bravely gave up her longed-for visit to her old home. "It wouldn't be right for you."

"But you were so longing to go to Dublin."

"I know, but it's not worth the risk now. I'll get a chance to go another time, I expect." She spoke with a cheerfulness she didn't feel. "We'll go back to London instead. Won't Father be pleased to have us back. I'll wire him straight away to let him know we're coming. It'll be a lovely surprise for him."

Mr. Kay was at the station to meet them. It was easy to pick out his tall slim figure among the crowd. After the first delighted rush of reunion, Mrs. Kay noticed suddenly that her husband's face looked pale and drawn.

"Are you all right, my dear?" She still had both her hands on his arms. "You're not ill, are you?"

"No. I'm all right," he told her. "Come along, we must get a cab before they're all taken."

She frowned. She didn't like the tone of his voice; it sounded flat and strange.

As the taxi rattled through the familiar London streets, Pat, sitting opposite his mother and father, felt too that something was terribly wrong. He listened with growing fear to his father's painful efforts to make casual conversation.

The house itself seemed empty and unfamiliar.

"Where are the servants?" Mrs. Kay stood in the hall, looking round, sensing the strangeness.

"They're in the kitchen," said Mr. Kay haltingly. "Perhaps Pat wouldn't mind taking some of the luggage up."

Pat reluctantly climbed the stairs. He saw his father and mother go into the study. Unknown fear beat in his heart as he heard the murmur of voices. What dreadful secret was his father telling his mother? Would they tell him too?

He went up to his room and dropped a suitcase on the bed. He hadn't the heart to unpack. He prowled about the upper landing and came to lean over the banisters. All about him was eerie silence. It seemed hours before he heard the study door open.

"I'll go up to him," he heard his father say, and Pat, hearing his approaching steps, fled into the bedroom.

Here, at last, he was told. Mr. Kay broke the news as gently as he could, but the cruel core of truth could not be softened. His brother Philip was dead. He had died in Egypt.

Pat sat on his bed, stunned. Philip, his beloved elder brother, dead. He tried to picture him as he had last seen him on leave. No. Pat shook his head. Not Philip in khaki; that Philip was a man, who was almost a stranger, for his leaves at home were too short to catch up the threads again. No, the Philip he knew and loved was a boy still, and the best friend and brother in the world. Philip had been part of his life ever since he could remember. Vividly there formed in his mind the swift, bright picture of their home at Felpham. Philip and himself romping in the garden with the dogs, their bird-nesting expeditions, games on the beach, glorious adventures, rock-climbing and swimming, picnics out in the country. The day Philip had helped him ride his first bicycle and they had got into such trouble. There was that wonderful holiday on the farm, the last one and the best of all. He could see Philip again, standing in the sunlight by the orchard fence, laughing as he shot bullets at the old fat pig. How strong and alive he had been, and now he was dead. Pat would never see him laugh again or hear his voice. Death had laid its cold hands on his warm body. Philip was gone for ever. The devastating sense of loss flooded over him. He fell face down on the pillow and the tears came.

Those two weeks in London were heavy with sorrow. Mrs. Kay suffered deeply. Pat and his father found courage themselves in trying to help her. They tried to persuade her to remain at home and give up the tour, but she insisted on returning with Pat to join the company at Leeds.

It was the beginning of November.

A few days later huge headlines in the papers blazoned the news: "Peace." "Armistice." It was the 11th of November 1918. Four terrible years of war had ended. All over the country bells, bonfires, fireworks, shouting, cheering crowds signalled the people's relief and joy.

On the stage of the theatre in Leeds a hastily improvised party started up the moment the curtain had rung down at the end of the show.

Tables were set up on the stage among the scenery. There was laughter and songs; the popping of wine corks, the hiss of beer. Everyone in the place, actors, musicians, stage hands, gathered to drink to the peace of the world. There were speeches and toasts.

Through the clink of glasses, and the splash of wine, Pat looked at his mother. In the hearts of both was the same aching thought. The armistice had come three weeks too late.

17 Acting and Dancing

There was a knock on the door.

"Come in," barked Mr. Boucicault. He looked up from his paper-smothered desk as the door opened. "Ah, yes! Pat Kay." His shrewd eyes watched the boy cross the room. "You came to see me in Manchester."

"Yes, sir."

"Do you remember your part in *Peter Pan?*" the questions rattled out.

"Yes, sir."

"Have you grown since last year?"

"No, sir."

"All right." Mr. Boucicault was a busy man. Already the coming production of *Peter Pan* was weighing heavily on him. "Be ready for rehearsal next week."

In this off-hand manner was Pat welcomed back into the *Peter Pan* family for the second year.

It was very different in the studio in the King's Road. Madame Astafieva was in a good mood and delighted to see him again.

"Patté," she called across the studio. "I am pleased to see you in my class again." Her dark eyes were alight with pleasure. "Yes, I know," she waved his words of excuse aside before he had a chance to say them. "You have been on tour; you wrote to me." She put her hands on his shoulders, looking him up and down. "You have grown a little, not too much, that is good. So, you have been in musical comedy." Her voice was deep with scorn. "You, who say you want to be a dancer, you work in musical comedy. Tell me, you have practised your ballet, yes?"

Pat shook his head.

"Not very often, we didn't get time."

"Patté." She looked at him in despair. "To be a dancer you must work, do exercises, two, three hours every day." Her hands gestured. "But now you come back, you work hard to make up."

"I'll come as often as I can," said Pat nervously, and explained that he was about to start working in *Peter Pan* again. This did not please Madame. She tapped her foot impatiently on the floor, her face darkened.

"You children, you are all alike," a sweeping gesture condemned all her pupils. "The only thing you think of is to get jobs now; to earn money at once. Never mind how; pantomime, musical comedy, chorus work." Her class seemed to wither under her scornful eyes. "Cheap, bad dancing. So you get bad habits, bad style, and then you find out it is no good, there is no future in it, and it is too late for you to start again to learn to be real dancers. No, you must work now, while you are young, there is no time to waste. In Russia a child goes into the Imperial Ballet School at eight years old, and there he stays until he is seventeen or eighteen. Think of it, nine, ten years of training. He lives for nothing but the dance. And when he has finished all this, do you think he is a star, as you call them? No, he is put in the *corps de ballet*. Yes, after ten years' training the dancer is just good enough to be in the chorus. From there, if he shows he has real talent, he may be given a small part of his own, and then . . ."

Madame was well launched on one of her favourite subjects. She had forgotten about Pat who eased his way, unnoticed, into the protecting shelter of the crowd of pupils.

A subdued class took its place at the bar, making private resolutions to devote itself to a life of ballet. The work began.

Madame, fired anew with memories of her own training at the Imperial School at St. Petersburg, was even stricter than usual. The jewelled stick darted mercilessly among the moving legs; and this was the moment an unlucky mother arrived at the studio to present her small daughter to Astafieva as a possible pupil.

The class watched curiously as a lady was shown into the studio. With her came a small, timid little girl.

"I am Astafieva, what do you want?" She frowned at the small white card which had been handed to her. "What is this? Alice Marks, the Miniature Pavlova."

Everyone's attention was suddenly focused on the frail, dark-haired child. Her small, serious face was turned to Astafieva in grave-eyed wonder.

"Miniature Pavlova!" Astafieva jerked the card about angrily. "You mothers, you are all the same," her scorn broke loose. "You are idiots. Yes. You think because your daughter can stand on her toes and wobble she is a Pavlova. Yes? You don't know how long it takes to make a Pavlova, what work, what tears, what art. You don't know what it means . . ."

The little Alice Marks' big dark eyes went on looking gravely at this beautiful, angry Russian lady, who wore such funny, shapeless clothes, but who had such perfect arms and legs.

Mrs. Marks beat an embarrassed retreat, taking Alice with her. (They were soon back again and Alice duly became a pupil.) Meanwhile, Astafieva, who had just banished the future Alicia Markova from her studio, spent the rest of the class delivering a long tirade against all dancing mothers.

"Not one of Madame's good days after all," Pat thought as he came out into the King's Road after the class.

As the tube rattled him across London he thought over what she had said. He wished with all his heart that he could have gone to the Imperial Ballet School in St. Petersburg. How wonderful it must be to give one's whole time to dancing, and not to be pulled about in all directions, trying to fit in dancing, acting, schooling and jobs as well.

"If I was in Russia, my training would be finished in three more years," he said to himself as he came up to the surface of the earth again.

He made his way through Russell Square to the Conti School in Great Ormond Street.

"Did you practise your elocution and voice production?" Italia Conti wanted to know.

Pat shook his head.

"Not very often. We didn't get time."

"Pat," she looked at him in despair. "You'll never get on in this profession unless you practise every day. But now you are back you must come to as many classes as you can to catch up."

Pat felt he had heard this conversation somewhere before.

He explained about *Peter Pan*.

"Yes, I know, dear. Mr. Boucicault told me he wanted you for John again. I'll get in touch with your mother about the contract."

Peter Pan, dancing classes, acting classes. What about school lessons? Pat was very relieved when his parents agreed that it wasn't worth going back to his tutor for only the last two or three weeks of the term.

Rehearsals started.

At the New Theatre there was a joyful reunion of the *Peter Pan* family. There were not many changes. John, Michael, Wendy and Mrs. Darling were all old friends. Most of the Lost Boys and Pirates had been in last year's company. A new Peter had joined them, however. Faith Celli was stepping, for the first time, into Peter Pan's brown leather jerkin and long brown tights, with all the bewildering business of the part to learn.

This year John faced Mr. Boucicault with all the confidence of a veteran actor who knew his part, while poor Peter, to whom it was all strange and new, became the target for the producer's temperament. The New Theatre rocked with shouts directed at the unhappy newcomer.

There were many tears before Faith was turned into a Peter that satisfied Mr. Boucicault's ideas. As before, though, once the curtain had gone up on the first night, the fiery temper went down and they settled into their happy, back-stage family life.

"Are you two coming down to tea?" Stella Patrick Campbell whispered to John and Michael in the wings as they waited for their entrance.

"Are you starting tea-parties again?" Michael was delighted. "How lovely. Thank you very much."

"Come down in the second interval as usual," she told them.

Pat, however, had an idea of his own to pursue. During the interval he tracked down the Kirby flying men to their lair below stage and held a long and earnest conversation with Tom, the man who flew him.

"I don't mind doing it for you just once," said Tom as they went on stage for the Underground Scene.

Pat felt he could hardly wait for the end of the play.

The curtain came down on the last scene. The theatre emptied. On stage, the men set up the Nursery Scene, ready for the evening show, and went off to their tea. The stage was deserted, until a soft padding of feet sounded on the boards and a white figure appeared, coming through the Nursery door.

"Are you there?"

"Yes, I'm here." The whisper came from the dark shadows of the prompt corner. Tom appeared.

"Now, tell me exactly what you want." He clipped on the flying wire.

Pat, a ghostly-looking figure in pyjamas, stood in the unlighted Nursery set.

"Will you take me straight up and down first." He placed his feet ready in the fifth position. Tom pulled on the rope and, as Pat went up in the air, his feet moved in a series of beautiful *entrechats*.

"I want to try some *grand jetés* now," he told Tom when the *entrechats* possibilities had been exhausted. "I'll run across, jump, and turn on landing."

Tom rapidly got the idea, and Pat had the unique sensation of leaping in the air and sailing across the stage in a series of perfect *grand jetés*. At least, they felt perfect.

"Here, young fellow, that's enough for now." Tom, out of breath, slackened off the wire.

"It was wonderful," Pat presented his back to be unhooked. "You see, on the wire I can do all the difficult things I've seen dancers do on the stage. Thank you very much, Tom." A packet of cigarettes changed hands. It was the first of several more, as Tom good-naturedly allowed himself to be bribed, and Pat's flying ballet practice became a regular event after the matinée, until the stage manager, returning early from tea one day, found them at it. This put an end to Pat's idea.

"Well, it was wonderful while it lasted." Pat had to content himself with reliving the glorious feeling of floating through the air. He wondered how long it would be before his muscles would be trained and strong enough to send him up in great leaps as he had seen other dancers do. What was the name of the famous Russian who jumped and flew like a bird? Pat leaned his elbow on his dressing-table and searched for the answer in his reflected face. Nijinsky! That was it. He could hear again Astafieva's clear voice telling him about this great artist.

"The most wonderful dancer of the age," she had said. "I have seen Nijinsky dance *Le Spectre de la Rose* with Karsavina." Astafieva had made the scene relive for him. He could see the spectacular leap through the open window.

"Right across the stage he is carried, in a single movement. He appears to fly without effort. No other dancer could ever dance that role as Nijinsky did," Astafieva's eyes would light up as she spoke of it. "Yes, when Karsavina and Nijinsky first danced *Le Spectre de la Rose*, they took Paris by storm. Nothing like it had ever been seen before . . ." Her voice faded away into her memories of those glittering pre-war days, when she too was dancing in Paris with the Ballets Russes, and Pat, looking in his mirror, saw his own image blur and fade. Through his eyes seemed to appear those legendary dancing figures shining like distant flames lighting the way he was to follow. Could he follow? Would he ever be a dancer in his own right, or would he merely be an actor who danced?

Every instinct in him urged him to dance, but cold reason held him back, telling him that acting should be his career on the stage.

Which should he follow? Instinct or reason?

Which way did his future lie? To act? Or to dance?

18 Break

"I think you need a holiday, Pat," Mrs. Kay announced when the six weeks of *Peter Pan* were over. "You're looking very tired, darling. After all, you have been working without a break since last August."

"What's the use of a holiday in February?" he grumbled.

"I think you ought to have a change of air and a complete rest." His mother had been worrying about his pale, drawn face. He had been through a great strain during the last six months. The shock of the news of Philip's death coming on top of the exhausting tour of *Betty* and followed by the hard work in *Peter Pan* had made him very run down.

"Will you come too?" he wanted to know.

"I wish I could, darling, but I'm afraid I can't leave the house now."

An unwilling Pat was dispatched to Brighton alone, where he spent four weeks missing his dancing and acting, and busy London life. The enforced holiday, however, had its effect. It brought back the old mischief and sparkle in his eyes. He came home in March with a new store of energy. He was going to need it too as he started on a strenuous, triple training. Dancing classes with Astafieva, acting classes with Miss Conti, and, instead of school, secretarial classes.

This last was his mother's idea.

"It will be much more useful than school lessons," she had argued. So, at fourteen and a half, Pat left his schoolroom education behind him and went off to daily classes in shorthand and typing. At least, that is what his mother fondly thought. More often than not, however, he never arrived at his destination, and a young boy who should have been pounding a typewriter might have been seen giving himself another sort of education, browsing round the exhibits in the British Museum.

"You don't seem to be getting on very fast, darling," his mother remarked, when the first test results came in. Pat hastily became engrossed in a large volume of Shakespeare.

"I've got such a lot of other work to think about." He rattled the pages impressively. "Mrs. Murray wants to send me in for a competition. It's an elocution competition," he went on.

"That's interesting. Who's organising it?"

Pat felt he was steering her safely past the dangerous subjects of shorthand and typing.

"It's for a prize given by the British Empire Shakespeare

Society." He rolled out the title importantly. "I've got ever such a long scene to learn out of *Romeo and Juliet*, and a lot of it is so difficult." He looked at her hopefully.

"Would you like me to help you with it?" She took her cue beautifully. The shorthand and typing crisis was successfully averted. *Romeo and Juliet* kept their attention fully occupied.

Mrs. Murray was a hard taskmaster. During the long summer weeks, Pat, encouraged by his mother and driven by Mrs. Murray, slogged away at the unnatural occupation of mastering a scene from Shakespeare.

"I know you can do it if you try," Mrs. Murray kept telling him.

She was right. He tried really hard and was rewarded for his effort. He won the Elocution Competition. On the stage of the Haymarket Theatre he received his prize from the hands of the great Ellen Terry herself.

"You must be feeling so proud." His mother shared his great moment. "You certainly did deserve it."

"I think Mrs. Murray ought to have the prize," said Pat. "It was all her doing."

"It was your own hard work."

"I suppose so," replied Pat, and found nothing else to say. It was, of course, a nice feeling to win a competition one had worked hard for. He wondered why he didn't feel more thrilled about it. He had felt far more elated that day at the studio when he had mastered his first *Tours en l'air* and Astafieva's praise had warmed him to delight. Acting was his profession, however, he told himself, and the prize he had won was another step on the way up. He was deeply grateful to Mrs. Murray who had made it possible, and his mother's delight in his success gave him pleasure in it too.

"Do you think I'll get lots of offers of good parts now?" he asked her.

"I hope so."

All that happened, however, was *Peter Pan* again three months later.

This third year, John's Eton suit sat tightly across Pat's broadening shoulders and pulled short in the sleeves. He had grown.

"This time it really is good-bye," he told Michael who had

looked in to his dressing-room on the last night to see if he was ready. "Next year I shall be too big to play John, and not big enough to play Mr. Darling," he added swiftly. A great sadness came over him.

"You're lucky, you've had three years running," Michael stood in the doorway pulling up her socks.

"That's true," Pat stared at his reflection and thought over those three years. How long it seemed since a frightened boy of thirteen had faced that terrifying audition. He remembered the excitement of being offered the part; the awful, never-ending misery of those first rehearsals, and then, the six happy weeks of the run of the play.

What a busy year had followed that first *Peter Pan*, joining the Conti School, the first acting lessons, the first long tour with *Betty*, and then the second *Peter Pan*.

"I don't seem to have done anything much this year," he said aloud as he thought over the long vista of weeks that stretched between his second and third *Peter Pan*. He saw only classes and more classes; acting, dancing, shorthand and typing.

"My mother says it's always like that in the profession," said Michael sympathetically. "One gets nothing for weeks and then everything happens at once."

"I wonder what'll happen to me next." Pat leaned forward and traced the date on his mirror in black greasepaint. 30th January, 1920. "I wonder what I'll be doing by January 1921 and who'll be wearing this Eton suit and sitting in this chair?" He suddenly felt very old.

"I'm fifteen," he told himself. "I've been on the stage since I was twelve, and where has it got me?"

"Overture and beginners, please!" The call-boy's sing-song voice echoing down the corridor put an abrupt end to these morbid thoughts.

The sadness returned that night as he said good-bye to "John" and the happy *Peter Pan* family for ever.

Eight months were to pass before he was to hear a call-boy's voice sing out as he sat in a dressing-room, making up in the glaring light of the big naked bulbs over the mirror.

"Your call, please, Mr. Kay." The door rattled.

"Thank you."

"Mr. Kay" got up and looked at himself in the mirror. This

time he was seeing, not the boy John Darling in an Eton suit, but a young man of sixteen, slim-hipped and broad-shouldered in his close-fitting uniform of a page. He tipped a jaunty pill-box at a rakish angle on his dark hair, took a close view of his make-up, gave a last tug to the immaculate tunic with its rows of gleaming brass buttons, and made his way down to the stage, to be Dimitri, the Russian Page, who stood very stiffly holding the door open for the lovely young actress, Marie Lohr.

Outside in the grey dusk of an October evening, the pulsing traffic streamed up and down Shaftesbury Avenue, passing the lighted entrance above which gilded letters spelled the name "Globe Theatre", and high overhead flashed the title *Fedora* into the evening sky, with the names "Marie Lohr" and "Basil Rathbone", while down below on the posters, in very small letters near the bottom of the list, might be seen the name Pat Kay.

"Dear Dimitri," Marie Lohr wrote in her Russian Page's autograph book on the last night of the play. "You have held the door open for me 111 times. I will always hold the door of the Globe open for you."

"What a lovely person she is," Pat thought as he hugged his autograph book and his happy memories of his four months in *Fedora*.

It was December 1920.

"I want you to go for an audition, Pat." Italia Conti sent for him soon afterwards. "Evelyn, where's that thing from the St. James's Theatre?" She churned over the tumbled papers on the desk.

"Do you mean this?" Evelyn produced a letter from a drawer.

"That's it." Italia, unwilling to admit that she needed glasses, held the paper at arm's length. "It's a play called *Threads*."

Pat got the part and was called for rehearsal at the St. James's Theatre.

Vivid memories came crowding back as he turned into the quiet street where the little theatre stood. The stage door keeper challenged him at the entrance. Was it the same man who had let them through two years ago? He couldn't be sure. Inside nothing had changed. It was all just as he remembered it.

"Not that way," the doorkeeper called after him, but Pat didn't listen. He was making his way to a certain door. It was shut fast.

He stood staring at it, wondering what lay the other side now. Was the furniture still there, gleaming darkly in the firelight, and the screen and the photographs? Surely the door would open and he would see the handsome figure of the great actor, as he had stood saying good-bye to them. He could hear again the measured tones of that beautiful speaking voice.

The door did open. An entirely strange face appeared, and a hostile voice asked what the blazes he thought he was doing there.

Pat fled on to the stage. Rehearsals began. The theatre echoed to the sound of the modern, strident voices of 1920, and maybe the gentle ghost of Sir George Alexander lingered in the empty stalls watching his successors at work and mourning silently for the good old days.

They had been rehearsing a week. *Threads* was beginning to take some sort of shape.

"What's the matter with you this morning?" the producer called up to Pat as he started on his lines. "Can't hear you."

"I'm sorry." Pat stepped up the pressure, but his voice was husky, he couldn't get the volume out.

"Have you got a sore throat?" the producer asked. "Thought you've been sounding rather rough this last day or two."

"No. I haven't got a sore throat," Pat replied, and his voice sounded strangely hoarse to himself now. "I'm all right."

There was a startled giggle from those round him, for the last bit came out in a shrill squeak.

Pat blushed scarlet, and put his hand to his throat. What horrible disease was lurking there?

"Come here, lad." The producer beckoned him down to the footlights. "How old are you?"

"Sixteen." Pat, taking no more risks, whispered the answer.

The producer looked at the others and then back at Pat.

"That's it," he said. "Voice breaking."

Pat had a great deal to think about as he left the theatre that day. This was to be a break in more ways than one. It was going to mean giving up his part in *Threads*. "Broken Threads," he smiled to himself. It was also going to mean the end of his acting career for the time being.

"How long does it take for one's voice to finish breaking?" he asked his mother when he got home.

"It depends. It may be three months, six months, or even a year. Some take longer to settle than others." She shared his disappointment, understanding so well what he was feeling. After all these months of work and struggle, now, just as he was beginning to make a small success and be in demand by producers and managers, it was suddenly ended.

"By the time I can get jobs again, everyone will have forgotten me," Pat croaked gloomily. "I'll have to start all over again."

It was curious, he thought suddenly, how fate seemed to turn in a circle. It was from St. James's Theatre he had started out on his serious acting career, to follow Sir George Alexander's advice by joining the Conti School. Now, two years later, the same theatre had seen the end of it, anyway for the time being.

"I shan't go back to Conti's," he told his mother. "I mean, there's no point in going on with elocution and voice production with a cracked voice."

Mrs. Kay hid the sudden stab of disappointment his words gave her. She supposed he was right and that it was unreasonable of her to have expected him to go on there. After all, he would go back to the stage later on, she told herself. He had worked too hard on it to throw it all away.

"You must do what you think best, dear," she told him gently. "One thing, you have still got your dancing."

"Yes," said Pat slowly. "I have still got my dancing." With that thought in mind he left her to wander out of the house and down the road, for the urge to be alone had come upon him.

He went down to the river and sat on the rails at the end of the park, just as he had done on his first day in London. That day had been a milestone in his life, this, he felt, was another. Five years had passed since he had first sat here looking down at the water. It had been summer then, and the sun had sparkled on its surface. He had sent his hopes and ambitions out on that moving current. What had he achieved in five years? The beginning of an acting career? Already it seemed to be finished.

To-day, the river was cold and brown in the dull winter light. Pat's eyes followed the flowing current. Had he really wanted to be an actor? he asked himself, or had he forced himself along that path to please his mother and father? Did he really want to take up his acting career again?

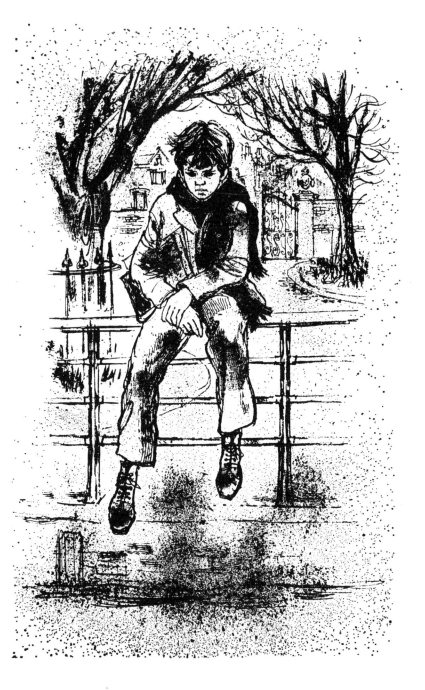

The wind rippled the surface of the water and the shadows moved and danced. As he watched them it seemed that the shadows in his heart lightened and lifted. Yes, he still had his dancing. More than that, he was now free to give his whole mind and body to it. No more would he be pulled in two directions, torn between acting and dancing, wondering which he should choose. His breaking voice had, for the present, made the decision for him. He could devote all his energy to dancing.

The thought sent the blood pulsing swiftly through his veins again. Hope and ambition went out once more on that swift current. He renewed his resolution to be someone who counted in the world.

The run of Pat Kay the actor had finished. The curtain was now to rise on Pat Kay the dancer.

19 The Russian Tradition

"One and two, three and four . . ." Madame's deep Russian voice chanted the time. "Keep your body straight, head up. One and two . . ." The long jewelled stick tapped the floor. "Yes. That will do. Turn. Now on the other foot. One and two . . . No!" The stick flashed out. "Keep your leg turned out. You—Jois, knee straight. Patté, stretch your foot more." Madame walked along the line of pupils working at the bar.

"All right," she clapped her hands. "In the centre, everyone."

The tall mirrors against the wall reflected the graceful figures moving to the insistent beat of the piano and Madame's clear voice.

Pliés, battements, ronds de jambe, arabesques, jetés, entrechats, fouettés. These things formed the whole pattern of Pat's life in the days that followed the end of his acting activities.

"Don't you get sick of doing nothing but dance?" Anthony, home for the Christmas holidays, sympathised over Pat's breaking voice.

"No, I don't," replied Pat. "I love it."

"Don't you miss the stage?" his young brother persisted.

"No, I don't think so," and now he came to think about it, Pat realised that, already, he had left acting very far behind him.

"It'll be the first Christmas for a long time that you haven't been working." Mrs. Kay smiled, happy to have both her sons at home. How different they were, she thought. Anthony, very much the schoolboy, concerned with football and cricket and winning his house colours. Pat, half boy, half man, had not yet found himself. He was still reaching out after his dream, the half-formed vision that had haunted him ever since he was a little boy, and still eluded him.

"As I'm not working, let's have a party at Christmas," Pat was saying. "Let's ask lots of people. We haven't had any real family parties for ages . . ." He suddenly fell silent, remembering their parties in the old days, when Philip had been there to share them.

"I don't think we can, darling," Mrs. Kay reminded him gently. "You see, Father really can't stand much noise."

"Oh yes!" and Pat was moved to swift shame for he had forgotten about his father. Mr. Kay hadn't been very well for some time now.

"What's the matter with Father?" Anthony wanted to know.

"I'm afraid your father isn't as young as he was," Mrs. Kay explained. "He's not very strong these days, and the doctor says he must lead a very quiet life."

"How dreadful to be ill and getting old," thought Pat, and his bounding youth and vitality revolted against the idea of the creeping weight of years on his body. Would the time really come when his own strong legs became feeble and he could no longer command his muscles and know the joy of dancing? He chased the thought away.

"Yes," Mrs. Kay was saying. "The doctor thinks we should move to a quieter district."

"A new house! That'll be exciting," both the boys decided. "Where shall we go?" They spent the rest of the evening discussing places to live.

Mrs. Kay had not told them all that the doctor had said.

"He may last for many years yet," the doctor had told her, and she knew that meant he never would get better. Meanwhile he must be kept quiet and free from noise. The most she could hope for was to prolong his life by careful nursing.

So it came about that, early in 1921, once again the big vans stood outside 49 Bishops Mansions while a team of men slowly emptied the house of its contents. This time, however, Pat was not going with them. The labels on his trunk read: King's Road, Chelsea.

"Good-bye, darling," his mother saw him into a cab. "We'll see you on Sunday, shan't we?"

"Yes, of course you will." He kissed her, and she sighed a little as she watched him being driven away. She hated letting him go, but she knew it was the only thing to do. She couldn't keep a high-spirited boy like her Pat in the sick-room atmosphere of a hushed house. She knew that all her patience and courage belonged now to her husband, and Pat must fend for himself for a while.

"After all, we shall see him quite often," she tried to console herself. "Hampstead isn't all that far away from Chelsea." But she sighed again, for she knew that this break from home marked the real end of Pat's childhood. This sixteen-year-old son of hers, with his deepening, husky voice, was a man now, starting on his own independent life; and though the love and understanding between them would never be spoiled, he could never be her little boy again, running to her to be taken in her arms and comforted, nor share all the treasured, small things of everyday life together, and her heart was sad, as all mothers' hearts are, for the young days that will never come back.

"Excuse me, Mum! but Cook wants to know if you're taking the fish kettle, she says it's got a 'ole in it." An anxious man in overalls breathed heavily over her shoulder.

"The fish kettle!" She laughed suddenly, and let the crowding business of the move chase away her dark thoughts. "I'll come and see."

"The past," she told herself as she went in to deal with Cook and her problem, "remains buried in our memories. The present belongs to my husband. And the future?"

The future was rattling along in the cab wondering what his new life would be like.

He was going to live with Astafieva. She kept a few rooms at the studios for resident pupils, and Pat, half pleased, half fearful at the prospect, was going to be one of them. What would it be like living in daily contact with that vivid, difficult, turbulent personality? He stared out of the cab windows with unseeing eyes, thinking what a

EXOTICS

Dance outside the ballet tradition photographed by Baron

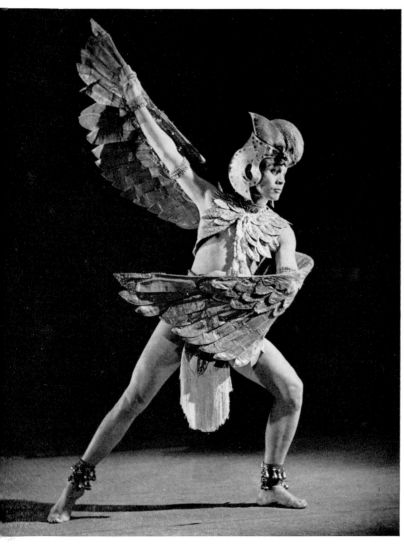

Ram Gopal who was a pioneer in bringing the
elegance and beauty of Indian dancing to this country,
in his Golden Eagle Dance.

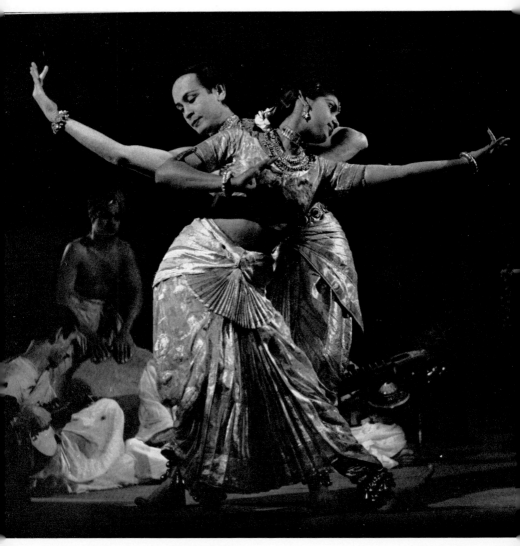

Kumudini and Ram Gopal

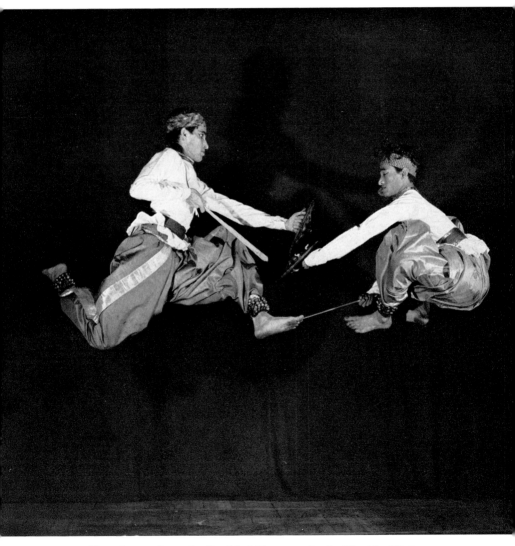

Two dancers from the Sarabhai Company in the Bhaddo Nittham, a warrior dance of Malabar

Mrinalini Sarabhai one of the greatest Indian dancers, demonstrating the beautiful formalised gesture language of the Indian dance.

a lotus flower in full bloom

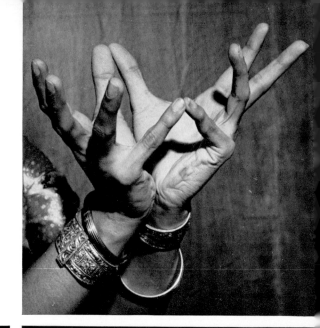

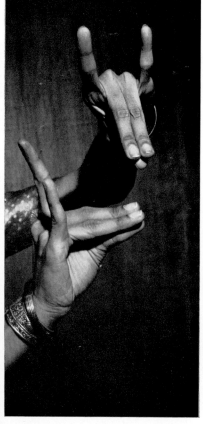

a deer

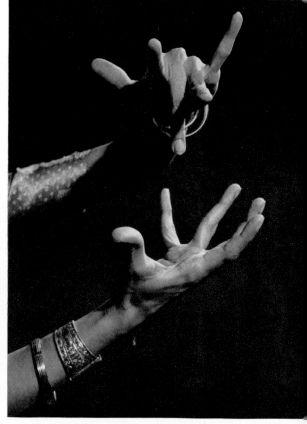

a bee taking nectar from a flower

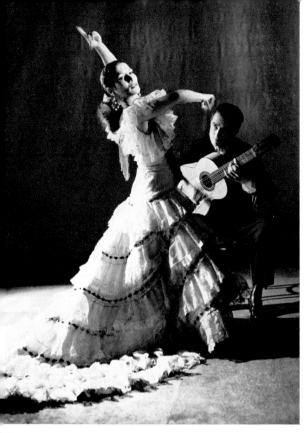

Carmen Amaya a dancer with a strong personality. Jean Cocteau described her as "hail beating down on window panes, the cry of a swallow, a black cigar smoked by a brooding woman, the thunder of applause."

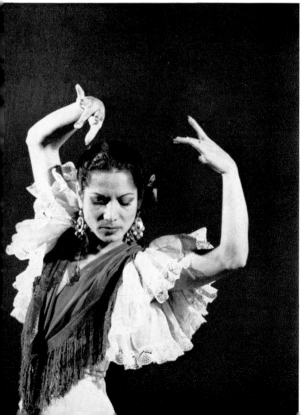

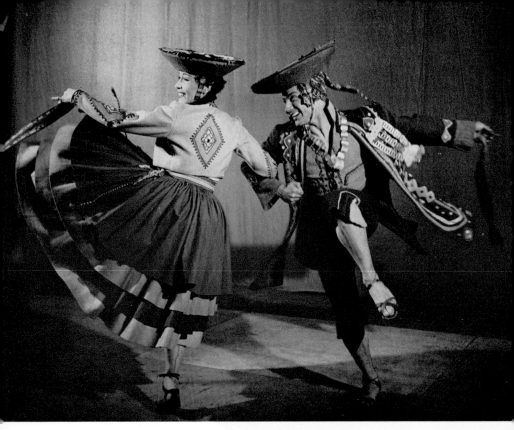

Rosario and Antonio, two popular and lively classical Spanish dancers who have brought Spanish dancing to a wide audience.

Above   Rosario and Antonio

Right   Antonio

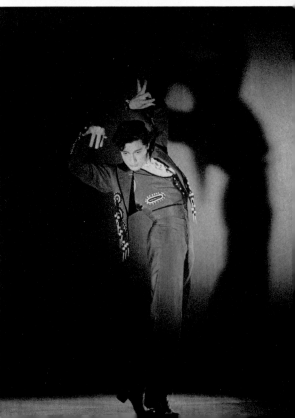

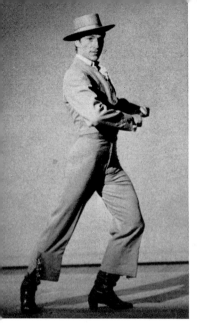

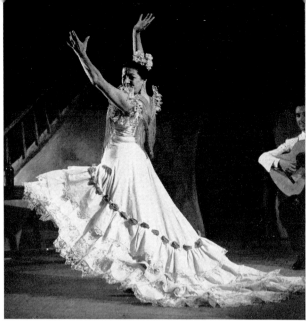

se Greco's name is almost
nonymous with Spanish dancing
day through the great traditions
his company.

Left	Jose Greco in *En El Cortijo*
Right	His wife, Nila Amparo in a Flamenco finale
Below	La Quica, one of the greatest teachers and exponents of Flamenco dancing

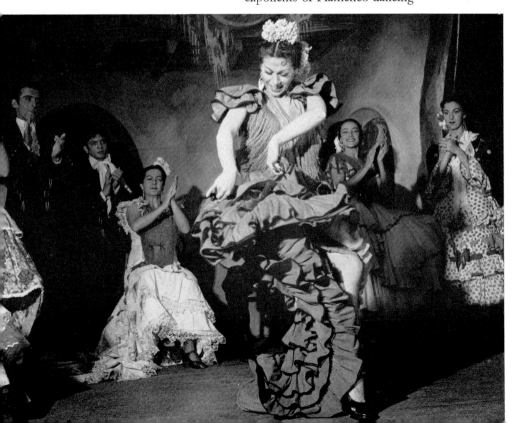

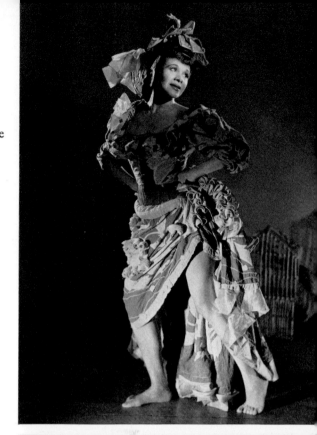

Katherine Dunham, the first, and perhaps the greatest exponent of the African dance on the stage. A choreographer and a dancer, she created this particular school of dancing, and for the first time brought the excitement of African dancing into the theatre.

Katherine Dunham

In her most moving role in *L'Ag'ya*, with Vanoye Aikens

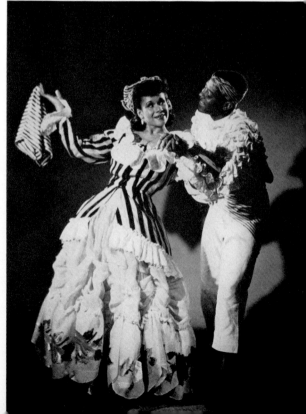

wonderful teacher Madame was and wondering what she really thought of his dancing.

It was a question he had often asked himself. For two and a half years now he had been going to her classes. People had told him that her favourite pupils were the ones whose legs carried the most bruises. If that were true, Madame must love him very much, for his legs were always black and blue from that flashing stick. Does she really think I have talent? Pat asked himself. She had never shown that she did, or singled him out for special encouragement in any way. As far as he could see she had always treated him like all her other pupils. He came for his lesson; if he worked well she smiled and said "good"; if he worked badly, there was the stick to make another bruise on his legs. That was as it should be, but there were the days when he wanted something more, the days when he felt discouraged and wondered if he was really going to get any-where. "Is it enough to want to dance and to work hard?" he asked himself in his black moments of doubt. "Do I really have the talent to go to the top?"

This question was becoming more and more insistent. He wished again that he knew what Astafieva really thought of his work. She would never tell him if he asked her. Now, however, though he did not yet realise it, he was slowly to discover the answer for himself.

They were a small, happy family, that handful of resident pupils in the studio in the King's Road. Astafieva created about her the warm Russian atmosphere of her own lively temperament, and Pat, ever sensitive to his surroundings, adapted himself swiftly to this new way of living and loved it. He ate strange Russian dishes, he learned Russian words, he absorbed the traditions of the Russian ballet.

Best moments of all, he found, were the evenings, when work was over for the day and the big studios were empty and silent. The door of Madame's sitting-room stood open, and her clear voice would call to them to come in.

It was warm and bright in this room with the thick curtains drawn, shutting out the grey London winter. In here was Russia. The firelight leaped on silk shawls that splashed bright colour across the chairs. It shone on the gold and blue of a Russian ikon, and on the polished curves of the steaming samovar that stood ready on the table. It glittered among the photographs, ornaments and souvenirs crowding the furniture. Every corner of that room was stamped with the vivid personality of its owner, and in the pool of light from the tall, shaded lamp, there she was, Madame herself, as Pat was always to remember that well-loved figure. Her black hair swathed in the folds of a coloured bandeau, the ropes of pearls round her neck gleaming milky white against the ivory of her skin. Those beautiful hands with long polished nails; the inevitable cigarette; the quick, mischievous smile and the sparkle in her dark eyes as she welcomed them in.

They sat round the fire drinking tea the Russian way, in tall glasses. The smoke from Madame's cigarette curled up in slow, blue-grey shapes, and the photographs seemed to smile down on the circle of young faces. It was very still and very peaceful.

"Who is that?" Pat's attention was caught one evening by the fading picture of a dancer, a man in a curious-looking costume of leaves—or were they petals?

"That, Patté, is the great Nijinsky." Astafieva watched his face as she told him. "He is photographed there in his costume for the *Spectre de la Rose.*"

Pat started, and looked again. *Le Spectre de la Rose*, that almost legendary dream ballet created by Nijinsky and Karsavina. Since Madame had described it to him, how often he had imagined the miraculous leap through the window. So this was what the great dancer actually looked like. He studied the photograph more closely, and saw a man of middle height, thick set, with a strong neck and powerful-looking legs. So this was Vaslav Nijinsky! How different he was from what Pat had imagined.

"Ah, Patté! No photograph can show you Nijinsky as he was." Astafieva had seen the disappointment in his face. "A picture, it is a dead thing. Only those who have been lucky enough to see Nijinsky dance can know what he really was. Nijinsky the man, he is nothing, he is shy, dull, he has nothing to say, you are disappointed, but Nijinsky the artist, let him put on his costume and dance for you and he is transformed, as though another spirit, the spirit of his role, had entered his body and taken possession of him. That is the genius of Nijinsky. I know, I tell you, I have been on the stage with him, I have seen this happen with my own eyes."

"You have danced on the same stage as Nijinsky," Pat repeated slowly, and looking at her, he envied her memories.

"Is he dead?" one of the girls wanted to know.

"No. He is alive. If you can call it that. How shall I say it?" Her hands moved in a tiny broken gesture. "He is ill."

"He is very old, I suppose."

"He is not too old to dance," said Madame sadly. "That is the tragedy. It is his mind that is ill." Her fingers tapped the side of her head. "Something here has broken. Everything has been tried to cure him." Her hands fluttered helplessly on to her lap. "Now, we can only pray that a great artist may be given back to the world again."

They stared in silent awe at the photograph that had caught one fleeting moment of his life and recorded for ever the great dancer as he was in all his beauty and strength.

"Who is that?" One of the girls noticed another photograph nearby. "It looks as though it was taken a very long time ago." She studied the picture of a young slender girl in a classical white tutu.

"It is very old!" Astafieva's merry laugh drove out the brooding shadow of Nijinsky's tragedy. "That was me! It was taken at St. Petersburg when I graduated."

"I say, I am sorry!" The girl blushed. "I thought it was old because it's faded."

"It has travelled about a great deal," said Astafieva with her mischievous smile. "I like to have it with me to remind me that I too was once young and beautiful."

"How did you become a dancer?" they asked her. "Did your father and mother dance?"

"No," she shook her head. "I was the only one in the family. It was my idea alone." Looking round at the eager young faces her own memories became young again. "My father was a soldier," she told them, "an officer in the Czar's army. When I was a little girl we lived in St. Petersburg, and I was sent to a school in a convent. I hated it. I wanted to dance, but my father and mother would not let me. Then, one day, I became very ill. I had typhoid fever. Everyone thought I would die, but me, I wanted to live! I made my father promise me that if I should get better he would take me away from the convent and let me be a dancer. Then the miracle happened, and I got better!"

"And your father kept his promise."

"Yes," she smiled at their impatience. "He engaged a dancing master for me, from the Imperial Theatre. Mr. Pichot his name was. He came to our house twice a week and gave me lessons."

"I suppose you were very good at dancing right from the start?"

"No. Just the opposite. My master did not like me at all. I was ugly and I was thin, and I was always crying." She laughed at the memory. "Mr. Pichot lost his temper with me and said I would never be a dancer, but still I wanted to go on. When I was eight, I was old enough to be taken to the Imperial Ballet School in St. Petersburg. Once a year all the professors, directors and physicians assemble to choose their new pupils. From all over Russia the children come, hoping to be accepted. It makes no difference if you are the child of rich parents or come from a poor peasant's home, if they think you will make a dancer they will take you, and train you. The year I went there were only seven vacancies, and in the big hall there were three hundred children assembled. My parents thought they were wasting their time, bringing me, so thin and so ugly. We were lined up and examined by the doctors. We were questioned by stern-looking men, we were made to walk, to run . . ."

"And you were chosen?" They couldn't bear the suspense.

"Yes. I was lucky. I was chosen." She laughed gaily. "You should have seen my parents' faces, their surprise that their ugly little daughter had been accepted as a pupil in the great Imperial Ballet School. As for me, I was the happiest person in the world. I joined the school and put on my uniform, a pink dress. All the new pupils wear pink. Later on you have a grey dress, and then, if you pass all your exams, a white dress. You are a very important person in the school when you have a white dress."

"Then you did nothing but dancing?"

"Of course not, we were educated too. We studied languages, literature, music, history, everything."

"Did you get holidays?"

"Yes. We were allowed home for Easter and Christmas, and for a holiday in the summer. Not too long, though, for we mustn't get out of training. After five or six years we might, perhaps, be allowed to see a ballet at the Maryinsky Theatre, by standing in a crowd scene at the back of the stage or walking across, but never more, for nobody may dance in the Imperial Theatre until the training is finished. Then the dancer may graduate into the *corps de ballet*."

"Did you still live at the school after you graduated?"

"No. We were allowed to go back home, but we still belonged to the Imperial Theatre. I enjoyed this new life." She glanced up at her photograph. "Do you know, people said I had changed and become quite beautiful. I can't think why, for I was still so thin, I weighed only six stone, and my waist," she spread out her hands, "it measured only sixteen and a half inches. But my parents were proud of me again." Her black eyes sparkled. "Admirers sent me flowers and presents, there were invitations to dinners and balls. How gay it all was, but always there was work as well, exercises and practice, for a dancer can never rest."

"Why did you ever leave the theatre?" they asked her.

"Ah!" she smiled at them. "I fell in love. It does not do for a dancer to fall in love," she went on sadly. "He was the Chamberlain of the Emperor's Court. He saw me dance at the Maryinsky, he sent me flowers, we met, we fell in love. The Emperor approved. Everything was happy and then war came. War between Russia and Japan. He had to leave quickly to go to the war. I left the theatre and followed him to Japan. There we were married. I gave up my dancing and trained as a nurse. I worked in army hospitals." Her hands swiftly closed up the ugly memories of those years: the young dancer and bride, in a squalid army hospital. Nor did she tell them of the private tragedy of her marriage, seeing an adored husband take to drink and turn into a brute who ill-treated her.

"I left my husband," she said briefly. "I escaped from him and fled to Russia where I hid in a convent. I thought my life was finished," she went on. "I could never go back to the Imperial Theatre now."

"Why not?"

"Because I divorced my husband."

"What has that got to do with your dancing?"

"The Emperor was very strict. Divorce was a scandal in those days. It was not permitted for dancers to have any scandal attached to their name. No, the Imperial Theatre was closed to me for ever.

What was I to do? My parents had died. I had no money. How was
I to earn my living, I who had only been trained to dance? Friends
helped me. They were so good to me. Then one day I met Serge
Diaghilev. He knew me from the old days at the Maryinsky. He
had often seen me dance and he asked me to come now and join
his company, the Ballets Russes. They had their headquarters at
Monte Carlo. There I went, to start once again to dance." She stared
into the fire, reliving those days. "Serge Diaghilev had collected in
his company some of the finest artists ever trained by the Imperial
Schools. Nijinsky, Karsavina, Tchernicheva, Lopokova, Fokine."
The mighty names rolled out. "Pavlova, too, had been with them,
but she had left to form her own company. The Ballets Russes
under Diaghilev toured all the capitals of Europe, and everywhere,
success. It was like the old days at St. Petersburg come back again.
What triumphs. It would have gone on, too, but war came." Her
face grew sad. "Yes, always, in my life it seems, war comes to ruin
everything. It was 1914. Two years later there was worse news
for us Russians. Revolution broke out. The Emperor was driven
from his throne. The Bolshevik Peasants came to power and ruled
the country."

"What happened to the Imperial Dancing Schools?"

"Who knows?" she shrugged her shoulders. "The Bolsheviks,
they have destroyed everything in my poor country. Those too,
no doubt."

"What about Diaghilev and the Ballets Russes?"

"We were in Europe, cut off from our country. We had to
survive as best we could. Poor Serge, he did what he could to keep
his dancers together during four years of war. Poor big Serge. How
he suffered to keep the ballet alive. How we all suffered. He had
spent his own fortune and his friends' money; all that he could
borrow or beg. He was penniless, but somehow he kept going with
a few dancers, giving seasons where he could."

"You left him?"

"Yes," she smiled sadly. "I had to, for even a dancer must eat.
I came to London and started my school."

"What does Diaghilev do now?" It was Pat who asked.

"Since the war finished he is building up the Ballets Russes once
more."

"Don't you want to go back to him?"

"No!" She looked up swiftly. "It is too late. Serge will find new dancers for his company. My work is here, in my school." She smiled at them. "You must understand, for many, many years Russia has been the home of the great tradition of the ballet. Now, since the Revolution, that home is broken up, the dancers scattered. It is for us few who are left to hand on our great tradition, now, before it is lost. We are the last of a great line. The future of the ballet now must be in the hands of you young people, you English dancers."

Pat looked at her, hardly daring to ask the question that lay so close to his heart.

"Can we ever become as great artists as those who trained in the Imperial Schools?"

She was silent, looking at this boy, whose hopes and ambitions were shining in his eyes.

"Why not, Patté?" she said softly. "If you go on working hard, everything is possible." And her eyes held for him both a challenge and a promise.

20 *Serge Diaghilev*

"Go on working hard," Madame had said, and her implied encouragement had sent Pat's ambition soaring.

"One day," he announced in all the pride of his sixteen years, "I, too, shall dance with the Diaghilev Ballet."

Madame had not laughed at him.

"You are right, Patté," she told him. "You work for only the highest prize. Diaghilev's Ballets Russes are the finest artistic organisation in Europe to-day."

Could Madame's far-seeing eyes look into the future, then, and see him fulfil his ambition? She said nothing, and for Pat himself the Ballets Russes remained a distant goal, as he practised and struggled and fought his way to achieve technical perfection.

As a dancer he was still concerned with technique, with the mastery of each classical movement, and the control of each muscle in his body. The artist in him had not yet been stirred into life. The full awakening of the soul of the dancer was to come later.

Meanwhile, the winter days lengthened into spring and summer. The flower barrows in the King's Road were a riot of colour. Madame flung open the tall windows of her studio, letting in the warm sunshine and letting out the cascading music of her classes, to mingle with the hum of passing traffic.

It was not only ballet music that joined the noisy bustle of the King's Road. Often the syncopated beat of a foxtrot, or a throbbing tango, went out through those open windows, as dancing couples gyrated over the studio floor. Under Madame's skilled training young and unknown names were growing up to fame as exhibition dancers. Moss and Fontana, Robert Sieller and Annette Mills, as well as others, went spinning up to success.

Madame was tireless. She held special classes also for acrobatic dancing. Sometimes Pat was allowed to watch a training that brought all his old delight in acrobatics flooding back. He felt rather guilty about this and would creep away on his own into a deserted corner afterwards to try out some of the things he had seen.

Madame caught him one day.

"What are you doing?" she screamed at him. "You, a classical dancer, standing on your 'ands? The good God gave you feet to dance." The storm raged in a torrent of broken English and Russian, but Pat's heart leaped in him for joy, for every angry word showed how much his dancing mattered to her.

"Go away," she raged at him. "Go and watch real dancing. 'Ere," she fumbled in the sagging pocket of her jacket. "You go to the ballet to-night. Go and watch Karsavina dance, and put these other ideas out of your 'ead."

Pat, clutching the coin she had given him, happily joined the gallery queue that was forming outside the Coliseum on that warm summer evening.

"Hallo!" He was greeted by the familiar faces of the "regulars". Many were young dancers and ballet pupils like himself. There were others, of indeterminate occupation; pale, ascetic young men, whose hair was too long and clothes too bright; lank-haired girls with large red mouths and clothes they had designed themselves. Serious-faced students; underfed and underwashed intellectuals in drab mackintoshes. They were a curious collection of penniless young enthusiasts, united in a fervent worship of the ballet.

The whole cult of the dance was taken very seriously. Pat, who went to see every ballet he could, had spent many hours in gallery queues engaged in hot argument over the rival merits of Karsavina and Pavlova, or the music of Tchaikovsky versus that of Stravinsky.

They were noisy, young and enthusiastic, and wherever ballet was performed its followers would be found, faithfully queueing to fill the gallery and shout their praise or disapproval.

It was in this high perch that Pat had spent enchanted hours. From the gallery of the Prince's Theatre he had seen the tiny figure of Pavlova floating across the great stage, and the spell of the beauty she wove about her had reached up even there, and caught him in it. Pavlova was something out of this world.

Now the doors of the Coliseum were swung open. Coins rattled down on the wooden ledge of the box office, and the noisy, cheerful crowd went surging up the stairs to scramble for the best places on the hard benches.

The theatre was filling. Somewhere behind the heavy curtain that hid the stage the great Russian ballerina was preparing to enchant them with the beauty of her art.

Pat remembered his first experience of such beauty, the night he had seen Astafieva dance on this very stage. As long as he lived he would remember the deep emotion her dancing had aroused in him, as though she had opened a door, showing him all the loveliness that lay in an enchanted world the other side of it. He could still feel the driving urge that had made him determined to learn from Astafieva herself and none else. How blindly right he had been.

Since then he had seen much dancing, but only two dancers could move him in the same way. The divine Pavlova, and Karsavina. How often he had seen Karsavina already, when she made those all-too-brief appearances at the Coliseum. He never lost the thrill of seeing the houselights fade, feeling his heart beat faster to know that she was there, poised in the wings, waiting.

The voices around him hushed and died. The moment had come again.

To Pat, Karsavina was a flame. She moved with a faultless beauty as swift and sure as a bird in flight. What a technique, what a style, born of those long years of training in the Imperial School. Through the music he seemed to hear Astafieva's deep voice telling the story of those years of training, the flowering of talent, and the young Karsavina's triumph in Paris; the immortal partnership with Nijinsky; the pair of them dancing their way to the glittering pinnacle of success in the Ballets Russes. But behind them there stood always the figure of the man who had made their triumph possible; who had brought the Russian Ballet to Europe; the man who, to Pat, was still a mysterious, shadowy figure, an unknown power—Serge Diaghilev.

"Bravo! Bravo!" A sallow young woman sitting next to Pat came noisily to life as the curtain came down for the interval. "Did you see those *fouettés*?" she shouted at him through the racket of the gallery's approval. "Perfect. Never seen her do them better. Bravo!"

But Pat, who was thinking into the great dancer's past, said: "How I wish I could have seen her dance with Nijinsky."

"Nijinsky?" The name brought into view a pale young man in a yellow pullover on the other side of the sallow girl. "People exaggerate the artistry of Nijinsky." He leaned across to argue. "What else could he do but leap? Now the real dancer to see is Massine."

"Nonsense," the sallow girl shook her lanky brown hair. "Massine hasn't half the technique."

"Have you seen Nijinsky dance?" Pat inquired.

"I saw Massine dance here, with the Diaghilev Ballet . . ." the young man began.

"Diaghilev?" A voice interrupted from the row behind. "Is it true that Diaghilev is bringing his Ballets Russes to London for a season?"

Pat twisted round on his hard bench, ears and senses alert.

"Yes, it is true." A man's voice shouted along the row. "They are coming here in September."

The distant voice broadcast the information round the gallery. "Diaghilev is planning to stage a revival of the *Sleeping Princess*."

"What, the whole of it?"

"Yes, it's a full-length ballet. Never been seen outside Russia."

"And Diaghilev is going to do it in London?"

"So I heard."

Pat sat in a dream as the young voices chattered on round him. Diaghilev coming to London with his whole company. He would see these fabulous Russian dancers at last. Perhaps he would see the great man himself. He was filled with an intense curiosity and desire to see this Serge Diaghilev. The Ballets Russes were coming to London. His whole body tingled with excitement.

"Do you think it's true?" he pestered Astafieva afterwards.

"Patté, darling. How should I know what big Serge is doing?" she laughed at him. "You will see soon enough when the time comes if it is true."

He did.

Towards the middle of September paragraphs in the papers carried the news that the Russian Ballet had arrived in London to start rehearsing for the *Sleeping Princess*.

There was great excitement among Astafieva's pupils.

"Does it give the date of the opening night?"

A whole bunch of them had gathered round a newspaper just before the morning class was due to begin.

"No. It only says they'll be at the Alhambra. Sh! Here comes Madame."

The newspaper was hurriedly bundled out of sight.

Astafieva was smiling as she came in. This was a good sign.

"To-day, my children," she told them gaily, "you must work extra well. We are expecting a very important visitor. Yes." Her eyes sparkled mischievously. "You have seen in the papers that the Ballets Russes are here in London. Well, they need extra dancers to take part in the *Sleeping Princess* and they are coming here to find them."

"Who is coming?" Pat had to ask.

Astafieva looked at him a moment.

"Serge Diaghilev is coming himself," she told him.

Diaghilev looking for extra dancers! Diaghilev coming to the studio to choose them himself!

They looked at each other and a sudden fever of excitement went pulsing through them all. They were to have a chance to be chosen to dance with the Russian Ballet.

"He may come to-day, or he may come to-morrow," Madame went on. "He told me he was not sure. Meanwhile we must be ready to show him what we can do."

Work started. How hard it was to concentrate on the preliminary exercises, *ronds de jambe* and *battements*. The bell rang.

"Pay attention, will you." Madame's stick tapped the floor angrily. "Think what you are doing."

It was all right, the bell was a false alarm.

"One and two and three and four . . ." Madame's voice dominated the class, demanding concentration.

"Will he come to-day?" Pat's legs moved mechanically. "What did he look like this great man who owned a ballet? Madame had spoken of 'Big Serge', so he must be tall."

"Patté! Patté!" The stick smacked on his legs. "Pay attention. Tempo. Two and three and four . . ."

The bell rang again. Pat's heart raced. This must be him.

No. He relaxed again.

"One and two . . . Would he come to-day . . . ? Three and four . . ." The question beat in his brain. "Would he come? Would he really see Serge Diaghilev to-day?" There was the bell again. Another false alarm, and a stab of disappointment. Surely the studio bell never rang so often on other mornings.

"All right. That will do." Madame released them from the bar. "Into the centre. *Petit Adagio*."

"Perhaps he'll come now," Pat watched the big hands of the clock move round.

"*Grand Adagio . . . Allegro*." It was after 12.30 now. The class would soon be finished. He hadn't come after all. Wait! Was that the bell? No. It would be for to-morrow.

"Go back and do that *enchaînement* again," Madame called out to two of the girls; and at that moment came a loud knock, as though someone had struck the door with a heavy stick. It opened. In the doorway stood a group of people.

No need to ask who was the big man in the black fur-collared overcoat, who led the way into the studio, swinging a gold-mounted cane.

The girls swept down in a curtsy; the boys bowed, low.

"Serge!" Astafieva greeted him with open arms.

Serge Diaghilev stooped to kiss her affectionately, and the studio was suddenly filled with strong Russian voices.

The pupils, forgotten for the moment, effaced themselves against the wall, watching, listening, and wondering who were the other three people who accompanied Diaghilev. It was only later they were to learn that the slim young man was his secretary, Boris Kochno. No ordinary secretary this, but an intellectual and a poet. The tall, suave man who swept his arms in wide, graceful gestures when he spoke, was Serge Grigorieff, a trained dancer from the Imperial School, and now Diaghilev's right-hand man and stage manager. Beside him stood a beautiful and distinguished-looking lady, whose poise and classic features bore the unmistakable stamp of the dancer. This was Grigorieff's lovely and talented wife, Lubov Tchernicheva, première danseuse of the Ballets Russes.

They stood in a group talking and laughing with Astafieva. Pat, however, had eyes for the central figure alone. It was he who dominated the room. Everything about Serge Diaghilev was unusual. His powerful physique, that massive head with its noble breadth of forehead, the curious white streak in his dark hair; the monocle that gave him such a look of arrogant power. He had a short, wide nose, typically Russian, a sensual mouth under a small dark moustache. He had the heavy jaw of a fighter and, by contrast, the white, sensitive hands of a man of culture and taste. He was laughing as he spoke with Astafieva. They spoke in Russian, his voice had a lazy, caressing quality that was strangely attractive. Pat wondered what they were saying.

They moved down to the end of the studio. Chairs were quickly brought.

Madame called out her pupils. In one's, two's and three's they danced. Pat, waiting with the other two boys in the class for their turn, saw Diaghilev's cane swing up and point to a small serious-faced girl who had just finished her dance. He said something in Russian, and Madame beckoned to the child to come up.

"This is Alice Marks," they heard Madame say in English. "She is only twelve." She went on to speak in Russian, and Pat wondered whether she was telling him of the first day that Alice Marks had appeared in the studio; the awful scene when her mother had introduced the "Miniature Pavlova" and an enraged Astafieva had slammed the door on them. That had not been the end of it, though, for nothing was going to stop Alice Marks wanting to dance. The offending cards had been torn up, and back she had come, this time to be admitted to Madame's classes and to prove herself one of the most promising pupils. Now, here she was singled out by Diaghilev himself. What an unerring eye for talent he had. Could they have looked into the future, they would have seen that in two short years this little girl, standing now so gravely before him, would join the ranks of his Ballets Russes as the youngest dancer ever to be engaged.

Diaghilev was leaning forward, smiling at his future Alicia Markova. They couldn't hear what he was saying, but they saw her curtsy and run to join the others.

The dancing went on, watched by those expert eyes. Grigorieff's calm and wise. Tchernicheva's dark and critical. Diaghilev's inscrutable, half-hidden behind that glinting monocle. From time to time he leaned over and spoke to his companions, and the stick singled out the lucky ones.

"Patté," Madame called him out at last. "We want to see you dance alone. You do 'Humoresque'."

Alone! His chance had come. His heart was thumping fast as he moved out to take his place. This dance was the only one he knew. Madame had arranged it for him to the famous music of Dvorak. It was a dance they had both seen executed by Volinin when he had appeared with Pavlova at the Prince's Theatre.

The piano began, and Pat, in all the innocence and audacity of youth, now danced this elegant and difficult solo before these most expert and critical judges.

Diaghilev was smiling as Pat finished, a big, lazy smile that showed a glint of gold in his white teeth. Was he impressed by Pat's performance or by the sheer audacity of a boy attempting so difficult a dance?

Madame signed to Pat to approach. Diaghilev rose and stood looking down at this young dancer.

"How old are you?" His voice had a soft burr as he spoke in English.

"I am sixteen." Pat was staring, fascinated, at the great man, now so close to him.

"One day you will dance." Diaghilev's hand rested on Pat's head and for a moment he looked full at him. What a curious, compelling power shone in his eyes, as though there was a light behind them, and he could see right into one's innermost thoughts. "Now you shall come and watch my dancers."

He turned away swiftly. The moment was over. Pat went to

join the others, shaking with emotion. It was all finished, he had been picked. He was going to dance with the Ballets Russes in the *Sleeping Princess*.

21 Rehearsals of the Sleeping Princess

The Alhambra Theatre, Leicester Square, seethed with life, and the young dancer Pat Kay was caught up and lost in the turmoil of preparation. Yet how few of them could realise the full scope of this gigantic undertaking in which they had a part?

Nearly thirty years had passed since the *Sleeping Princess* had been first performed on the stage of the Maryinsky Theatre, St. Petersburg. Now, Diaghilev was staging a sumptuous revival of this single, three-hour ballet in the pure classical tradition, a ballet that had never been seen in its entirety outside Russia.

The *Sleeping Princess* was to be awakened and brought to Europe to herald the triumphant return to the pre-war glories of the Ballets Russes. Diaghilev had assembled round himself the most famous team of artists of the day.

The Russian painter, Bakst, had designed the costumes and seven great scenes; a riot of pageantry and colour. It was to be his last and perhaps his greatest work for Diaghilev. In Stravinsky's master hands lay the score of Tchaikovsky's beautiful music, especially written for this ballet. Sergeyeff, trained in the classical tradition, handled the choreography that had been first evolved by Petipa, the great Maître de Ballet of the Imperial School.

This superb classical ballet had been created to revolve about one person, the central, dazzling figure of Aurora, the Sleeping Princess. For Diaghilev, however, one ballerina was not enough, and for his production no less than three top-ranking ballerinas were brought in especially to share the honours of this great role. Olga Spessiva and Lubov Egorova had arrived in London. Soon Vera Trefilova was to join them.

Behind these queens of the dance gathered Diaghilev's own famous dancers of his Ballets Russes, and around them swarmed the crowd of extras, and walkers-on, especially engaged for the production. Altogether a cast of two hundred people collected in the Alhambra Theatre. The opening date was fixed for the 2nd November.

All day and frequently all night the work went on. Russian voices dominated the turmoil as Diaghilev's key men took over. Chief machinist, Koristoff, a tall Russian with a startling red beard, took charge of an army of English stage hands, carpenters and property men. In the labyrinth of passages and rooms at the back, Vassily reigned over his kingdom of wardrobe assistants, sewing machines, ironing boards and costumes. The whole building echoed to the sound of musical instruments as the orchestra rehearsed under Stravinsky.

For Pat, a tiny cog in this vast machinery, the first days were spent in the cold, bare rehearsal room with a crowd of other extras learning steps under the stern eye of the choreographer Sergeyeff. He was a short, spare man with a grim expression and a fixed purpose, perfection, even for so straightforward a matter as walking across the stage.

Occasionally during rehearsal the door would be unexpectedly flung open and the big figure of Diaghilev would be there, watching. His visits always spurred them on to greater efforts, and even when he had gone the feeling of his watching presence remained.

This one powerful man was the central focus of all the activity that went on during those chaotic days. Everyone in the theatre was aware of him. He had an uncanny way of making each of them feel that they were working for him alone.

One day he came into the rehearsal room to speak to Sergeyeff. Pat was called out.

"Try him," said Diaghilev in English, and Pat discovered that he had been chosen to dance in a waltz.

"We need four male dancers for the waltz," Sergeyeff explained afterwards. "Only three can be spared from the company."

Pat didn't need to be told what an honour it was to be singled out for this. His only fear was that he should not prove good enough.

"Don't worry so much, Pat," his waltz partner Hilda Bewicke calmed him down as he muddled his steps. "I tell you what, we'll stay behind after rehearsal and go over it again by ourselves."

How comforting she was and how hard Pat worked at his little dance.

Soon they were all ready to come out of the preparatory school of the rehearsal rooms to work in big groups on the stage itself. How vast and bleak it was on the first evening they assembled on that empty stage. Down in the cold, gloomy auditorium a group of people sat in the unlit stalls. The broad shoulders of Big Serge were easy to pick out. Beside him sat the dapper, trim Leon Bakst. Nearby was the familiar grim figure of Sergeyeff, and with them two dancers wrapped in furs. On the side of the stage by the piano Pat recognised the tall, graceful stage manager, Grigorieff. He was talking to a woman wrapped in a long dark cloak.

Pat wondered who she was. She half turned and he saw her face, a curious face, pale and rather heavy, with big slanting eyes and an untidy mop of yellow hair.

"I say," Pat nudged one of the extras near him. "Who's that?"

"It's Nijinska. She is helping Sergeyeff with the choreography."

"So that is the sister of the famous Nijinsky." Pat, looking at her, felt a pang of cold disappointment. She wasn't beautiful, she didn't even look like a classical dancer—or did she? Nijinska had suddenly flung her cloak back. She was moving, demonstrating something to Grigorieff. Training and style showed in every line.

A voice of authority called out suddenly from the stalls. Grigorieff hurried to receive Diaghilev's instructions. Rehearsal began. They were to feel the difference now for the master himself had taken over. It was patient, tiring work. Every few minutes the dancers were interrupted.

"Wait," Diaghilev would call up, and they waited while he consulted with Sergeyeff or Stravinsky. Others would join in, there would be argument and gestures, while everyone on stage hung about getting cold and bored.

"All right, do it again with the quicker tempo." Diaghilev would get up and stride towards the footlights. There he stood, his long overcoat thrown over his shoulders, his head curiously tilted as he watched.

"No." He clapped his hands. Back they went over it again, once, twice, or as many as twenty times until it was artistically right.

"That will do. Rest." Tired dancers moved away to the wings, forming little whispering groups. Diaghilev went back to his seat.

It was the turn of Aurora's *pas seul*. The whispering groups fell silent, and all turned to watch as the principal figure came on to the stage. In her plain practice costume, Olga Spessiva looked little different from the other *danseuses*. She stood, waiting for her music, looking, with her frail beauty like a slender, ivory statuette. Then she danced. That graceful delicate body had muscles of steel. What a style, and what a technique! Her dancing was the finished, perfect product of the Russian School.

"Bravo!" The élite in the stalls called out as her dance came to an end. Spessiva, smiling, made a mock curtsy to them and ran off. The *corps de ballet* moved in once more. The work went on. For Pat, the ordeal of the waltz passed off without special incident. The ordeal of the mazurka was still to come. This dance was in the finale of the ballet. Pat felt happy enough as long as he was hidden in the back row. The moment arrived, however, when the long line of dancers circled round the stage. This meant coming across the front in full view of those critical eyes.

"Patrickieff!" Diaghilev suddenly called out. "Awful! Patrick-ieff, what are you doing?"

Pat suddenly registered the fact that he was hearing his own name. Diaghilev had Russianised it for him.

"Patrickieff!" the deep voice called out again. "Tempo! Tempo!" and his stick beat the floor.

"That's done it," Pat decided as the mazurka finished. "They'll throw me out. He said I was awful."

The rehearsal was nearly over. Tired and miserable, Pat waited to be dismissed and told not to come again. He saw the short, spare figure of Sergeyeff hurrying through the pass-door on to the stage. He stopped short as he caught sight of Pat.

"Ah!" he said. "I was looking for you."

The tone of his voice sent Pat cold all over.

"We want you to stay behind after the rehearsal," Sergeyeff told him. "You are to go through the mazurka again." He passed on quickly.

"That is all for to-day, thank you." Dimly, Pat heard the stage manager's voice dismissing the company. "Rehearsal to-morrow at the same time." The dancers drifted away. Pat was left alone on the stage.

"Now, then." Sergeyeff suddenly reappeared. "We will work at this step." Patiently, clearly, he showed Pat how it was to be fitted into the music.

The small solitary figure went dancing round the empty stage. Pat, intent on his work, did not see a silent, dark silhouette standing in the shadows at the back of the stalls.

"That will do for now." Sergeyeff released him at last. From the depths of the theatre came the soft sound of a door closing.

"How late you are, my poor Patté," Astafieva called out as she heard him come past her door. "Why do you come in after all the others?"

"I had to stay behind and practise." Pat felt rather guilty having to admit this. There was a pause, and then:

"Come in!" Astafieva called out sharply. "What did you say? They made you stay behind?"

"Yes." Pat stood in the doorway and bowed his head waiting for a deluge of reproach. "I was in the mazurka and Diaghilev called out in front of everyone that I was awful."

"And he kept you afterwards?"

"Yes."

"But that is wonderful!" Astafieva beamed. "Wonderful, Patté."

Pat gave up all hope of understanding these people.

"Don't you see, you stupid boy." She laughed at him. "It means they take an interest in your dancing. Do you think they would waste their time to give you extra practice unless they thought you were worth it?"

"Oh!" This was a new idea to Pat. Perhaps Astafieva was right. He thought things over. Diaghilev had picked him out of the studio class here; he had picked him out at rehearsal to take part in the waltz; and now he had been picked out to stay behind and rehearse.

"Does it really mean that he thinks I have talent as a dancer?" Pat asked himself. "Will I get the chance, perhaps, to join the company of the Ballets Russes permanently?"

The hope formed in his mind and grew there.

22 First Night

Diaghilev had set his publicity agents to work and seen to it that everyone was talking about this fabulous ballet that was in preparation behind the closed doors of the Alhambra. As a result, the restless, post-war London of 1921, with its short skirts and long cigarette holders, with its convulsive Charleston and strident jazz, scrambled for first-night seats at a romantic, classical ballet. Advance booking boomed.

The days passed swiftly to the evening of the 2nd November. Outside the Alhambra ballet enthusiasts had been queueing since the early hours for gallery seats. The stage door was besieged all day with messengers, errand boys, pages, workroom girls. Boxes, parcels, letters, telegrams, last minute costumes and wigs, presents, flowers and laurel wreaths poured through. Inside, the stairs and corridors seethed with hurrying figures. Away in silent hotel bedrooms principal dancers rested with their legs up. At all costs they must be calm and relaxed before their exacting work tonight.

As dusk drew over the city someone turned a switch and the dark front of the theatre was suddenly a blaze of light, flashing the *Sleeping Princess* into the darkening sky, and cheering the patient gallery queue below. While they waited in the cold, a group of men were dining at the Savoy. Diaghilev, Stravinsky, Bakst, Boris Kochno and several more sat down to caviare and smoked salmon, and drank champagne to the success of the Princess. Diaghilev was pale, there were deep shadows under his eyes. He had spent most of the previous night in the theatre, working without rest to ensure the perfect working of scenery and lighting. The strain of the weeks of preparation showed in the tired lines of his face, and his friends were aware of the tense undercurrent of anxiety, of nerves strung to fever pitch.

At the theatre the fashionable public were beginning to arrive. A Diaghilev first night never failed to attract a brilliant audience. Leicester Square was jammed with cars and taxis moving slowly up to the lighted entrance. A crowd gathered to watch, and in the brilliant, flower-decked foyer, critics and faithful first-nighters jostled with the rich and the successful, the well born and the talented.

The gallery door opened and the patient queue was suddenly brought to life and swallowed up through the dingy side entrance.

"Overture and beginners, please." The call-boys hurried round. Dressing-room doors opened and down the stairs they thronged, to crowd in the wings waiting and whispering, listening to the hum of that unseen audience on the other side of the great velvet curtains.

It was nearly time. The theatre was packed. Only one box still remained empty. Heads were turned as the door at the back of it opened. There was a gleam of white shirt front as a big man in immaculate evening dress came through, folllowed by a group of others. He took his place in the centre of the box, his monocle flashed as he looked round. There was a stir; people nudged each other.

"That's Serge Diaghilev who has just come in."

The lights dimmed, and the talk died. The conductor raised his baton and the glorious music of Tchaikovsky filled the house. Smoothly the heavy curtain rose on a scene of breathtaking grandeur. The Palace of the King and Queen at the birth of Aurora. Soaring columns reaching for the sky, the vast sweep of marble staircases curving majestically into distant space, and on whose white steps were ranged tier upon tier of motionless, living figures, the scarlet and gold Negro guards of the King's Household.

To the music of a march the stage filled with the glittering figures of the King's Court. It was a wealth of colour and pageantry, centring round the golden cradle of the baby Princess. Here came the fairies with their gifts. Ballerinas in white tutus decorated with the emblems of their power, and accompanied by their pages, carried out a series of brilliant *pas de deux*.

The dark-eyed Tchernicheva, who had come to Astafieva's studio on the famous day of Diaghilev's visit, was now a lovely vision in the white and scarlet costume of the Mountain Ash Fairy.

The Cherry Blossom Fairy, a graceful fair-haired dancer who hid an English birth under her Russian name, Sokolova, brought her gift to the cradle.

Nijinska, transformed into the Humming Bird Fairy, took the stage, dancing with a style and power that evoked memories of her famous brother.

The Pine Tree Fairy, the Song Bird Fairy, they all came, and after them the sinister entrance of the wicked fairy Carabosse, whose ugly, wrinkled make-up covered the faded beauty of an ageing dancer named Carlotta Brianza. She had been specially brought from Russia for this part. Perhaps as she danced her wicked role this night, her thoughts went back to an evening at the Maryinsky Theatre nearly thirty years ago in 1892 when the curtain had gone up on the first performance of the new ballet the *Sleeping Princess*, and the applause had rung out for the young and lovely ballerina Carlotta Brianza, who had danced the role of Aurora before the Czar himself and all the élite of the old Russian nobility.

A last brilliant dance from the belated Lilac Fairy, Lopokova, and the curtain came down at the end of the scene.

In her dressing-room the Aurora of 1921 waited for her entrance. To Olga Spessiva had fallen the honour of dancing the great role on the first night. The mirror reflected a radiant vision in a deep rose-coloured tutu, whose bodice was laced with gold. On her head she wore a wonderful pale gold wig. The dresser placed a shawl round her delicate shoulders.

On stage a sweating team of stage-hands swept away the palace to replace it by the Royal Gardens. There was some delay in getting the heavy scenery shifted into place. Friendly applause, however, greeted the rustic celebrations of Aurora's sixteenth birthday. A circle of peasants in red and green costumes were dancing about the stage. Out of the romping music grew the celebrated village waltz. Four couples detached themselves from the throng to hold the attention for a brief few minutes.

"Well done, Pat." Hilda Bewicke whispered to him as they whirled to a finish, and the new dancer who appeared in the programme as "Patrickieff" smiled back at her. At least that bit was successfully over. He was hot and shaking as they passed into the shadows of the wings, crowded with courtiers standing ready for their entrance. There waited Aurora herself, glorious in white, red and gold.

Pat slowly made his way to gaze at the loveliness of Olga Spessiva. As the moment of her first entrance neared, she slid the shawl from her shoulders. Pat saw his opportunity. He hurried forward and took it. She gave him a fleeting smile over her shoulder as she moved away. He saw her bow her head and cross herself three times. The next moment Aurora floated into the brilliant lights.

Pat stood hugging the soft, scented shawl as he watched her.

He was still there, waiting, when she came off. Greatly daring, he put the shawl over her shoulders, but was too overawed to find the words to tell her how her dancing had moved him.

The applause from the audience was warm and heartening. All was going well until the scene shifting broke down badly. The mechanism that worked the Lilac Fairy's spell became jammed. The curtain remained down for long tedious minutes while stagehands worked frantically to get it right, and dancers stood about nervy and worried. The audience grew restive.

After this, the whole complicated stage machinery seemed to be thrown out of gear. Another long delay preceded the rise of the curtain on the Prince's Hunting Scene. The evening was not half-way through yet. There was still the scene of the Enchanted Palace to come and the scene of the Awakening. In a room deep in shadow, a single shaft of light shone on the golden-haired Princess, asleep on a gigantic canopied bed, veiled by a monstrous web guarded by two enormous spiders.

They were running nearly an hour late now. At last the curtain came up on the final brilliant spectacle. The scene of Aurora's wedding.

Vast colonnades, open to the sky, curved into the distance. Spiral pillars of white and gold, entwined with flowers, made a fairy-like setting of space and beauty. It was perhaps one of the most successful sets that Bakst ever designed.

The action of the story was finished, and the scene given over to a spectacular ball, led by Aurora and Prince Charming.

There was a series of brilliant *divertissements*.

The last mazurka. "Tempo. Tempo, Patrickieff!" Pat could almost hear Diaghilev's voice calling out as he danced across the stage. Swiftly came the grand finale, and the audience were cheering and calling out. The gallery were wild with enthusiasm. The unlucky delays had already been forgotten and forgiven, it seemed, in their crescendo of clapping.

The curtain came down at last, and for the company there was the sudden bubbling up of relief and excitement that the first night was safely over.

Back to the dressing-rooms they went, while autograph hunters massed at the stage door and privileged visitors pushed their way in to find their friends. Parties started up, champagne corks popped.

There was laughter and gaiety backstage for success seemed to smile at them. Life was wonderful, or so thought a very tired young man, letting himself into the studio in the King's Road in the early hours of the morning.

23 Good-bye

The *Princess* had been rapturously received by the first-night public, but the critics, bored by the unfortunate delays, had not been kind in the papers next day. Although the scene-changing machinery was in perfect order by the end of the week, the poor *Princess* never recovered from her bad start.

More than that, the public could not get used to the idea of the same full-length ballet night after night. They lost interest. Box office receipts began to fall off.

"Another bad house to-night, I hear." A group of extras were standing in the wings.

"Expect it'll pick up a bit over Christmas," another was saying.

"Hope so. I can't afford to be out of work yet."

"Excuse me."

They moved aside at the sound of a soft voice. The pale, golden wig of Aurora shone among the coloured costumes of the courtiers. How small and frail Olga Spessiva looked among the men.

She smiled as she saw Pat standing near.

"My little boy with the shawl," she said as she handed it to him.

Since that first night he had never missed his self-appointed task of holding Spessiva's shawl. Always he was there, in the wings, to watch her performance. He watched Trefilova too and Egorova when they danced Aurora in their turn, but Spessiva remained always his first love.

What a lot Pat learned as he stood in the wings night after night, watching the great dancers. He studied the men; and seeing the performance of the leading dancers Vladimiroff, Wilzac, Idzikowsky and Woizikowsky made him realise how little he himself knew. He also realised for the first time what art and skill lay in a male partner's role. He had never given much thought to this before, but now he began to see for himself how important it was, and how a partner could make or mar a ballerina's performance. He watched Vladimiroff as Prince Charming partnering Aurora. How beautifully he handled her, always effacing himself, timing every move to blend with hers. How easily he lifted her, without sight of strain. He made her look as light as a bird in his arms. How gently he controlled her descent, to land her softly on one pointed toe. Pat's imagination leaped forward to the day when he too would partner a ballerina.

As he placed the shawl over Spessiva's beautiful shoulders again he longed suddenly to put his hands round that tiny waist and raise her shoulder-high. How angry she would be.

"Thank you, Patrickieff." She smiled at him and he blushed, glad that she could not read his thoughts. She turned away to speak to Vladimiroff. How Pat wished he could understand their language. The few words he had picked up from Astafieva were soon drowned and lost in this sea of Russian that surrounded him.

A group of the regular *corps de ballet* of Diaghilev's company were gathering near him now. He gazed at them wistfully, wishing he could be one of them. He used to watch them practise on the side of the stage, or exercise in the rehearsal room. They worked in little groups on their own. At first Pat had hoped he might be allowed to join them, but he soon realised that this was not to happen. A barrier seemed to stand between him and them. Was it language only? Or was it the pride of artists who knew they belonged to the finest ballet company in Europe, a team that had no place for untried strangers?

"They will recognise me one day," his ambition beat strongly in him, and he turned again to the stage to watch Lopokova and Idzikowsky dance the Bluebird, one of the most thrilling and difficult *pas de deux* ever created. The Bluebird called for brilliance, strength and an impeccable technique.

Pat forgot his disappointment as he stood now absorbed by the beauty of the music and the brilliance of the performance. Slowly, however, he became aware of a presence near him. There was a scent of almond oil; the weight of a hand on his shoulder. He looked round and his heart beat faster, for Serge Diaghilev was looking down at him.

"And when are you going to dance the Bluebird?" There was a smile in his eyes.

"When you want me to." There was no hesitation about the reply. The hand on his shoulder tightened as though this was the answer Diaghilev wanted to hear.

It was the first time he had taken any notice of Pat since the rehearsal. Both of them, however, were to remember this little incident which had its strange sequel three years later. The night Anton Dolin danced the Bluebird for the first time in London he received a laurel wreath, and on the card, in Diaghilev's own hand, was written: "When will you dance the Bluebird? 1921-1924." The amazing man had not forgotten.

Did he foresee that night already in 1921 as he stood beside Pat in the wings of the Alhambra? The dance finished. Pat watched him move away to speak to someone else. What thoughts and plans went on in that powerful head? Was it possible that he would want Pat to join his company after this? The secret hope throbbed with quick life.

Whatever plans Diaghilev might have had, nothing could come of them, for all too soon it became obvious to everyone that the days of the *Princess* were numbered. She would never run six months. By the New Year it was doubtful if she would last three. In the middle of January the notices went up on the boards, announcing that the run of the *Sleeping Princess* would finish in two weeks' time.

The great experiment, though artistically successful, was a disastrous financial failure. Diaghilev had run up huge debts to put on this ballet. When the curtain came down for the last time, the pack of creditors closed in on their prey. The *Sleeping Princess* was to be torn apart.

The cast disbanded. Principals returned to Russia. The extras disappeared into the oblivion from which they had come. Diaghilev, hounded and worried by debts, fought to keep his own company together. Many of them, fearing to be out of work, left him to join Massine at Covent Garden.

Most tragic of all, Bakst's glorious scenery and costumes, which had cost thousands of pounds, and for which there was no money to pay, had to be abandoned, to fall into the hands of creditors and be lost or irretrievably destroyed.

Diaghilev gathered the faithful remnants of his company round him and prepared to leave. Their destination was the South of France, the sunshine of Monte Carlo, headquarters of the Ballets Russes.

On a dark February morning in 1921 a very sad-hearted young man watched the long boat train pull out of Victoria Station, carrying away Diaghilev and his dancers. With it seemed to go all Pat's hopes and dreams. He was left with a sense of emptiness and desolation.

Would he ever see Spessiva dance again? Would he watch Idzikowsky and Lopokova in the Bluebird? Would he ever see Diaghilev, that strange and powerful man who could build a dancer's career and create a ballet that was a piece of sheer, living beauty?

Pat felt like a child who has been shown a glimpse of fairyland, a place full of beautiful, dancing figures who had beckoned him and lured him in to dance with them in their enchanted world, and now he had been pushed back, the door had been slammed and he was left on the outside, alone.

"If only I could have gone with them," he thought in the desperation of his loneliness, and he suddenly wanted sympathy. He wanted to talk to someone. Not Astafieva, she had too much courage, and Pat felt at this moment he had none at all.

He took the tube for Hampstead.

His mother welcomed him home. He realised guiltily how little he had seen of her since he had been caught up in the glamorous spell of the *Sleeping Princess*. Hurried visits, scribbled postcards, rare telephone calls. She had been to some of the rehearsals, and of course she had seen the finished performance, but their moments together had been rare. He had grown out of the way of talking everything over with her. Since living on his own he had got used to keeping things to himself and working out his own problems. Could she understand now what he was feeling, inside? Could she know without his having to put it into words? It seemed she could and she did understand.

How good it was to be with her again. She looked tired and worn though. Her husband's failing health was taking all her strength. He had his good days when he went out and about. There were more frequently his bad times when he stayed in the house, or remained in bed.

"Go into the sitting-room and talk to him, darling, he'll be so pleased."

Pat, seeing his father in the arm-chair by the fire, thought how old he had become, and was touched with deep pity that he could not express. He felt embarrassed and talked of trivial things, wishing there could be between his father and himself that sure, deep understanding that had always existed with his mother. He knew that it was his own "demon of the dance" that had brought this about. His father, puzzled and bewildered, could never get used to the idea of having a son who was a professional dancer. His mother had always understood and believed in his dancing with all her heart. How lucky he was to have such a wonderful mother.

He came away from her comforted and reassured, able once more to face the future. She gave him back his courage to match Astafieva's indomitable spirit, and to listen also to the quiet voice that spoke deep inside telling him that, as a dancer, he was not yet ready to take his place in a company like the Ballets Russes.

Pat shook off his depression, faced up to reality, and went back to Astafieva's studio to work.

24 Creation

The music of Beethoven's "Pastoral Symphony" poured out of the battered gramophone perched precariously on a chair. Sprawling on the floor beside it, Pat listened in a rapt stillness until the last chords, changing abruptly into the ugly hiss of a scraping needle, broke the enchantment.

The young people in the room stirred and came to life.

"All right, I'll take it off," Molly Grosvenor reached out and picked off the soundbox.

"Now let's listen to something more modern," her friend Poppœa Vanda began sorting over the pile of records.

"No, put on something by Tchaikovsky." Pat struggled into a sitting position.

"The greatest composer who ever wrote for the ballet,"

Poppœa waved a record about to emphasise the point, "let's see what we've got of his."

"I've found something," Molly Grosvenor interrupted suddenly. "We must listen to this." She put on Borodin's *Prince Igor*.

Impossible to lie still and relaxed to the music of the Polovtsian dances. The stirring music seemed to bring wild Cossacks right into the room. Pat's eyes glittered as he listened. He felt his muscles grow taut for action.

In the middle of it the door opened. It was Astafieva.

"I hear *Prince Igor*, I come in," she whispered. "No! No! Don't move." But Pat had already jumped up to find a chair for her. When the record was over she stayed on, talking with them.

"Patté, you are growing up." She sent him a mischievous smile.

Pat wasn't sure he approved of this.

"I am grown up," he said in his deepest man's voice. "I shall be eighteen next month."

"You are growing up as a dancer as well as a man," she told him.

"How do you mean?"

She looked round the room, at the table strewn with records and books, at his friends, Poppœa Vanda and Molly Grosvenor.

"You reach out beyond the studio and the bar," she said. "Until now you think that to be a dancer is to have technique. That once you have learned all the steps, to do them perfectly, there is nothing more to learn. Now I see that since you have been with Diaghilev you have other ideas. You have seen that to be a great dancer you must have more than a fine technique, you must have—how shall I say it?—a dancer's soul. So, Patté, I am happy that nowadays you think about things, you listen to great music. You see how you grow up? You read books too!" She picked up a stray volume lying on a chair. *History of the Ballet*.

"That's mine," said Molly Grosvenor. "I brought it along to lend Pat."

"That reminds me," put in Poppœa. "We brought along something else for you too, Pat. We've got a new record that you must listen to. It's Rimsky-Korsakov's 'Hymn to the Sun'."

"Who's playing?" asked Pat.

"Isolde Menges," Poppœa told him as she wound up the gramophone.

It was strange and beautiful music. There was a pagan, primitive spirit in it that matched the mood of modern life. Pat listened to it, thinking over what Madame had said to him.

It was true, he was now reaching out beyond the studio and the mere perfection of technique. What did he hope to reach? What did he want? The questions floated formless in his mind on the surging tide of the music. As he listened, strange emotions moved in him. He was suddenly linked across the years to his own childhood. He felt himself a little boy once more, listening to the music of his mother's piano, and unbearably moved by it. There rose in him the urge to put into movement all the feelings that the music aroused. It was an urge that had lain dormant, forgotten for years under the strict discipline of his training.

"What a lovely violinist she is," Poppœa's voice brought Pat to the reality of his surroundings again. The record was over.

"I say, do you think I could borrow that record, Poppœa?" he asked. "I'd like to play it over again."

"You can keep it," said Poppœa, swiftly generous. "We brought it for you." She turned away to ask Madame for news of Diaghilev. It was four months since the *Sleeping Princess* had finished.

"Poor Serge, he is having a hard time," Madame told them. "He is still in Monte Carlo. The *Sleeping Princess* ruined him. He has no money to put on a Paris season. This summer he does only Ballets Chantés in the Monte Carlo Opera House." She shook her head, grieving for the troubles of Big Serge.

"I wonder if there is a future for ballets with singing?" said Molly Grosvenor thoughtfully.

"Why not?" Poppœa pushed aside the records and leaned over the table ready for a discussion. "They have ballets in opera, why not singing in ballet?"

"But surely it can never be justified, artistically."

The argument started up. Pat joined in, Madame left them to it, and the three of them went on arguing and talking late into the night.

After Poppœa and Molly Grosvenor had gone, however, and Pat was alone in his room, he picked up the record of the "Hymn to the Sun" and stood a long time, staring down at the shining black surface, while an idea slowly formed in his mind.

Pat loved these evenings in his room when friends came in and sat listening to fine music or talking, discussing books and articles they had read, or ballets they had seen. Sometimes when Madame joined them she would start telling them stories of Russia and the great dancers, till Pat, unable to sit still another minute, would jump up and dance himself. Or, if the mood was on him, he would get a pair of old toe shoes from the dressing-room and dance the solos from the *Sleeping Princess* while Madame sang.

It was an atmosphere of youth and hope, of preparation for things to come.

But while Pat's life stretched ahead, full of promise and a world waited to be conquered, another life had nearly run its course.

In the quiet house in Hampstead the flame of this life was burning low. It flickered and went out.

The news of his father's death sent Pat hurrying to his mother's side. Sharing her sorrow, he wished again that he and his father had been able to understand each other better. He was old enough now to realise what a bitter disappointment it must have been to his father to have a son who danced. It was so far removed from everything he had been brought up to value. Pat loved his father for the sincere and simple man he was; a true sportsman of the old school. How empty his life must have been these last few years, living in London, cut off from everything that had made his life worth living. "And all because of me," Pat realised. The family had come to London because of his dancing. His father had made that sacrifice so that his son should be able to do something he neither understood nor really approved of, and the sorrow welled up in Pat afresh for all the things that were gone and could never be brought back, and because his father had died too soon without seeing his son fulfil his destiny. "But you shall be proud of me yet," Pat vowed to the spirit of his father, and it came to him that he was now the head of the family, the eldest son. He would take care of his mother and Anthony now, he was eighteen and a man. As though she knew what he was thinking, his mother smiled at him through her tears. He found her hand and held it fast in his, and perhaps at that moment the thought of Philip came to them both and sorrow tore anew at their hearts.

This was the final break-up of the family home. The house in Hampstead was given up, the furniture stored. Mrs. Kay, drained

of strength after months of devoted nursing, went to the country
to stay with relatives. Pat took a small studio of his own in Molly
Grosvenor's house in Belsize Park, and went back to his dancing,
back to the world that he belonged to now, and loved.

Astafieva had been right when she told him he was growing up.
A change was coming over his work. He began to understand
what he was doing and to be aware of the possibilities of his body.
Now, when he danced before the big mirrors in the studio, he was
not looking to see if a leg were properly turned out or a foot
correctly placed, he was watching the lines that his body could
create, discovering for himself what was beautiful and what was
ugly.

He tried experiments on his own before the mirror, with different positions and steps. The idea that had formed in his mind grew
insistent, and one evening in his own studio in Belsize Park he
brought out the gramophone.

In the twilight of an autumn dusk the music of the "Hymn to
the Sun" flooded the small room. Once, twice, the record played
through before the crouching figure beside the gramophone came
to life and began to move. He stretched up his arms and let his
body respond to the music that swept through him.

The mirrors reflected a dancing figure glimmering in the half-
light, and as Pat danced the blood seemed to course through his
veins like fire. The record finished. Now to remember those
movements, to try them again. The urge to create was on him and
the hours fled by.

When Pat finally stumbled into his bedroom and flung himself
down, his strength was spent, but in his exhaustion was a deep
content that he had not known before.

"Patté. Patté. That is careless work," Astafieva's stick landed
heavily on his legs in class next morning. "What 'ave you been
doing that you work so badly?" She came close to him, peering at
his pale face and the dark shadows under his eyes. "Ah! Late
nights. You sit talking to your friends Poppœa and Molly Grosvenor." There followed the usual lecture about dancers getting
plenty of sleep.

"You go to bed early to-night. I don't want to see a face like
that in my class to-morrow," was Madame's parting remark to Pat
that evening as she herself went out to dinner. A few minutes

later, as she passed some people coming up the stairs, he heard her say loudly, "and you, don't you keep 'im up late again."

"What's the matter with Madame?" His friends came into the dressing-room to see if he was ready. "What's all this about keeping you up late?"

"We didn't," added Molly Grosvenor. "We left you on your own last night as you said you didn't want to come out."

"I worked badly in class to-day," said Pat, "and she thinks I look tired."

"Oh!" Poppœa investigated. "She's right, Pat. You look awful. What have you been up to?"

"Nothing." Pat was unwilling to part with his secret.

"Do you think you had better not come to the theatre with us to-night?" Molly Grosvenor was looking at him with a puzzled frown.

"Why, Pat!" Poppœa burst out laughing. "You do look guilty. I believe you'd forgotten all about it."

"No, I hadn't," said Pat. "But . . ."

"But what?"

"What is all this mystery?" They closed in and got the story out of him.

Pat expected them to laugh at him, but it was just the opposite.

"I think it's thrilling." Poppœa was enthusiastic. "You must let us see what you've done."

"Let's go back home straight away," added Molly Grosvenor.

"What about the theatre?" Pat hedged.

"Never mind about that," Poppœa retorted. "This is important."

Back in his own studio, Pat danced, and they treated his work with the sincerity and seriousness that all true creative effort commands. He warmed to their encouragement and interest. They praised and criticised; suggestions were made, new ideas tried out.

The "Hymn to the Sun" began to take shape. Pat's confidence in himself grew, and the day arrived when Astafieva came upon him rehearsing his new dance in her Chelsea studio.

"So," she looked at him intently. "You too, you will create a dance?"

"You must see it, Madame," Poppœa told her.

"But it's not finished," Pat protested.

"No matter, let me see what you have done," Madame's interest was aroused.

The studio was cleared. The other students collected to watch. Pat danced to his first audience.

There was light and excitement in Astafieva's eyes as she watched.

"Bravo, Patté," she clapped her hands as he finished. "You begin to dance, really to dance." There was pride and delight in her voice. This young plant she had tended for so long was grown into a bud ready to open into full flower. He was ready now to receive all the great treasures of knowledge that she could give him. He was no longer just a talented pupil. He had become a fellow-artist. The soul of the dancer was stirring into life.

25 Anton Dolin

The summer had come round again. It was the summer of 1922. Over a year of solid work lay behind Pat. Long weeks of routine daily classes, his technique growing under Madame's patient, brilliant teaching. Side by side with this, his creative dancing had developed by watching others and by trying new experiments himself. Helped and encouraged by those who surrounded him and believed in his future, the artist in him grew.

The "Hymn to the Sun" was completed. Hardened and shaped in the fire of criticism, the first rough dance, sketched out on that autumn evening nearly a year ago, had been hammered and polished into a finished, shining thing.

Out of the welter of experiments another dance had grown to completion. "Dance Russe" gave expression to the young dancer's love and admiration for the great people who had passed on to him their art. Perhaps as he danced it he was aware also of a shadowy figure in the background of his mind, a man with a curious white streak in his hair, and an enigmatic expression in his eyes. Did the future lie in this direction? Or was the "Dance Russe" a tribute to past things?

Diaghilev had once described Pat as the "little boy with brown ever". There was nothing of the little boy left now. The last shreds of childhood had fallen from him during this past year. In the place of the uncertain boy who had fought and struggled blindly along the path of his destiny stood a young man, strong in the quiet confidence of his own growing powers. At eighteen Pat was slim and muscular. The years of his training had moulded his body to the supple grace of a dancer. There was love and pride in the eyes of his "dancing mother" Astafieva as she saw this "child" of hers grown into all the vigour and beauty of a young male dancer. Soon he would be ready to leave her, to make his own career in the world. Could either of them guess how soon?

Certainly neither of them could guess that it was the finger of fate pressing the studio bell during class one morning in June. The finger in question belonged to a Mr. Charguine. His card carried the information that he was an Impresario.

Madame returned from the interview with the light of battle in her eyes.

"I 'ave just promised that we shall put on a dancing exhibition," she looked round the class, pausing to give the full effect to her news. "We dance in the Albert Hall on the 26th June."

There was a stunned silence.

"The Albert Hall!" They looked at each other, "And by the end of the month."

"It appears that another dancing performance was booked for that date," Madame explained, "but something 'appened and they cannot do it, so I am asked if I will provide an entertainment, and I say 'yes'," she told them airily. "There is not much time so we must work quickly."

From that moment the Albert Hall loomed largely in everybody's life. The school had, of course, given displays and taken part in charity shows many times before. From the existing repertoire Madame began to compile the programme. This, however, was no hired hall and piano effort; this was to be a dancing exhibition on a grand scale.

"We shall 'ave an orchestra," Madame announced. "A large orchestra. The costumes we shall hire or have made." She scratched about on the littered table in her room looking for the first draft of the programme.

"Patté!" she called him in. "Come 'ere and see the dances you 'ave to do." She waved the paper at him.

Pat looked down the list and saw the familiar items, extracts from classical repertoire, one or two modern arrangements and mime. For him it was the usual group work and partnering, with a short solo or two among the *divertissements*. He handed back the list.

"I should like to have a dance of my own to do," he said.

"But you 'ave a solo in the *divertissement*."

"I mean an item of my own," Pat explained. "I would like to dance the 'Hymn to the Sun' and the 'Dance Russe'."

Astafieva looked up at him swiftly.

"I arrange the programme," she said. "If I 'ad wanted to put them in, I would 'ave done so."

Her voice and words sent a sudden tide of revolt surging up in Pat. Why shouldn't he be allowed to do his dances? Madame herself had said they were good. As though a voice within him was telling him that his whole future depended on it, his determination hardened.

"Why shouldn't I dance them?" he argued.

Unfortunately Astafieva was accustomed to have her own way in these matters.

"If you dance a solo it will be something that I choose." She spoke in a hard, clear voice and her words were the spark that sent Pat's Irish temper raging up inside him.

"I will not dance what you choose," he shouted at her suddenly. "I will do my own dances."

"You will dance what I say." She banged her fist down on the table.

"I will do my own numbers." Both temper and temperament had taken possession of him like a demon, and he no longer cared what he said. "I will not be dictated to by you," he screamed at her. "I shall dance what I think is best for me, and if not I shan't take part at all in your exhibition."

"You will learn to do what you are told," Madame screamed back. "Get out and go into the studio for your rehearsal."

He went, slamming the door.

Pat's temper cooled but his determination remained. He was now resolved to have his own way over this. Rehearsals became a battleground. Pat, still possessed by his demon, either sulked or screamed. A deep instinct in him was driving him on to fight for his right to do his own dances. He was long past caring what he said.

In his cooler moments he half-expected Madame to turn him out of the school altogether, or at least to forbid him to speak like that to her, but strangely enough she did neither. She put up with his temper. She seemed, even, to understand. She let him scream and give full voice to his feelings, but she was too obstinate and her own fiery independent nature was not ready to give in. The whole school was awed by the din of battle.

"I tell you, I will not 'ave my pupils telling me what they will or will not dance," Madame yelled at him across the studio.

"Why not? It is we who dance." Pat worked into a blind rage, knocked himself against the wall, fell over and rolled on the floor, refusing to get up.

"That's right. You knock your head. It is good for you. You knock some sense in it maybe."

Madame's full, rich laugh suddenly went ringing out. Pat sat up, purged of rage, and feeling rather foolish. Her laugh had brought him to his senses.

"Come on, Patté, it is finished now, you work," she told him.

Pat got up and they looked at each other. He knew without being told that it was truly over, he had made a fool of himself and he had won. The "Hymn to the Sun" and the "Dance Russe" would be put in the programme.

No more was said. The rehearsals went on quietly, and Pat, as though he wanted to make up for his display of temperament, went enthusiastically to work to help in any way he could. Night after night he stayed up late helping to copy out extra parts for the orchestra.

"I don't know what I should do without you all." Madame came into her room one evening to find half a dozen of them sitting round the table strewn with musical scores. "Patté, you are a great help to me." She came and leaned over him, a paper in her hand. "Would you look at this now and see that I 'ave spelled these names as they should be." She put the final draft of the programme before him. "Mon Dieu, these English names, they are so difficult."

Pat smiled as he took the paper. He looked down the list. There were "Dance Russe" and "Hymn to the Sun" with his own name staring back at him.

"I don't think Pat Kay will look very good in print," he said thoughtfully. "It doesn't sound like a dancer, does it?"

"We can put Patrickieff if you like, as you had for the *Sleeping Princess*?" Madame suggested.

Pat considered this. It was, in fact, the first time he had really thought about his name.

"No, I don't think Patrickieff is right," he frowned. "I must find something else. Yes," he warmed to the idea. "I'll disguise myself under a completely new name. It'll be fun, I'll mystify all my friends."

"You do what you like with your name," Madame told him, "but this list must go to the printers in the morning, early."

"What sort of a name do you want, Pat?" One of the others asked him.

"I don't know exactly. Something very Russian but not too difficult." He went over to the shelf and found a volume of Tchekov.

"Let's see if we can get any ideas out of here." He flipped over the pages. The name Anton stared up at him from the printed page.

"Anton," he said out loud. "I like that. What do you think?"

The jury round the table stopped copying band parts and decided that they liked it too.

"Now for something to go with it," said Pat, but Tchekov could only suggest long and complicated surnames.

"There's nothing here under five syllables." Pat pushed the book aside. "Nobody would remember them, let alone spell them." He appealed to Madame. "Haven't you any simple surnames in Russia?"

The answer to this question was a knock on the door. Mr. Charguine the Impresario had arrived to see how the preparations for the show were getting on. He was rapidly drawn into the discussion.

"So you want a name to go with Anton," he looked at Pat. "What about Dolin?" he suggested at length.

"Dolin?" Pat frowned. "That doesn't sound very Russian."

"But it is," replied Mr. Charguine. "Anton Dolin is a very good Russian name."

"Yes, and it is a good name for the stage." Madame was

becoming quite enthusiastic about the idea. "I can 'ear the public call out, 'Bravo, Dolin.' "

"Anton Dolin," Pat tried it out rather doubtfully. "I suppose it does sound foreign. Anyway, it's easy to spell."

"Anton Dolin", he wrote it down with a flourish.

"Anton Dolin", people read in the printed programmes as they took their places in the Albert Hall on 26th June, and in a dressing-room at the back Anton Dolin was putting on his ballet shoes and getting ready amid the turmoil that is an inescapable part of a one-night show.

Out in front the boxes and seats were far from full. A dancing exhibition was not a powerful magnet for the mass of the public, and the Albert Hall itself, vast, gloomy and circular, was not the ideal setting in which to stage ballet.

A bored sprinkling of men and women with notebooks occupied seats labelled "press". To them, this was just another routine job.

The performance began.

It was a pleasant entertainment. Madame's pupils in their classical white tutus looked young and lovely and they danced with precision and style, the hallmark of their famous teacher. The audience appreciated it and clapped politely. A short modern piece by six of the students was well received, and then came the moment for which one small group of people in the audience was anxiously waiting.

A stirring Russian rhythm that sent the blood tingling brought a whirling, leaping figure on to the stage. The fire and vigour of his dance stirred the imagination of those who saw him. Even the critics sat up and looked interested. That bounding dancer on the stage seemed to embody the very spirit of Russia.

Applause broke out, spontaneous and full.

"Who is that young man?" people asked each other as he ran back to take his bow. The programme told them it was Anton Dolin.

"I don't seem to have heard that name before," they told each other. Which was hardly surprising.

"What a remarkable agility."

"He hardly touches the ground."

Comments like these reached the ears of Mrs. Kay who sat

with a group of her friends. They looked at each other and smiled triumphantly. It was a proud moment.

The display continued. As it drew near the end of the show people began to say:

"What comes next?" Programmes rustled again.

"Hymn to the Sun", they read. "Anton Dolin."

"That was the young man who did the 'Dance Russe' so well." A sense of eager anticipation surged through the audience.

They were not prepared, however, for what they did see. The dramatic opening bars of Rimsky-Korsakov's music echoed through the hall. A magnificent young pagan appeared on the stage. From that first moment he held his audience. He carried them with him in the fiery, primitive dance of a pagan praying to the sun to pour down its warmth on his body. There was drama and power in every line of that splendid body, which lifted the dance right above the level of the rest.

The audience realised that they were witnessing something dramatically outstanding. The applause was thunderous.

As the whole performance came to an end and the dancers lined up for their bows, the shouts rang out for "Dolin".

"Bravo, Dolin!"

The stage was suddenly filled with a riot of flowers, but at Dolin's feet were green laurel wreaths, the first he had won.

"Bravo, Dolin!"

To the echo of applause the dancer Anton Dolin was born.

It was an unforgettable moment.

26 The Critics

"No, I'm not going to bed, we're going to celebrate." Pat's room was crowded with young people, and his mother, who wouldn't go to bed either, was installed in the best arm-chair, while Astafieva, who wouldn't even sit down, paced about restlessly, talking, re-living every moment of the evening. Champagne was fetched, toasts were drunk, and a sense of feverish gaiety laid hold of them. Pat hung up his laurel wreaths.

"I can't rest now till I've seen the papers," he declared, and they prepared for an all-night vigil.

When the champagne ran out they drank coffee, and sat about in quieter mood smoking and talking, until the dawn chorus of the London birds heralded a new day, and the early streaks of dawn lighting the sky sent young people hurrying out into the deserted streets in pursuit of first editions.

Before long, newspapers covered the furniture and floor of Pat's studio, and from the printed columns still damp from the press, there arose a unanimous chorus of praise:

"Last night at the Albert Hall . . . was a young man in advance of many of the established stars of the day."

"Dolin was as light as a feather, as graceful as a fawn."

"He combined the most marvellous agility with a true dramatic instinct."

"I, for one, believe that Dolin, ere long, will be proclaimed the rival and successor of Nijinsky."

"Pat! What wonderful notices," they all congratulated him.

"Every one of them is good."

"You've won over all the critics. There's not a single adverse notice."

Pat, dazed with happiness, tasted the first rewards of his long hard work. How worth while it all seemed now, and how he loved all these loyal friends who had helped him and were as pleased about his success as if it were their own.

There was one person, though, who mattered above all those who surrounded him. He sent a special look to his mother. Her happiness and pride in him glowed in her eyes. She was sharing this great moment to the full.

"Will you keep the name Anton Dolin?" someone was asking him.

"Of course I will, it's a lucky name." Superstition ran strong in Pat's Irish veins. "Anton Dolin brought me success."

So, the name that was chosen for fun, to mystify his friends, remained. It had brought him luck. It was to bring him something else as well. The echoes of his success were to reach out beyond the shores of England and across the Channel.

A letter arrived for Astafieva. It bore a Paris postmark, and bold foreign handwriting sprawled across the envelope.

"Patté." She called him excitedly. "Patté, come here."

"What is it?"

"I 'ave a letter from Serge Diaghilev." She waved the paper about. "He has seen in the papers that there is a new Russian dancer Anton Dolin. He writes to me to know who it is." Her dark eyes were sparkling with mischievous excitement. "Big Serge thinks he knows every dancer of note in Europe. 'E is curious about this Anton Dolin."

Pat's heart beat fast as he listened.

"I shall write and tell him," Astafieva went on. "I shall say that Anton Dolin is the little boy Patrickieff he engaged for the *Sleeping Princess*."

Like a door opening before him, Pat saw the opportunity he had been wanting. He had aroused Diaghilev's interest.

"Will you ask him, then, for an audition?" he begged her. "Ask him to see me dance again."

She did. She sent Pat's photograph as well.

The letter reached Diaghilev just before he left Paris.

What did he think as he sat with Astafieva's letter in his hand and the photograph of the "little boy with brown eyes" on the table in front of him?

Did it carry his thoughts back over the eighteen months that had passed since the *Sleeping Princess* had sent the Ballets Russes down to the very rockbottom of their fortunes?

A year of scraping and struggling to keep the company alive had followed that disaster. Diaghilev had held on. Then, six months ago, it began to look as though the tide of ill-luck was turning at last. The Princess of Monaco had graciously extended her patronage and the company now bore the official title of the "Ballets Russes de Monte Carlo". No empty honour this, but a title that carried with it the privilege of presenting each year a three-month season of their own ballets in the Royal Opera House.

Monte Carlo had become more than their headquarters, it had become their home.

Already this year 1923 had opened with a successful season there, bringing in enough money to enable Diaghilev to launch a Paris season. June and July had seen the Ballets Russes dancing to well-filled houses at the Théâtre Gaieté Lyrique in Paris. Now the company were having a six weeks' holiday, and after it, a tour planned for the autumn would take them to Belgium and Switzerland.

The Ballets Russes were very much alive again, and recovering rapidly, but the team was not complete. The place of the leading male dancer remained empty. Nijinsky had gone, his successor Massine had gone. As yet, no one had risen to take their place. True, there were good male dancers in the company. Idzikowsky, Woizikowsky, Svereff, were all first-class performers, but in Diaghilev's eyes they lacked the rare outstanding quality of genius that he looked for. Moreover, these men were fully mature artists, there was nothing further to be got from them. He wanted young talent that he could influence and inspire as he had done with Nijinsky and Massine. Under his guidance they had reached the full flowering of their individual genius.

The photograph of Anton Dolin still lay on the table before him. Was this the young dancer of the future that he so badly needed? Had this young man the stuff in him of which great artists are made? He had promised well. It might be worth seeing him, but not now, the holidays were here, and for Big Serge the month of August meant Italy and his beloved Venice. Time enough to see this young dancer later when he returned to Paris in September.

Diaghilev picked up a pen and answered Astafieva's letter.

It arrived in London just after Pat's eighteenth birthday.

"September!" Pat was disappointed. "That's nearly two months to wait. Even then he hasn't fixed a date."

" 'E will write again," Astafieva consoled him. "Of course he will see you. Do you think a man like Diaghilev troubles to write that 'e will see you when 'e does not mean it? Stupid boy. Now, we must prepare what you will dance for him."

While Diaghilev and his friends passed the golden hours of August in the sunshine of the Venice Lido, Pat worked on in the airless heat of a London studio.

September came and the anxiously awaited letter arrived.

"I told you Big Serge would not forget, Patté," Madame's clear voice called out to him. "You are to go to Paris."

"Did you say Paris?" Pat hurried in, hardly able to believe what he had heard.

"Yes. You will audition at the Théâtre Gaieté Lyrique in two weeks' time." They looked at each other. The great moment had come at last. An audition with Diaghilev was a golden opportunity. Was Pat now strong enough to grasp it?

27 Paris

Three excited people prepared to travel to Paris. Pat was accompanied by a young fellow-pupil, Jois Berry, who was to be his partner for the audition, and Madame herself who was to escort them both.

Ever since the arrival of Diaghilev's letter all three had been caught up in the whirl of preparations. There was the final polish to be put on the dances; the journey to be arranged; tickets and passports obtained; music to be sorted out; clothes packed. Finally the great day itself arrived.

The first journey to France.

For Pat a taxi to Victoria where the long boat-train waited. How important he felt as he made his way through the flood of people arriving from mere suburban trains, to reach the platform labelled "Continental Departures".

There at the barrier was Astafieva, looking quite strange in a hat, and Jois Berry, very young and pretty in a new outfit, standing with her mother.

As they went down the platform to find their reserved places on the train, they heard their names called. There was the sound of running steps. The next minute they were surrounded by familiar faces, friends and fellow-pupils who had come to see them off and wish them good luck.

The guard's whistle blew and the long train pulled slowly away from the platform, away from the group of smiling faces and waving arms, away from the grimy station. It gathered speed and went racketing past the packed, squalid houses of south London, and the thinning suburbs, till it shook itself free of the city and roared out into the open, green country.

They reached Dover where the air blew salt, the sun sparkled on the water, and the white-painted Channel steamer waited by the long customs sheds.

Soon they were leaning on the rail watching the coast of

England recede behind the creaming wake of the propellers. The white cliffs dwindled to a blue-grey outline that slowly disappeared into a misty horizon. The worrying thought that one would be seasick and perhaps too upset to dance was lulled by the calm sea and the sunlight on the water, another good omen.

At Calais an invasion of shouting porters in baggy blue tunics and an unfamiliar torrent of French pursued the passengers and their luggage through the customs shed and up into the high, waiting train, which was to race them through the flat farmlands of northern France towards the capital.

Not much longer now. As the daylight faded and the train roared through the darkening countryside, scattered lights twinkled out of the gathering dusk, the houses crowded in on either side of the carriage windows, and soon they were sliding under the high-domed roof of the Gare du Nord. They had arrived.

Paris, to new travellers emerging timidly from the Gare du Nord, presented a bewildering, rackety spectacle of noise and lights.

Through the lively, rowdy streets a perilous taxi screeched and blared its way to the Rue de Rivoli, to unload three weary but excited travellers at the door of the Savoy Hotel.

They were shown their rooms.

"I will go and let Diaghilev know we are arrived," Madame told Jois and Pat. "He is staying in this hotel himself."

They went to wash and change. Astafieva returned to tell them that the audition was to be at twelve o'clock the next day.

"As we're free this evening do let's go out and see the sights," Jois pleaded after dinner.

They were all of them as thrilled as children on that first evening in Paris, but Astafieva had to be strict.

"No, it is too late," she told them. "You go to bed early and get a good night's sleep so you dance well to-morrow."

Sleep! How could one sleep in this exciting city whose pulsing night life seemed to beat its way into one's room?

Sleep was a long way from Pat as he stood at the open window looking out into Paris. He leaned on the bar, surveying the long lighted street below, listening to the mingled sounds of traffic, music and voices; smelling the warm, heady night air of this glamorous city.

The impressions crowded in, but in the centre of the confused

thoughts that whirled round in his tired brain, the words "twelve
o'clock" shone like a white, blinding light. Twelve o'clock would
decide his future.

He went to bed at last, to a night of restless tossing and turning,
falling into an uneasy sleep at dawn.

Twelve o'clock. The hours passed somehow and Pat was
sitting with Jois in the hall of the hotel, his stomach turning over
as he watched the hands of the clock creep round. Beside him was
the little suitcase containing tights, ballet shoes, clean shirt and
socks.

"Ah! There you are." Astafieva came hurrying in. "The car is
here."

Outside the hotel entrance a large black limousine was waiting.
Pat's heart seemed to flutter like a trapped bird as he saw in the
back seat the broad shoulders and massive head of Serge Diaghilev.
Astafieva got in next to him. Pat and Jois sat on little seats facing
them. The sleek secretary Boris was in front beside the chauffeur.

Of what was said in that swift journey Pat remembered not a
word. Of the streets and buildings they passed he saw nothing.
He was seeing only the big man in front of him. Diaghilev was
talking and Pat was held by the compelling power of those wide-
set eyes that watched him so steadily. He was aware of their strange
light, which made him feel they were looking right through him,
laying bare all the secret places of his heart. Diaghilev smiled at
him suddenly and turned away to talk to Astafieva. As he spoke he
gestured with his hands, those sensitive surprisingly small hands
that held a dancer's future in their grasp. How vividly Pat remembered the lazy, caressing quality of his voice and the whole power
of this man to charm those around him and bend them to his
purpose.

The Théâtre Gaieté Lyrique was cold. They climbed endless
flights of stairs to the rehearsal room, a bare, draughty place at the
top of the building that served by day as a studio, by night as the
gallery bar.

In the middle of it a bunch of dancers were rehearsing. Pat's
teeth were chattering with cold and emotion as he changed. He
came to warm up at the bar, and the familiar exercises gave him
back his courage and confidence.

The rehearsal finished and the dancers drifted away. A row of chairs was placed across the room. Pat, looking over his shoulder as he worked, saw Diaghilev invite Astafieva to sit beside him. How serious she looked, she must be nervous too. A tall man hovered in the background. He recognised the stage manager Grigorieff. There was another woman with them, no mistaking those heavy features and pale, untidy hair. Nijinska was also to see him dance.

The pianist had sorted out the music and sat ready. This was it. Pat flexed his legs and feet. Jois gave him a wan smile. They took up their positions. There was a moment of horrible, empty silence. Diaghilev nodded his head. The music of the *Sleeping Princess* filled the studio.

Pat and Jois danced a *pas de deux*. It was the famous last act Adagio of the *Sleeping Princess* that had been performed by every leading artist since Petipa had created it thirty years before.

After this Jois's part in the audition was over, and Pat was alone. Before the silent scrutiny of those expert eyes he did a Russian dance that Astafieva had chosen and arranged for him.

He was well warmed up to his work now and ready for the third and final dance, his own creation.

The familiar and inspiring music of the "Hymn to the Sun" lifted him out of his surroundings. As he danced he was no longer playing the role of a pagan praying to the sun, he was himself, a young dancer stretching out his arms to the great power who ruled the destiny of the Ballets Russes, imploring it to open its doors to him, a foreigner. It was a passionate prayer into which he poured every feeling that was in him.

There was silence as he finished. The echoes of the piano died away. He saw Diaghilev turn to Astafieva and say something.

He went over to Jois, and they stood together in the corner whispering and watching.

Diaghilev rose to go. The audition was over.

What had the great man thought of it?

Pat was to be kept in suspense for another twenty-four hours.

"I cannot tell you," was all that Astafieva would say.

It was not until the next morning that she came to find him.

"Diaghilev will see you in his apartment now." Even then he could not guess from her voice what this meant. She would tell him no more.

Diaghilev's room was, as usual, overheated and overcrowded.

There were Boris and Grigorieff on a sofa; one or two strange men lurked in the background, and the atmosphere was heavy with cigarette smoke and the scent of almond oil. The windows were shut as always, for Diaghilev lived in terror of draughts.

The big man was sitting at a table smiling as he looked at Pat.

"I want you to join my ballet," he said. His words sent the room spinning round in a mad whirl. Dimly Pat heard the soft deep voice saying in English to Astafieva, "I want him to join as soon as possible. He must go to Monte Carlo without delay to study with Nijinska. Do you hear that, young man?"

Pat shook himself back to reality.

"Nijinska will prepare you for the roles you are to dance." The lazy voice went on to spread the glittering carpet of his future before him. No *corps de ballet* work for Anton Dolin. He was joining as a dancer in his own right, to dance his own roles. He was to take part in the next Monte Carlo season in December, and prepare from there to take over leading roles.

"It is most important that you should begin work with Nijinska as soon as possible." He turned to his secretary, "Boris, when does our tour finish?"

"The end of October."

"That will give us not quite a month." Diaghilev looked thoughtful. "It is not long but it will have to do. Yes." He looked full at Pat. "You will join us in Monte Carlo at the beginning of November. You will have to work very hard."

"I will," said Pat, and he meant it with all his heart. The passionate prayer he had poured into his dance had been answered.

The next day they left Paris to return to London. Pat carried a contract in his pocket. To him it was the most precious document in the world. He, an Englishman, was to be a member of Diaghilev's famous company. He, an Englishman, was to dance leading roles in the great Ballets Russes.

28 Monte Carlo

November 1923. A train roared through the night hauling its freight of human lives across the sleeping land of France. Southward they sped through the hours of darkness. As dawn was breaking the long line of coaches slowed and jolted to a halt. Heavy-eyed passengers, grimy and unshaven, rubbed the steam from the windows to read the name Marseilles in staring white letters on the station boards. They had reached the south coast. The long night was over and the grey autumn skies of northern France lay far behind them. This was like waking into another world.

As the train left Marseilles and wound its way along the coast, the sun rose up brilliant and warm in a blue sky. From the carriage windows they looked out on to tumbled red rocks and golden sand thrust out into the sparkling waters of the Mediterranean.

So this was the famous Côte d'Azur. Pat watched the scenes roll by in a series of vivid and beautiful pictures. From time to time they stopped at sunlit, flower-decked stations, Juan les Pins, Cannes, Antibes, romantic names that he had only heard of, appeared now in the unfolding reality of this fairy-tale journey.

It was after midday when they halted at a tiny wayside station perched on a ledge of rock with a precipitous drop to the sea sparkling below. Monte Carlo. They had arrived.

Pat and his luggage stood on the little platform. The train steamed away and was lost to sight round a bend. A small boy rushed into view.

"*Ascenseur*," he screamed.

Pat was still puzzling it out when a leisurely, baggy-bloused porter took charge of the situation. As Pat followed his luggage into the station yard to be put into a cab, he suddenly saw the explanation. Set against the rock face was a large iron lift cage. Looking up he had a glimpse of a white balustrade and palm trees overhead, and above them the soaring pile of a massive ornate building whose gleaming white pinnacles reared up against the blue sky.

"Casino et Théâtre de l'Opera," the porter jerked a horny thumb in its direction.

The Opera House! So this was to be the scene of his work. In this great white building that overlooked the sea.

The cab took him through climbing, twisting streets to his hotel. It was a quiet, pleasant place, too quiet he found as he stood alone in his room, for the grinding rattle of the train still sounded in his head. The silence of the room was oppressive. The flame of excitement that burned in him demanded noise, bustle and restless activity. He paced up and down. For days and weeks past every thought and every plan had been centred on this day. The audition in Paris, the contract, the preparations, the last part at home, the great send-off by his friends, the thrill of the journey, and it had all led up to—what? To this quiet hotel bedroom? What an anti-climax.

A sense of loneliness took hold of Pat. He felt suddenly shut off and imprisoned in this room. He went out quickly. At least he would move about and have a look at this place that was to be his home. What day of the week was it? Friday. He wondered what the others in the company were doing at this moment, and where they all lived. Perhaps there were some in his hotel. If only he had some-one to talk to. Then he remembered with a jolt that he didn't know enough Russian to talk to anyone for long, and he didn't speak a word of French. The sense of loneliness deepened. He wandered disconsolately round the town and went to bed early that night a discouraged, disappointed young man.

The next day, Saturday, stretched bleak and empty before him. Not until Sunday were Diaghilev and his friends due to return. He spent two of the loneliest days he had ever known. He had his solitary meals at the hotel and longed for the haphazard companion-ship of the studio in London.

On Sunday afternoon arrived a message for Mr. Dolin. He was to dine with Diaghilev that evening!

The loneliness was over.

Dining with Diaghilev meant sitting down to table with six or eight other people as well, a bewildering cosmopolitan crowd of celebrities. Pat, floundering in a conversation of mixed French and Russian, strained to pick up a word here and there, and wondered who they all were.

Big Serge was in great spirits. A successful year lay behind him. His ballets had done well and made money. Now, with pockets full, he could plan boldly for the future. He called Pat over to sit beside him and spoke to him of the work he was to do, of the future plans for the Ballets Russes, clever far-seeing plans that opened a glitter-ing prospect before the young dancer. They were to start with a three months' winter season of classical ballets here in the Opera House. It was to be a safe, money-making season, and a trial run for the new dancer. After that, a tour, and then, if Anton Dolin justified the faith placed in him, he would be launched in Paris, making his big début as a leading dancer of the Ballets Russes.

The hotel bedroom was no longer lonely when Pat returned to it. His mind reeled with the things he had heard. He realised what a great treasure of golden opportunity Diaghilev was holding out to him. There was more than just personal success too. He felt that on him had fallen the responsibility to show the world that an English dancer could uphold the tradition of the Russian Ballet.

Pat looked at himself in the mirror.

"I will prove to the world that an Englishman can dance as well as a Russian," he vowed.

Meanwhile to-morrow still lay ahead, and with it the ordeal of taking his place in the company. He would meet them all at the morning class with Nijinska. Diaghilev had made him understand that he must be very tactful with Nijinska for she was not altogether pleased to have a foreigner coming into the company.

"You must give her time to get used to you," Diaghilev had said. "To begin with you will work under her in the general class with the rest of the company. Later we shall see about private lessons." He had not explained that Nijinska had flatly refused to give private lessons to "the foreigner". Neither did he mention that the company did not exactly welcome strangers in their midst. These things Pat was to find out for himself.

The rehearsal room in the Opera House was underground. It was long and low-ceilinged. The class was at nine. By half past eight on that first morning Pat was already there warming up at the bar and feeling as shy and anxious as a new boy on his first day in boarding-school.

In one's and two's the company arrived. They all stared curiously at this new dancer who had appeared among them. A few recognised him from the *Sleeping Princess* days and smiled. The girls were more friendly than the men.

Sokolova came over to him. Here at least was a fellow-countryman. They talked together until Nijinska arrived.

The class began and Pat forgot the unspoken hostility about him in the effort of work. He was so used to Astafieva that he found it difficult at first to adapt himself to Nijinska's style of teaching. The principle, of course, was the same, but the handling of it strange and new, and the exercises they did were advanced and complicated. The standard set was very high.

"We have a break now," Sokolova told him as they were dismissed. "Rehearsal this afternoon."

"Does Nijinska take all the rehearsals too?" Pat wanted to know.

"Not all of them, Duckie." Sokolova smiled at him with wise understanding. "Don't worry if she doesn't take much notice of you at first, she will get used to you."

Would she? Pat began to wonder as the days settled down into the routine of work and Nijinska still treated him with a marked lack of interest. He felt that she was merely carrying out instructions that Diaghilev had given her, resenting his presence in the company. As he worked, sweated and strained under Nijinska's indifferent eyes, he mourned for the friendly encouragement of Astafieva.

Three ballets were to open the season on the 25th November.

"You will dance in *Prince Igor* and in *Cleopatra*," Diaghilev had told Pat. "Small *corps de ballet* roles only to begin with for there is not much time."

As the ballets took shape on the studio floor, Diaghilev and his friends frequently came to watch the rehearsals. On one occasion Pat was beckoned over.

"I want to present you to a cousin of mine," said Diaghilev. "Paul Koriboute."

Pat bowed politely before the elderly, aristocratic-looking man who stood beside Big Serge.

"I thought it was time you two knew each other." There was an amused twinkle in Diaghilev's eyes. "You are both at the same hotel."

It was the beginning of a pleasant and profitable friendship. Mr. Koriboute was a charming, cultured man, and a lonely one. Like many other Russian aristocrats he was a refugee from the horrors of the Russian Revolution. He and Pat were soon sharing a table at the hotel.

"I do wish you would teach me your language," Pat said to him one day.

"Shall we make a bargain?" Mr. Koriboute suggested in his formal, stilted English. "I teach you Russian, you teach me English.

At meal times we must promise that neither of us shall speak his own language."

It was a bargain they both kept. Pat was seriously determined to master this difficult language. Curious Anglo-Russian conversations took place, but they had results. Pat at last began to acquire a certain fluency, and with it he began better to understand the people with whom he was working.

Slowly, gradually, the atmosphere of unspoken hostility began to lift. They became accustomed to the foreigner who worked as one of them, and Diaghilev, who saw and understood everything that went on in his company, judged that this was the moment to approach Nijinska again about private lessons for Pat. It was not easy. Nijinska still obstinately insisted that there was plenty of young talent in the company which could be brought on. There was the young Serge Lifar, for instance, who showed great promise. Why not train him instead of wasting time on "the foreigner"?

Diaghilev, the diplomat, did not remind her that when Lifar had joined them at the beginning of the year she had been furious that she should be expected to teach an almost untrained young refugee from Communist Russia. The temperamental Nijinska would not be ordered about or bullied, and Diaghilev, with infinite charm and tact, patiently persuaded her that Lifar, who had been dancing seriously for less than a year, was not yet ready for big roles and that Anton Dolin, who had been five years with Astafieva, was. He flattered her into understanding how important it was that this young English dancer should be trained to express her ideas in the ballets she created. How could he do justice to her choreography unless she taught him herself?

Diaghilev's charm was irresistible. Grudgingly Nijinska agreed to give Pat a daily private lesson.

"But not in the rehearsal room," she declared. "I don't want the company to know of this, it will make jealousy."

She agreed that Pat's private lesson should take place in the afternoon on the stage of the local cinema.

"But not at once," was her parting shot. "I am too busy. Not until after the opening of the season." Diaghilev, smiling, let her have her way.

The November days drew on and the opening date loomed near.

Rich and fashionable society gathered in Monte Carlo for the winter. The hotels filled, the Casino gambling tables were crowded, and on the 25th November the Opera House opened its doors and the curtain went up on the first performance of the season's ballets; the white, classical purity of *Les Sylphides*, the richly beautiful spectacle of *Cleopatra*, and the blood-stirring dances of *Prince Igor*. Three safe, well-tried favourites, for Big Serge was taking no chances—yet.

Pat's part in them was small, but he put all his heart into his work, and on that first evening he knew the exhilaration of dancing in the perfect conditions Diaghilev created for his ballets. Magnificent artists, beautiful décors, faultlessly lit, and impeccable music blended into a complete and satisfying work of art.

The fiery dances of *Prince Igor* brought the evening to a dramatic finish, and the dancers lined up to take their bow. Down came the curtain. As it fell, however, the applause was suddenly mingled with laughter. Out in front, cut off from the others, stood an embarrassed young man. Anton Dolin stood acknowledging the applause as though he had provided the whole evening's entertainment.

"A good omen," Diaghilev said to him afterwards. "Yes, a good omen for the future." He drew Pat aside. "Early in the New Year you will make your real début here. I am reviving *Daphnis and Chloe*. You will dance the lead, partnering Sokolova. Nijinska will teach you your role." He added in a low voice. "You will begin your private lessons with her to-morrow."

"To-morrow!" Pat looked up swiftly as though he would ask how this miracle had come about.

"I persuaded her," Diaghilev smiled, sketching a swift gesture with his hand. "She will take you in the cinema to-morrow afternoon. It is better if you do not mention these lessons to anyone yet." He put his hand on Pat's shoulder, "Nijinska can teach you a great deal," he looked at him intently. "It is for you now to win her over to your side."

One morning early in December a notice appeared on the board that set tongues wagging.

"Have you seen the latest notice?" People passed the news on to each other. "There's a rehearsal call for *Daphnis and Chloe* this afternoon, and guess who's dancing Daphnis?"

"I don't know. Idzikowsky, I suppose, or Vilzak?"

"It's Dolin. He's chosen for the lead to partner Sokolova."

Heads came together to talk over this startling development.

"Let them talk," said Diaghilev when he heard. "They will learn soon enough that this is only the beginning."

Meanwhile Pat had to face renewed hostility from jealous rivals who had imagined that they would be chosen for the part.

"They will get over it," Diaghilev haughtily disregarded the jealousies that threaded like turbulent dark currents below the surface. "If they don't like my decisions they can leave."

To make matters worse, the newcomer had been taken up into the circle of Diaghilev's intimate friends. Anton Dolin was a frequent guest at the table of the great. Jealous eyes saw him placed among the rising young celebrities whom Diaghilev had gathered round him.

A new team of talent was forming here in Monte Carlo during this winter. A new chapter in the story of the Ballets Russes was opening. The old purely Russian regime was dead, for the Revolution had severed the life-stream that fed the Ballets Russes with dancers, artists and musicians. Now Diaghilev was looking to the West, to Europe, for the new young talent he needed.

Very few were left of the original team that had blazed the way to fame. The Russian artist Bakst was dead, and the glorious riot of colour he had created for so many ballets passed into history. In his place came Marie Laurencin, with pale clear hues, and the dark-eyed Spaniard Picasso, with his bold modern handling of pure line and colour. Stravinsky had gone his own way, and in his place gathered young French composers, Auric and Poulene, to be joined soon by Darius Milhaud. With them too came the French writer

Jean Cocteau, a restless, witty, brilliant young man already famous.

These were the people in whose hands lay the creation of future ballets. It was an intellectual and highly-cultured group of people, but the young Englishman was at a disadvantage for the sparkling, witty talk going on round him was a mixture of French and Russian and he could only listen, struggling to understand.

"What's the matter?" Nijinska asked him as he came to his private lesson after one of these lunch parties.

"Language!" Pat pressed his hands to his aching head.

"Ah! You have been with Serge Pavlovitch and his friends?"

"Yes. Nothing but French and Russian, and they talk of politics and art, of books and music, and Diaghilev expects me to follow for he suddenly asks what I think." Pat shook his head despairingly.

"Understanding will come," Nijinska told him. "Already you have learned much Russian. French will follow."

Pat looked at her swiftly, for her voice was unusually warm and friendly.

"I do want to understand," he said. "For there is so much to learn."

"So! You are beginning to find that out."

"What do you mean?" He was puzzled by her tone.

"I mean that you are beginning to realise at last that you have things to learn outside ballet. You find out that to be a great artist you must have knowledge and culture. You English you have no culture. Now you are with the great Diaghilev he educates you. He teaches you that it is not enough to live in a world of ballet shoes. To be great yourself you must appreciate greatness in others, and have knowledge of other arts. Like that he trained my brother, Vaslav. He took him to the great cities in Europe, he showed him the finest paintings and sculptures; he made him listen to concerts and operas, and study books; he let him meet all the most interesting people of the day. That is how he trains his chosen young artists. He did the same for Leonide Massine, he will do the same for you. He trains the mind and the spirit of the dancer, while I," she smiled, "I train the feet!"

They both laughed.

"Come now, enough talk. To work. Let me see you first walk across the stage and stand in the centre there."

To walk and to stand had been the first lesson Nijinska had

given him. Pat, astonished and indignant, had been informed that he didn't know how to do either of these things.

"You walk like a tired old woman." Nijinska had given him a cruel imitation of a slouching gait. "You learn to walk straight. Not to strut like a turkey cock, but to be tall and proud like a young god, and stand strongly with your head held well."

At first Pat had thought she was doing this out of spite, but he soon realised he was wrong and that these things were vitally important, to give style and finish to a dancer. Strange that no one had thought to teach him so before, he thought, as he crossed the stage with firm, measured tread.

"That is better," Nijinska told him, and they passed to more difficult work.

Pat loved his lessons with her for she taught him so much. Undeterred by her sulks, tempers and indifference, he had worked hard and enthusiastically, and Nijinska, on her side, began to admit to herself that this young man was really sincere and serious about his dancing.

"No." She checked him after he had done a high leap across the stage. "That is not good. The jump should be higher, and spread out." Her hands described a long curve.

"I've tried so often," Pat despaired. "I suppose my muscles are not powerful enough. I haven't the feet and legs of Nijinsky."

"It is not only the feet and legs that make a jump." Nijinska looked at him out of the corners of her slanting eyes. She was silent as though she were deciding whether to say more.

"Yes." She turned her head and looked full at Pat. "I will tell you how my brother did his great jumps. It was by the control of breathing, here." She tapped her chest. "You prepare to jump, you breathe deeply, your body is full of air, and you stay up. Look, I show you. First I breathe as you do, anyhow." Nijinska ran across the stage and demonstrated. "You see, I am heavy, my muscles must do all the work, it seems to be a great effort, that is bad."

Pat thought it was wonderful but said nothing.

"Now. I do it our way. I control my breathing." She seemed to sail up into the air in an effortless movement. What tremendous power she had for a woman.

"Now." Nijinska came back to him. "I teach you to do the same." Pat looked at her with sudden emotion, realising that she was passing on to him the secret of her brother's famous elevation. He knew then that the last barriers were broken down between them. At last Nijinska was on his side.

The bright sunny days passed swiftly for Pat in a mounting pressure of work. The routine of each day following its inexorable rhythm; the morning class, the afternoon rehearsal, the private lesson, the evening performance. Lunches and dinners with Diaghilev and his friends, and all the time a growing knowledge of French and Russian. It was a hard, exacting life, but Pat was utterly happy in it.

The opening of *Daphnis and Chloe* was fixed for the 1st January.

On New Year's Eve the dancers were in the theatre getting ready for the last dress rehearsal when startling news broke.

"Idzikowsky is gone!" It passed from mouth to mouth like a fire spreading consternation in the dressing-rooms. Doors were opened and little knots of people gathered in the corridors.

There was a further wave of excitement as Nijinska arrived.

"All is well." Pat's dresser brought him the news. "Madame Nijinska is dancing Idzikowsky's role herself. The situation is saved."

"A man's role?" Pat frowned.

"It will not be noticed in that costume," the dresser chuckled, thinking of Nijinska stepping, literally, into Idzikowsky's discarded trousers.

"That's all right then." Pat, putting the finishing touches to his make-up, was more concerned with his own coming ordeal than the drama going on round him.

Later, on thinking it over, he was to realise that the unceremonious departure of Idzikowsky would mean that many important roles would fall vacant and that probably he would have the chance to take them on.

There was a knock on the door.

"It is a lady to see you," his dresser told him. "She would not give her name."

Pat frowned, trying to guess who it could be.

"No," he said. "I can't see anyone now. Ask her to come after the rehearsal . . ." he broke off, hearing a noise, and turned round. The door of the dressing-room was open. There, standing smiling at him, was Astafieva.

"Madame!" Pat ran to greet her with open arms. Surprise and delight were complete. Out of the torrent of broken English and Russian, he gathered that this was all Diaghilev's idea. He had invited Astafieva to come from London as his guest so that she could see her pupil's début.

"Dear Big Serge, he thinks of everything."

Dear Madame! Her familiar reassuring presence seemed to fill Pat's dressing-room. How lovely she looked. The wonderful hands, the vivid face. What a lot they had to say to each other.

Pat danced the dress rehearsal that night on winged feet. Time enough for nerves at the opening to-morrow. They danced to a privileged group of people in the stalls whom Diaghilev had invited. After it was over Sokolova and Pat were summoned round to the front. Here they were presented to a distinguished-looking gentleman. There was a twinkle in Diaghilev's eyes as Sokolova curtsied and Anton Dolin bowed low before his Royal Highness the Duke of Connaught, who discovered, to his surprise, that the two leading dancers of the Russian Ballet were fellow-countrymen.

He was friendly and charming and they withdrew from his presence with royal wishes for a Happy New Year.

In the stress of the dress rehearsal they had almost forgotten that to-morrow would be 1924. For Pat, though he could not know it yet, those good wishes were to be royally fulfilled. Nineteen twenty-four was, indeed, to be a very happy year.

30 The New Year

On the first day of the New Year the second ballet of the evening introduced for the first time a young English dancer in a leading role.

It was twelve years since the curtain had gone up on *Daphnis and Chloe*. Those years, however, had not dimmed the glorious colours of Bakst's scenery, and the audience of 1924 saw the same green and leafy grove sacred to the God Pan, and luminous with sunshine and blue sky. They heard the music that Ravel had written weaving the same enchantment into this pagan setting of old Greek Mythology. In place of the legendary figures of Karsavina and Nijinski, though, there now stood the English dancers of the new generation, Sokolova and Anton Dolin.

Anton Dolin and Nijinsky. Did Diaghilev realise the ordeal he had set his young Dolin by bringing him for the first time before an expert and critical public to dance almost literally in Nijinsky's shoes? Since the great Russian had created the role of Daphnis, no one else had danced it. To-night, therefore, the young Englishman would be measured against the standard set by a man who was acknowledged to be the greatest dancer of his day and, some people considered, of all time. There never would be another Nijinsky, they said—or would there?

The overture was finishing and in the wings stood Anton Dolin, a graceful, boyish figure in Daphnis's short white tunic. He waited for his entrance, a prey to first-night nerves, trying not to let himself think of failure, or of the critics who were waiting out there like harpies, he imagined, to tear him to pieces. It was only the thought of his friends, the people who had helped him and believed in him, that gave him the courage to go out on to that stage—to be judged.

The judgment was summed up by one of the critics afterwards. The great André Levinson wrote:

"Anton Dolin, that strong and beautiful young man, has made a promising beginning, though rather a premature one. His professional skill is rudimentary. He does, however, execute high leaps quite well. If his miming lacks subtlety, it is, nevertheless, not clumsy. Without being expressive, his acting is anything but stilted, and his youth, well in evidence, is on his side."

"What an unkind write-up," was Pat's first indignant reaction. He read it again and took comfort by realising that it might have been much worse. He had made a "promising beginning". Enough that he had come through the first trial and survived. "A promising beginning"—Pat took heart again. He was further encouraged when he learned that Diaghilev was pleased, Nijinska was pleased, Astafieva was proud and delighted, and in the eyes of the company he had done well. Anton Dolin, they considered, had deserved the laurel wreaths he had won. They accepted him as one of them and warmed to friendliness.

Pat felt that he had passed another milestone on his hard upward journey. It was indeed a happy beginning to the New Year.

After this things were to go more easily. He was now living and working in an atmosphere of friendliness and encouragement. *Daphnis and Chloe* passed into the regular repertoire, and already Diaghilev was planning three new ballets to follow on.

"I want you to dance in two of them," he told Pat. "Small parts only. That will be enough while you still study with Nijinska."

Pat understood clearly now that his training and career were in master hands. He was being steadily and skilfully prepared for great things. Success in Paris was the ultimate goal. Diaghilev was a dictator where his company were concerned. He had made it clear to Pat from the beginning that he was the master, that he made his dancers and ruled their destinies. Not until later would Pat's proud and independent spirit rebel. For the present he was grateful for all the things Diaghilev was doing for him, and content that it should be so.

Diaghilev had told him that he would make his début in Paris in *Daphnis and Chloe* some time in the summer. Meanwhile the Monte Carlo winter season was in full swing. New rehearsals started in the long underground room.

The first of the new ballets, *Les Tentations de la Bergère*, was a fragile Dresden shepherdess creation. Pat found he was partnering Tchernicheva.

"You are a God and Goddess," Nijinska set them to work to learn their *pas de deux*.

They were hard at work on it when the door from the office opened. A thin, lively face appeared.

"Ah! I see you are busy with La Bergère." Jean Cocteau came tripping gaily into the room. "Have you seen the costumes these two are to wear?"

"No," said Nijinska, concentrating on her dancers.

"I saw the designs this morning," Jean Cocteau perambulated round the piano. "Would you believe it, the God and Goddess are to be dressed exactly alike." He came across the studio imitating the steps they had just been doing.

"Jean, go away. I want to get on with my rehearsal." Nijinska was trying not to laugh at his antics.

"In pink rosebuds!" Jean cocked a mischievous eye in her direction. "We shan't know which is Tchernicheva and which is Dolin! Think of the possibilities that creates," and the *enfant terrible* of the place darted round in a circle making them all laugh.

"What is going on in here?" The broad figure of Diaghilev filled the open doorway. "Jean, it is you, up to your nonsense again!" He came into the studio followed by an artist who carried a portfolio under his arm.

"We were thinking of letting Tchernicheva lift Dolin on to her shoulder, the effect should be decidedly quaint." Jean was quite irrepressible. "Ah! Here are the designs." He went darting across to the artist, Juan Gris. Rehearsals were suspended while Nijinska joined a committee meeting that gathered over the sketches.

The dancers hung about waiting. Pat drifted away to the far end of the studio. For rehearsals the long room was divided across the middle by a curtain. Pat pushed his way through it to find three or four of the men leaning against the bar talking. He joined them, and found to his surprise they were discussing acrobatics.

"Of course, it will never take the place of ballet," one of them was saying. "This craze for modern acrobatic dancing is only a passing fashion."

"They are very clever, some of these people," another put in. "I saw a remarkable couple at the Casino at Nice last week. They had amazing balance and control."

"Those sort of things are only tricks," said one scornfully. "Any well-trained classical dancer could do them with a little practice."

"Try them yourself then," he was challenged.

"I used to do some of their tricks to amuse myself." Pat joined in the conversation. "They're not really difficult if you have a good sense of balance and don't mind falling over."

A few minutes later, if Diaghilev or Nijinska had looked round the curtain, they would have been greeted by the edifying sight of their classical dancers tumbling over the floor in a series of wild acrobatics.

"It is really much more difficult than it looks," they admitted, and it was not long before they had all given up to stand and admire Pat.

"How did you learn to do it?" they wanted to know as he stood on his hands and slowly shifted his balance till he was supported on one hand alone.

"I don't really know," Pat came the right way up again. "I used to practise for fun when I was a boy, and I found it came quite easily. There is one thing I'd like to try that I've never had the chance to do before and that is to be swung round."

"Oh yes, the couple at Nice did that."

"Come on, let's try it."

None of them saw the curtain move, and a bright inquiring face appear. Jean Cocteau, bored with the costume discussion, had come in search of other interest. He found it. He saw the body of Diaghilev's new leading dancer whirling round in the air, an arm and a leg held in the grip of a muscular member of the *corps de ballet*.

The rest of Jean Cocteau came round the curtain to see better.

He leaned against the bar watching intently as Pat followed it up with different tricks. For once Jean forgot to be witty or clever. He was quite silent, absorbed in the movements of that supple athletic body. Pat was realising just how much he had missed his "hobby" and was thoroughly enjoying himself. For long months these acrobatics of his had been forgotten in the stress of strict ballet training.

"What you do there is very interesting," said Jean as he finished.

"I'm out of practice," Pat told him.

"Then you must get in practice again," Jean replied seriously.

"As long as Nijinska doesn't see me!" Pat laughed.

He did practise again. Whenever there were spare moments at rehearsals he would disappear behind the curtain to the deserted half of the studio and amuse himself trying out different tricks. Whatever he did, though, he tried to carry out with the style and grace of a dancer. He wedded his acrobatics to his classical dancing.

Sometimes he was alone, more often, though, the still, silent figure of Jean Cocteau would be there, leaning against the bar, and as he watched the lively, brilliant brain was active, for the sight of a classical dancer doing acrobatics had struck a spark and given Jean Cocteau a powerful new idea. An idea that was to grow into *The Blue Train*.

In February the ballet season finished. Diaghilev and his friends
prepared to migrate to Paris. Only the *corps de ballet* were to remain
in Monte Carlo to take part in the opera season that was following
on.

"Nijinska will be too busy to give you lessons here," Diaghilev
told Pat. "She has to prepare the dances for the operas. I have
arranged for you to go to Paris. You will study with Trefilova."

Pat was delighted. He didn't want to be left behind in the south
of France after the others had gone.

So, once again, he stood on Monte Carlo's wayside station,
waiting, this time, for the "Paris Rapide". Was it only three months
since an excited young man had climbed down from the train at
this same station and had had his first glimpse of the theatre
towering up through the palm trees, dazzling white against the
blue sky? How strange and frightening everything had been. Now
the young leading dancer of the Russian Ballet could smile at that
other timid figure. He was no longer the "stranger" and the new
boy. He had made his successful début in Monte Carlo. Before him
now lay the final test of Paris. It was a challenge that made his
heart beat strongly.

The dusty green train came whistling and screeching round the
bend. Pat climbed up into it. In a few hours they had left the sunlit
Mediterranean and the palm trees and were headed north on the
long journey across France.

In Paris Pat found a message waiting for him at his hotel.

"Come to lunch to-morrow. D."

Boris Kochno met him in the foyer of the hotel.

"Serge Pavlovitch is full of plans for a new ballet." He linked
his arm through Pat's and the two young men made their way into
the dining-room. "It's been specially written for you."

Questions came piling into Pat's mind, but there was no time
to ask them, for he was face to face with Big Serge. Those strange
light eyes were looking deeply into him, as though Diaghilev

wanted to assure himself there was no change. Swiftly it was over and Pat was enfolded in a warm Russian greeting.

He shook hands with Igor Stravinsky.

"Now, I want you to meet another musician," Diaghilev still had his arm about Pat's shoulders as he presented him to a dark-haired man of massive build. It was Darius Milhaud, the French composer.

The others at table were old friends. Pablo Picasso was there with his beautiful Russian wife Olga, who had herself been a dancer in the Ballet Russes. Jean Cocteau too, mischievous and irrepressible as ever.

"Has le Grand told you?" he greeted Pat as they all sat down to lunch, "I have written a ballet for you. A new ballet in a new style. It will be the most modern thing ever seen."

Diaghilev leaned across to Pat.

"We want a ballet for your début in Paris."

"So I have created *Le Train Bleu* especially for the occasion!" Jean was bubbling with enthusiasm for his idea. "And Darius Milhaud here is to write the music."

"But I thought I was to dance in *Daphnis and Chloe*?"

"That is what I intended but we ran into trouble over the performing rights." Diaghilev turned to Boris. "What was it exactly?"

"It appears that we cannot put on a performance of *Daphnis and Chloe* in Paris," the smooth Boris explained. "It seems that the Paris Opera Ballet Company own the performing rights."

"So," Diaghilev gestured, "we must find another ballet to present you to the Paris public, and Jean, here, arrived with his idea for something entirely new."

"When is this to be?" Pat asked.

"In the early summer. I am arranging a season here for May," Diaghilev told him. "We go on tour to Spain first. We shall have about three months to prepare the Paris season, so we must get this new ballet *The Blue Train* into rehearsal as soon as we can."

"What! With the music not even written," remarked Stravinsky dryly.

"I have already one or two themes I have been working on," put in Darius Milhaud . . .

The Blue Train was the centre round which their talk revolved, while hovering waiters brought the caviare, the sole meunière, the entrecôtes, and the wines flowed. Pat listened and learned about this ballet that was being specially created for him.

"When I saw you doing your acrobatics down in the studio," Jean explained to him, "the idea came to me of acrobatics on the beach. I pictured the smart young people who go to the fashionable seaside places . . ."

"I think I shall get Chanel to design the costumes," Diaghilev interrupted.

"But she is not a stage designer," remarked Picasso.

"No, but she is the smartest woman in Paris, and a leader of fashion. She should be able to dress for the stage as well as *le monde*."

"Undress them," put in Jean swiftly. "It will be bathing costumes."

"You two must get together," Diaghilev turned to his secretary. "Boris, remind me to arrange a dinner so that Jean and Coco can fight about what the dancers are not to wear."

"What role am I dancing?" Pat tried to find out. "What is the story of the ballet?"

"There is no story," said Jean Cocteau airily. "That is the point. It is an expression of modern life. These young people are on the beach, by their attitudes and movements they symbolise modern life. They swim, they play tennis, golf and beach games. Their dances will express all these. You are the swimmer, the 'Beau Gosse', and the centre of attention."

"And my music will be modern, syncopated rhythm," Darius Milhaud joined in. "The music of the present day."

"*The Blue Train* will be the forerunner of the ballets of the future." The force of Diaghilev's enthusiasm infected them all. "We shall show people that the Ballets Russes lead the way. As soon as Nijinska has finished at Monte Carlo she must get to work on the choreography."

"What will Nijinska say when she learns that she has to do the choreography for modern acrobatics?" inquired Picasso.

"She will get used to it." Diaghilev's hand smoothed over Nijinska's feelings. "She will be dancing in it herself."

"There are four principal roles," Jean put in. "The Beau Gosse and Perlouse, that is you and Sokolova. The tennis champion and the golfer; Nijinska and Woicikowsky."

"It is the first time a ballet has ever been written round an individual dancer," remarked Stravinsky.

"Yes, that is true," said Serge. "You are a very honoured young man."

"It is not every day you find a classical dancer who is also a skilled acrobatic," put in Jean Cocteau swiftly.

"How many others will take part?" Darius Milhaud was asking.

"About a dozen? Twenty?" Jean shrugged his shoulders, looking at Diaghilev. "They are the casual, modern young people one finds on the smart beaches."

"I want Lifar to have a small role in this ballet." Diaghilev was speaking half to himself, staring into the glass of champagne he held in his hand.

"That young man is coming on well," said Jean. "I was noticing him in Monte Carlo. You have a future dancer there, Serge."

"The future of Lifar is for me to decide," said Diaghilev coldly. "Moreover, I will not have people spoiling members of my *corps de ballet*. You gave Serge Lifar a great deal more attention than was good for him. I want that young man kept in his place to work." Words which made Pat feel much better.

"There is the English girl," Diaghilev went on. "What's her name?"

"Ninette de Valois," suggested Jean.

"Yes. That's the one." Diaghilev made a point of not remembering her name as he disliked it. It annoyed him that she wouldn't Russianise it. "She will do perhaps to dance opposite Lifar."

"Why don't you use that girl for bigger roles?" asked Jean.

"She is not suitable," said Serge. "She is a nice dancer but not yet ready."

"I think you are very hard on her, to keep her in your *corps de ballet* after she has danced leading roles in London."

"She did not have to join my company," retorted Diaghilev, "and she does not have to stay in it."

"Why don't you give her a chance to show herself?"

"Are you trying to tell me how to run my company?" There was a dangerous light in Diaghilev's eyes.

"Yes," said Jean solemnly. "You know perfectly well I can run it better than you."

Big Serge laughed and they went on to discuss other dancers who would take part.

The lunch party broke up at last, with enthusiasm at fever heat for *The Blue Train*.

"No, young man," Diaghilev checked Pat as he was taking his leave with the others. "You are not to run away. You are coming with me this afternoon to visit the Louvre. While you are in Paris your artistic education shall be attended to."

They walked together through the long galleries of the massive grey palace that houses the collection of some of the world's greatest paintings. Diaghilev was a remarkable guide. Pat was impressed yet again by the profound culture and knowledge of this incredible man.

"Pictures were my first love," he told Pat as they came to stand before the "Mona Lisa". "In the years before the war I organised exhibitions of Russian art here in Paris. The public flocked to my salons. To them the works of our Russian painters were a revelation. After this I brought into Europe our Russian dancers, and they were an even greater sensation. Yes, with my ballets I bring the public living pictures." He leaned heavily on his stick and a sad expression came into his eyes as he looked at the smiling face of the "Mona Lisa".

"I am often envious of these painted canvases," he said slowly, "for their beauty can endure. The pictures an artist creates may hang on a wall for generations to see and love, while the pictures I create, my ballets, are but moments of passing beauty. They can live only in the fading memories of those who have seen them."

He looked away from the painted face on the canvas to the living face of the young dancer beside him, and his voice was deep with the yearning sadness that lies in every Russian heart.

"I would that I too could capture for ever in some enduring form the youth and beauty that I give to the world."

An express train rattled and roared through the night, its long string of dimly-lit coaches crowded with slumbering passengers. In the early hours of the morning they crossed the frontier and headed into Spain.

To the remorseless beat of the wheels, Pat's weary brain went over and over the steps he was to dance this very night. Steps that he had been rehearsing ceaselessly for days past. It was April now. Nearly a month ago he had been recalled suddenly from Paris to learn the leading roles in *Les Sylphides* and *Pulcinella*. As he had foreseen, Idzikowsky's dramatic departure from the company on the eve of *Daphnis and Chloe* had left a gap in the ranks of the leading male dancers, and Diaghilev had called on Pat to step into Idzi-kowsky's place. To-night, in Barcelona, he was to dance these two roles for the first time.

His role in *Pulcinella* was a long and exacting one. *Les Sylphides* he loved. He had the only male part in it and was partnering Nemchinova. As he thought of this ballet, through the thunder of the wheels, he seemed to hear again the swelling sounds of Chopin's lovely music. He could feel himself move across the stage, floating with Nemchinova in his arms, floating . . .

"Barcelona! Barcelona!" Shouting voices and stamping feet awoke Pat with a start. He had fallen asleep after all. Now the sun was shining. It was eight in the morning, the long night journey was over. They had arrived.

Barcelona, city of sunshine, dust and dirt; strange smells, strange language and strange rattling taxis that distributed the weary company and their luggage at their various hotels. Bath, breakfast and sleep before rehearsals. That very same afternoon the dancers gathered on the stage of the Liceo Theatre. Grigorieff was on the look-out for Pat.

"Ah! Dolin!" The tall stage manager came up to him. "I have a telegram," he waved the paper about in a wide sweep. "Nem-chinova, she is ill." He made poetic gestures in the direction of his neck and ears.

"He means she's got mumps," Sokolova translated.

A ballerina with mumps! How unromantic, but what a crisis for the company.

"You must dance *Les Sylphides* to-night with Sokolova," Grigorieff smiled and spread out his graceful hands, "we must rehearse now. Yes?"

Pat and Sokolova looked at each other. Pat thought of the hours he had practised this role with Nemchinova. Now, at the last minute, he had to start all over again with a new partner.

"Have you danced it before?" he asked her.

"Never," said Sokolova cheerfully. "I have been eleven years with the company and I have never danced the *pas de deux* in *Les Sylphides*."

"Then you will start now and learn it," said Grigorieff calmly. She did.

They worked almost until the curtain went up at ten o'clock. Somehow they got it ready and Sokolova and Dolin made their début together in *Les Sylphides*.

Between them they got through the ballet successfully and the rest of the programme went without a hitch.

It was one o'clock when the curtain came down.

"Do they always play as late as this?" Pat asked.

"Yes," he was told. "In Spain everything is much later. They seem to sleep in the day and come to life at night."

There was no sleeping in the day for the company, however. For them work started as usual at nine o'clock in the morning. The daily two-hour lesson was a rigorous part of their discipline from which no one could hope to escape.

On the second day a notice went up on the board at the theatre.

"First rehearsal of *The Blue Train*, 25th April, 2 o'clock." Underneath was pinned a list of names.

The dancers in practice clothes gathered on the bare stage. There was much talk and guessing about this new ballet that had suddenly come upon them.

Pat stood a little apart from the others listening and saying nothing. He was remembering the lunch in Paris when he had first heard of this ballet that was written for him. Later he had been invited to dine with Diaghilev to meet Coco Chanel who was to design the costumes, and Laurens, the sculptor, who was to do the décor. By then Milhaud's music was already written. They had all listened to this ultra modern score of syncopated rhythms and strange disharmonies. After it they had sat late into the night talking, planning and clothing the idea of *The Blue Train* with colour and movement.

He wondered what the company would think when they discovered that the ballet had been especially created for him.

The babble of talk died away to silence. Serge Diaghilev came on to the stage with Boris and Grigorieff.

A chair was brought, and Diaghilev signed to his dancers to gather round him.

He began to talk in Russian. In his deep, attractive voice that knew so well how to play on the minds and feelings of those who heard it, he spoke to them of modern music. He explained that the modern composers like Stravinsky and Strauss deliberately did away with the old-fashioned melody and theme, that in their work they went all out for colourful rhythms, for quick brusque movement and discords that expressed the restless, nervous pulse of modern life. Then he spoke of the music of Darius Milhaud.

"In his music you see the shape of things to come," the persuasive voice went on. "You are already familiar with the rhythm of the machine age, and the poetry of the transatlantic skyscraper. Now you must accept this new poetry, the music of the street. Yes, we must take it very seriously, this new music which comes from the streets. It is the music of to-morrow. My Russian Ballet is the artistic advance guard. We cannot mark time and live the life of yesterday. We cannot even live the life of to-day, we have to look to to-morrow, and see into the future, for we are the leaders of the world. It is for us to guide the crowd and reveal to them the things that no one else has seen yet. I attach a great importance to this new ballet, and I want you to do the same."

They stood around him, listening intently to this compelling, forceful man. His words aroused in them a tremendous urge to succeed, to carry this new ballet into the forefront of modern dancing.

Diaghilev went on to tell them of the general theme of the ballet, with details of the different roles in it. With his usual skill in handling people he whipped up their enthusiasm. They set to work with tremendous drive on the first rehearsal of *The Blue Train*.

May time in Paris. The broad avenue of the Champs Élysées was alive with movement and sunshine. Restless traffic passed in a glittering coloured stream flowing between the wide Place de la Concorde and the distant Arc de Triomphe, standing on the crest of the slope, aloof and beautiful against the skyline.

Under the bright awnings of the cafés the coloured tables were filled, for in Paris there is always time to sit at a terrace and watch the smart people strolling to and fro on the wide shady pavements. The sounds of tapping feet and quick French voices and the hum of traffic, swelling into a great symphony of springtime, as the colourful life of Paris beat and throbbed along this great artery.

Half-way along the Champs Élysées a quieter, tree-shaded avenue cuts a straight broad line through the tall grey houses to the river. Here on the spring days of 1924 there were cars parked in the shade of the trees outside the entrance of a tall new building. People came and went through the wide doorways above which the letters cut into the white stone spelled out "Théâtre des Champs Élysées". Already the posters were up on the boards outside, splashing the news that the Ballets Russes de Monte Carlo, under the direction of Serge Diaghilev, would shortly open their eighth Paris season. Two new ballets were listed for the opening. *Les Fâcheux* and *Les Biches*. No mention yet of *The Blue Train*, but the new name Anton Dolin figured prominently in bold black type.

"Who is this new dancer?" people were asking. What surprises had Diaghilev in store for them now? Curiosity and interest were aroused.

"Tell me, Mr. Dolin, is it true that you are an Englishman?" A newspaper reporter was sitting in the makeshift office at the back of the stage interviewing this rising new star of the Ballets Russes that was so soon to shine in Paris.

"Yes, I am English," Pat looked across at Diaghilev as though to say, "Please, release me from this," but the big man only leaned back in his chair, fanned himself with a programme, and smilingly told the reporter that it was the first time in the history of the Russian Ballet that leading roles were to be entrusted to an Englishman.

"And a very young one too," the reporter tactfully suggested.

"I am nineteen," said Pat, and watched the man write it down.

"Phenomenal young Englishman of nineteen makes his début with the Russian Ballet," the reporter was already seeing his article take shape.

Pat went on to answer endless personal questions about his home, his training, his life in England.

"Is it true that you are making your first appearance in Paris in a ballet that has been specially written for you?"

"Well, not exactly," Pat hesitated and looked to Diaghilev.

"It is correct that *The Blue Train* has been written for him." Big Serge screwed in his monocle and fixed the reporter with it. "But it will not be given until the second week. During the opening week of the season Anton Dolin will appear in *Les Fâcheux*."

Boris Kochno looked in.

"The photographer from *Paris Match* is here," he announced.

The reporter was rapidly disposed of and Pat was taken away to be put under glaring lights, posed and photographed from all angles.

When it was over Boris brought him back to the office where Diaghilev was deep in talk with Jean Cocteau.

"You have a costume fitting at four o'clock," Boris picked up the list of his appointments. "After that, an interview with *Samedi Soir*, they are probably sending a photographer too."

Pat made a face. More interviews, more silly questions. It had been amusing at first, but by now he was already bored with it.

Nijinska came in.

"Can I have Dolin for rehearsal now?" she inquired.

"I hope so." Pat longed to get away.

"To-morrow," Diaghilev turned round on them. "I have invited some important people to watch *The Blue Train* rehearsals in the afternoon."

"Oh!" said Nijinska blankly, "that means we get no work done."

Pat silently agreed with her. Important people to rehearsal

meant clean shirts, new shoes, being on one's best behaviour and giving a performance rather than having a rehearsal.

"What are you rehearsing with Dolin now?" Serge asked Nijinska.

"*Les Fâcheux*," she replied. "Our room is free. I have sent the rest of the company to lunch."

"Interviews, photographs, fittings, public rehearsals," Pat grumbled as he made his way to the room where he practised privately with Nijinska. "It never stops."

"That is the price you must pay for success," she told him. "The lights are on you all the time, and your life becomes public property."

"Yes, even rehearsals," Pat went on. "At least no one can see these." He prepared for his work.

Les Fâcheux was a ballet that Boris Kochno had adapted from Molière. It had been first performed in January at Monte Carlo, following *Les Tentations de la Bergère*. Now it was to open the Paris season.

Diaghilev had hoped to include *The Blue Train* in the opening night, but as it was not going to be ready in time he had had a special part written into *Les Fâcheux* for Pat. He was to play the role of "L'Élegant", appearing towards the end of the ballet in a short solo dance as the elegant, affected Dandy.

In this private room he and Nijinska were preparing a surprise for the rest of the company as well as for the public. Once again, Pat was making history.

For the first time a male dancer would appear on the stage dancing on his points.

"You will make the *danseuses* jealous," chuckled Nijinska, as Pat turned four neat pirouettes on his toes with the grace and accomplishment of a ballerina. "They will never believe that it comes to you naturally."

Her words sent Pat's thoughts back over the years to the little girl in the blonde wig who had made her first appearance on the stage of the Brighton Hippodrome on her toes. What a curious turn of the wheel of fate that he was to make his first appearance in Paris on his toes. It would be amusing, original, but that was all. For Pat, the affected, lace-ruffled Dandy in a long skirted coat and embroidered knee breeches, who appeared in *Les Fâcheux*, was but a prelude. The important work, the one thing that mattered and on which all his hopes and thoughts were focused, was his own ballet, *The Blue Train*.

Everything that had gone before, his successes in Monte Carlo and Barcelona, faded and dwindled into insignificance. He felt now that all these had been but a rehearsal, a preparation, for the big event.

The days went by and the opening night of the season was on them. The curtain went up on *Les Fâcheux*, and Anton Dolin made his début in Paris, on his toes.

The ballet itself did not arouse great enthusiasm among the critics. For them, only one thing stood out in it, and that was the performance of Anton Dolin.

One of them wrote afterwards:

"Only Dolin saved the ballet from complete insignificance by a brilliant effort in its final section."

The critics had called his first trial in Monte Carlo "a promising beginning". Now they called his prelude "a brilliant effort". What were they going to say about the real thing?

34 Last Rehearsals

"Rehearsal of *The Blue Train* 2.30." The daily notices went up. Only a week left now before its première. Everyone's thoughts and attention were centred on this new production. Time was running short and there was still much to be done.

By half past two on a sunny afternoon in June the temperature inside the theatre had risen uncomfortably. On the drab, bare stage thirty dancers worked and sweated in the heat. The iron safety curtain was down, shutting them off from the dark and empty auditorium, and against it stood a table and chairs. On one side was the piano, the young Russian accompanist frowning over the unfamiliar manuscript of Milhaud's music. In a corner Picasso stood talking to Grigorieff, and near them were Madame Picasso and her little son who watched the dancers, entranced. Jean Cocteau, nervy and anxious, hovered about ever on the alert, ready to jump in and find fault. In the centre, Nijinska, in a black practice dress, pale-faced and tired, her hair scratched up in an untidy bun, directed operations.

"No, Dolin, that is not what I want." A vivid gesture swept aside his movement. "It is not like that. See, I show you." Her tired face lit up and her whole body seemed transformed with new life as she danced the movement he was to copy.

"And then you do your jumps in this direction." She went round the stage in a series of high and beautiful leaps, and suddenly, through the silence, came a shrill childish voice.

"Look, Papa! Is she never going to come down again?" There was Picasso's small son tugging at his father's hand and staring open-mouthed at this magnificent sight.

Nijinska heard him and laughed, and they all forgot for a moment that they were hot, sweating and tired. Picasso Junior had a great deal more to say, but his running commentary was drowned in the noise of the piano and the beat of feet.

"Now, Dolin, this is where you come over," Nijinska called out, and Pat whirled across the stage in a series of cartwheels.

The music changed.

"Now the backfalls . . ."

As Pat stood ready to begin he became aware of a curious silence round him. The atmosphere had grown suddenly strange. Everyone seemed to be looking in the same direction. Pat turned too and saw that the large scenic door at the back had opened. Through it was coming a man, moving slowly towards them. It was a strange figure that glided rather than walked as though he were not sure of his feet.

A name was whispered from one to the other and a deep hush fell over the whole company, a tense, painful silence, centred on that gliding figure.

They were watching Vaslav Nijinsky move on to the stage. Behind him with Serge Diaghilev followed his wife and valet.

Slowly he walked down to the safety curtain and sat down.

In awe and pity the young Anton Dolin stared at this living tragedy of the great dancer on whom he had built all his ideals. The man whose achievements had inspired him and spurred him on. The face and body of Nijinsky still resembled the faded photograph that stood in Astafieva's room in London; the same shaped eyes, the same beautiful mouth; but there was a terrible blankness in the look, and his helpless hands moved and fidgeted continually.

Big Serge leaned over and said something. They saw Nijinsky smile and shake his head, but he didn't speak. Did he understand what that voice he knew so well was saying to him? He gave no sign. There was an infinite depth of sadness and tenderness in Big Serge's eyes as he looked at the pathetic, broken figure of this artist he had created. The magnificent body was there, if only the broken threads of the mind that controlled it could be mended. Diaghilev, hoping against hope, had poured out his own money to send Nijinsky to the greatest brain specialists in Europe, but none had been able to cure him. So he lived on, day after day, in his flat in Paris, tended by his devoted wife and valet, and seeing, without understanding, his daughter growing up into a lovely child. Would she too be a dancer? Had she inherited her father's genius? The years to come would show; meanwhile, Nijinsky sat staring in front of him and his restless hands were never still.

Unbearably moved, Pat looked away, and he saw the tragedy of that broken life reflected in the eyes of all those who looked on it. Sokolova's face was white, Nijinska's eyes were wet with tears.

"I can't go on," she leaned on Pat's shoulder. "I can't go on, it's too awful."

Pat, finding no words, put his arm about her to give her courage, and felt her body shaking with emotion, while her brother sat on the chair, as helpless as an invalid, staring at the dancers before him with eyes that saw but could convey nothing to that poor, dazed brain.

Somehow they got the rehearsal going again, and this god of the dance, he who did not jump but flew like a bird, sat and watched his successor Anton Dolin doing backfalls, cartwheels and classical acrobatics.

"What did he think of it all?" Pat wondered. What were his feelings as he watched, but no one would ever know, for Nijinsky did not speak, and presently he rose. His wife took his arm and, as quietly as he had come, he went out of the gloom of the theatre into the sunshine of Paris.

The work continued. *The Blue Train* struggled on into existence. It was a hard struggle, but out of the clash of temperament and conflicting ideas the new ballet was slowly forged.

Jean Cocteau and Nijinska quarrelled incessantly over the

scenario and choreography. Hours were wasted in discussion and argument that should have been spent rehearsing. Without Diaghilev the ballet would never have been completed.

"Of course it is difficult," he told Pat after he had been called in to smooth over yet another quarrel. "A new, original creation is always full of difficulties. I remember when we did *Petrouchka* we had the same troubles. Fokine, who was to do the choreography, found the music so difficult that he said it was impossible to arrange dancing movements to it. Stravinsky refused to alter his music and they would argue about it by the hour. In the end I managed to persuade Fokine that it could be done, that something great would come of it, so *Petrouchka* came through its difficulties and lived, just as *The Blue Train* will live. We shall overcome the obstacles."

It was during these stormy days that Pat realised fully where Diaghilev's own genius lay. It was by the power of his personality, by the unique mixture of bullying and charm, of brute force and tact, that he kept his difficult, brilliant team working together. No detail ever escaped him but, at the same time, he never lost sight of the whole conception of the ballet. It was his impeccable taste and sure artistic sense that guided them, often in spite of themselves, to the finished whole, to the result that they all wanted. Music, scenery, costume, choreography, all had to be blended into a single and perfect work of art.

"We shall overcome the difficulties," Diaghilev had said, but even Pat began to wonder as he scrapped or altered one décor after the other as Laurens produced them, and Chanel's costumes were repeatedly changed or redesigned. So things went on, right up to the dress rehearsal, the day before the première of the ballet. Even then they were not finished. They had rehearsed in costume and, after it, the whole thing was torn to pieces again. Jean Cocteau ran about the stalls in a mounting rage, shouting that this was wrong, and that was wrong. Nijinska shouted back from the stage. There were storms and tears, and more alterations, and a further rehearsal for the next morning, a rehearsal that went on all the afternoon and right up to the moment when the stage-hands arrived to set the scene for the first ballet of the evening.

"We must go through this new *pas de deux* once more," Nijinska led Pat away, and upstairs, in a large, empty dressing-room, they rehearsed.

It was here Diaghilev found them. He did not interrupt until they had finished.

"Now you have done enough," he came and put his arms around their shoulders. "You will rest. It will be all right to-night, you will see," but by that time they were almost too tired to care.

"I came to tell you," Diaghilev said to Pat, "there is someone in your dressing-room waiting to see you."

"Not another reporter," Pat groaned.

"No," Big Serge smiled at him, "not this time."

"Who is it then?"

"Go along and see."

Pat opened the door of his dressing-room and saw his dresser arranging a big basket of flowers on the table. There was someone else in the room too, on the sofa in the corner. She got up quickly as he came in.

"Pat, my darling!"

"Mother!" and he was hugging her tightly. She had come to see his success, and in the joy of that dear, familiar presence, the tiredness and worry all slipped away from him.

35 The Blue Train

Friday, 20th June, 1924. The public were filling the theatre. It was a brilliant public. Diaghilev had drawn all the chic and the intellectual of Paris to the Théâtre des Champs Élysées this night.

The seats filled and programmes rustled open. A classical ballet was to begin the evening. It would be followed by *Les Biches*, and lastly, the climax of the evening, *Le Train Bleu*.

In his dressing-room banked with flowers and smothered in telegrams, Anton Dolin wrapped in a dressing-gown paced to and fro wondering how he would live through the next hour and a half.

This walking about was no good, he told himself, he must rest and relax. He flung himself on the sofa.

"Curtain up!" The call-boy came round.

He pictured the scene out there, the crowded house, hushed to expectant silence, the immaculate black figure of the conductor outlined against the footlights, the orchestra watching that raised baton, and in the wings the dancers in classical white tutus, clustered like flowers, waiting.

Somehow the time passed. Soon now it would be his turn.

"I'm going to get dressed." Pat sprang up from the sofa. His dresser brought out his costume. The bathing suit of the Beau Gosse had the deceptive simplicity of colour and line that is the secret of the French "chic". Pat tied and retied his shoes, whatever happened they must not come off.

He fidgeted with his make-up, he did unnecessary warming-up exercises. He went in to find Woicikowsky already dressed in his golfer's costume; plus-fours, with pullover and socks of matching stripes.

The hands of the clock went slowly and remorselessly round. The dancers came up hot and sweating from *Les Biches*. Interval now while the stage-hands set the scene for *The Blue Train*.

The *corps de ballet* were changing quickly into their smart bathing costumes. Nijinska appeared in the passage in her white, short tennis frock.

"Where's my racket?" She sent people scurrying to and fro in a panic of searching.

Sokolova, in a bathing costume, came to find Pat.

"How are you, Duckie?"

"Awful."

"On stage for *The Blue Train*, please," the call-boy chanted. They went down together.

"I wonder how Big Serge is feeling," said Sokolova as they stood on the side of the stage dipping their feet in the rosin tray.

They thought of him out there in his box, the big man with the monocle and the white streak in his hair. He was the only person that really mattered to them, the one person the company danced for, the man who had been the driving power bringing this moment into being. On this occasion, sitting next to him, in the place of honour, was a grey-haired lady in evening dress.

"Who is she?" people asked each other, but Mrs. Kay was unaware of the staring eyes. Her thoughts were all linked to her son's. She was sharing vividly his first-night hopes and fears. On the other side of Diaghilev sat Jean Cocteau. His face, under its shock of dark hair, was as pale as his shirt front. Nearby was big Darius Milhaud and his wife, Picasso, too, with Olga. Chanel sat among her smart friends. There was Laurens with his wife. All the team, in fact, were in the house to-night, anxious and watchful, waiting for the moment when the curtain would rise on this new thing they had created.

While they waited the public read in their programmes what Diaghilev himself had written about *The Blue Train*:

"The first point about *Le Train Bleu* is that there is no blue train in it. This being the age of speed, it has already reached its destination and disembarked its passengers. These are to be seen on a beach, which does not exist, in front of a Casino which exists still less. Overhead passes an aeroplane which you do not see. And the plot represents nothing.

"Moreover, this ballet is not a ballet, it is an *operette dansé*. The music is composed by Darius Milhaud, but it has nothing in common with the music which we associate with Darius Milhaud. It is danced by the real Russian Ballet but it has nothing to do with the Russian Ballet. It was invented for Anton Dolin, a classical dancer who does nothing classical. The scenery is painted by a sculptor, and the costumes are by a great arbiter of fashion who has never made a costume."

Strange words these that whetted the curiosity.

The house-lights faded. The conductor mounted his rostrum. This was the moment they had all been waiting for. The hush was intense.

As the first harsh chords of the overture to *The Blue Train* filled the house, the velvet curtains swung silently upwards, revealing, not the scene, but a painted drop curtain. On it, Picasso's modern brush had sent two massive, surrealist figures with streaming hair racing across a tortured stormy background of rocks and sea. The feeling of the painting was matched by the strident, modern music which found its echo in the hearts of that modern audience.

The mood was set. Picasso's curtain rose on a bare and empty beach. Empty blue sky, empty, distant blue sea. Angular planes of rocks rising up on either side. Two vast modern fish standing on their heads. A pair of cubist bathing machines. The whole scene was lit with brilliant white sunshine.

A single dancer made his entrance and all over the house opera glasses were focused on him. No, it was not Anton Dolin.

From behind the rocks, from behind the giant fish, came the others, the strolling, casual smart crowd of young people who thronged the beach with youth, colour and movement. They smoked, and ground their cigarettes out under their heels. They looked at non-existent wrist-watches. They stared at an invisible aeroplane passing overhead.

In the wings stood Anton Dolin, the bronzed and muscular Beau Gosse. His breathing was quick and fitful as he gathered himself for his entrance, feeling the force of energy in him rise to such a pressure that if he couldn't release it in his dance his very heart would burst.

It was his music now. Someone was whispering something and he was on.

As he moved into the violent light of the projectors, a transformation took place. He felt light and strange as though he no longer belonged to himself, as though a spirit greater than he had taken control of his body, telling it what to do, lifting him off the ground.

The public saw a young giant who seemed to tread on air. This muscular and athletic young man appeared to grow in stature before them as he whirled across the stage in cartwheels and overs. Up on his hands he went, on one hand. What a perfect control he had of that beautiful body of his. Applause followed him as he ran off. They wanted more. They would get it.

The Beau Gosse waited for his next entrance while Sokolova danced with Woicikowsky.

More applause as the *corps de ballet* borrowed a startling trick from the cinema and danced in slow motion. How curiously effective it was.

The Beau Gosse again. *Pas de deux* with Nijinska. The swimmer and the tennis champion. Easy to see here that these two were classical dancers. What style and what grace they gave to these modern movements. The Beau Gosse had won over his audience. They waited eagerly for his next appearance. It was dramatic. Alone, he ran, and flung himself into the air, turning over. A thrill of horror ran through the house. He was falling, straight on to his back. No, he was up, on his toes, and doing the same thing. A series of sensational backfalls brought frenzied applause. Never

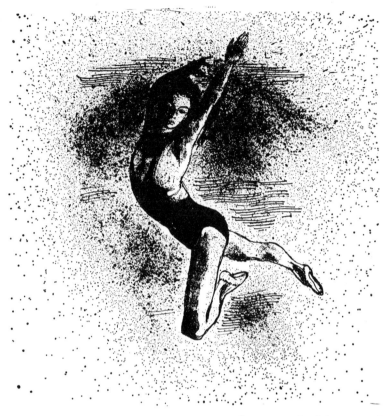

before had a classical dancer been seen doing such things, and he did them with such polish and style.

The climax was still to come. Hidden in the wings stood a spring-board. The music built up the moment. The crowd on the beach broke and grouped towards the rocks. A rising crescendo of chords drowned the sound of running feet and the take-off. The body of the Beau Gosse came hurtling through the air above their heads. It was a spectacular sight, and a thrill of fear shivered through those who watched, for below that flying body were the bare boards of the stage. His legs would be smashed to pieces when he landed.

People gasped. He was falling now, coming straight down on to his knees. How did he land? It was too quick to see. He was up on his toes, running forward, he's all right. Relief broke through in an outburst of applause.

The short half-hour of *The Blue Train* had run its course. The finale and it was over. The dancers lined up for the bow, and the curtain rose again to the thunder of applause. The four principals stepped forward, then Dolin alone, and a crescendo of enthusiasm brought the house to its feet calling out "Dolin! Dolin!" The stage was suddenly filled with laurel wreaths and flowers. Would the applause never tire?

Up in the box Serge Diaghilev's hands reached out for Jean Cocteau and Mrs. Kay. The bold experiment had succeeded. It was the triumph of *The Blue Train* and the Ballets Russes, and the personal triumph of the dancer Anton Dolin. He had won Paris to his feet, and his name was made.

There he stood, in the centre of the stage, a magnificent young dancer in all the glory and beauty of his nineteen years; still bowing and smiling. He turned now towards the box, his eyes seeking out the small figure of the one person in the world who mattered, his mother, whose steadfast belief had lighted him through all the darkness and doubt of his early years to this supreme moment.

"He is smiling to you," Big Serge leaned over to her, but Mrs. Kay could no longer see her famous son. The flower-filled stage had blurred, and her eyes were filled with tears of unbearable happiness. The shouting and the applause around her receded, and she was seeing her son Pat again through the groping years of his boyhood, through the years of courage and discipline that had led up to this triumph. To-night a new dancer had been given to the world, and his mother knew that he had overtaken at last the vision that had haunted him for so long. With *The Blue Train* the last veil had been pulled aside. Now clear and bright before him shone the glittering star of the Destiny of Anton Dolin.

Acknowledgments

I wish to express my acknowledgments to Cyril Beaumont for permission to use material from his *Complete Book of Ballets*, published by Messrs. Putnam; to Arnold Haskell for permission to quote from *Balletomania*; and to Mr. J. Kirby for allowing me to describe one of his flying rehearsals.

I am most grateful to Messrs. Hodder and Stoughton for their help and co-operation over the *Peter Pan* chapters. Under Sir James Barrie's great literary Bequest, the Copyright of *Peter Pan* is vested in the Great Ormonde Street Children's Hospital; I wish to express my sincere thanks to the Governors of the Hospital for so kindly allowing me to make use of material from the play.

Finally, I should like to thank Mr. Dolin for his help and co-operation over the book in manuscript.